CORRELATIVE PHYSIOLOGY
OF THE
NERVOUS SYSTEM

To
Brain Workers
everywhere

CORRELATIVE PHYSIOLOGY
OF THE
NERVOUS SYSTEM

H. J. CAMPBELL

Department of Neuroendocrinology, Institute of Psychiatry
The Maudsley Hospital, London, England

1965

ACADEMIC PRESS
LONDON and NEW YORK

ACADEMIC PRESS INC. (LONDON) LTD.
Berkeley Square House,
Berkeley Square,
London, W.1.

U.S. Edition published by
ACADEMIC PRESS INC.
111 Fifth Avenue,
New York, New York 10003

Library of Congress Catalog Card Number: 65–27737

PRINTED IN GREAT BRITAIN BY J. W. ARROWSMITH LTD., BRISTOL

PREFACE

Some ten years or so of teaching neurophysiology for the University of London Academic Postgraduate Diploma in Psychological Medicine is, perhaps, not a very high qualification for writing this book. However, the encouragement of my colleagues, coupled with the apparent lack of a text designed for such a course, has led to this small addition to the many volumes devoted to neurophysiology. No harm would come from using the book in preparation for such examinations as the B.Sc. (Special) in physiology. It is hoped that the functional as opposed to the structural approach will appeal to those who dislike to think of brain functions in terms of centres. The reader is assumed to possess or be in the process of acquiring a modicum of neuroanatomy. Likewise, he is expected to have followed a course in neurophysiology at about the level of the 2nd M.B., although allowances are made for lapses of memory. Each main section is followed by a supplement that is intended for those whose neurophysiological horizons are wider than the examination syllabus. Special care has been given to the preparation of the sections on higher functions, partly because so few textbooks deal with them at length and partly because these are the topics that interest the more mature student. The overall aim with these sections has not been to dogmatize about the neural basis of higher functions, but to show how expert evidence is confirming the view which some of us cherish—that mental phenomena have something to do with the brain.

No one would credit that the author wrote this book out of his own head. Nevertheless, it is still necessary and desirable that acknowledgements should be made to some of the sources of information that has been recast into this particular mould. Many original papers were consulted but references cannot be given to all of them without altering the character of the book. Happily, the investigators involved are more concerned with research than with public relations, so they are sure to forgive. The origin of illustrations is given where applicable. In the way of reviews, the section on the nervous system in Philip Bard's "Medical Physiology" has provided the collected wisdom of many contributors. More detailed treatment when required was readily to hand in the magnificent three-volume section on neurophysiology in the "Handbook of Physiology". Other books that have been consulted are listed in the Bibliography in the hope that some readers will pursue at least a few topics to levels beyond the scope of this book.

There has been no lack of people to give useful advice and criticism—too many to name here. Nevertheless, the encouragement and cogent wisdom of Professor J. T. Eayrs cannot pass unacknowledged, since they were so fundamental to the book's being. Wives play an important and many faceted role in the genesis of such a book; mine no less than others. Miss C. E. Harmer-Brown did magical things in the preparation of the manuscript, which was excellently typed by Mrs. J. King. Photographic services were freely given by Mr. S. A. Williams. To these and to those unnamed my gratitude is great.

August, 1965   H. J. CAMPBELL

CONTENTS

Part I

General Organization of the Nervous System

CHAPTER 1

INTRODUCTION

It is the purpose of this section to run very briefly over some of the general features of the nervous system. A good deal of it will be, it is hoped, more a reminder of things the reader has learned in the past —and is a little hazy about!—than topics completely new to him. Some of the matters dealt with will be hazier than others. The reader is recommended to turn back to his undergraduate textbooks for a fuller treatment of these. A good acquaintance with the elementary features of the nervous system is the only suitable foothold for the ladder of this book.

Stripped of all detail, the nervous system can be represented by a diagram in which an arrow points towards a circle and another arrow points away from the circle, back along the first arrow. This diagram shows that information is carried to a central region and instructions are carried away from the central region. Adding a little more detail, we could put in another arrow on the other side of the second one. This would represent the "feedback" of information that acquaints the central region with the extent to which its instructions have been carried out. Thus, the first arrow takes the place of peripheral nerve fibres running from sense organs to central nervous system (CNS); the second arrow represents peripheral nerve fibres running from the CNS to the effector organs—skeletal muscles, smooth muscles of blood vessels, viscera, etc., glands and suchlike. Without adding more detail, but devising a more realistic diagram, we would put in a great many more arrows of the same type as those already drawn. We would be showing more accurately how many fibres are running in and out of the CNS, but we would be showing nothing new in principle. To add new principles, we would have to take account of the inside of the circle. It would be necessary to fill this with a whole lot of little arrows pointing in all kinds of directions—and they would each represent something different, something of the manifold neural interactions of the CNS. This is about as far as we could usefully go with such a simple diagram. The next step would be to break up the circle into sections to represent the various functional levels of the CNS, but no great purpose would be served in doing that. For our present task, we have plenty to be going on with.

Beginning with the nerve fibre, any nerve fibre, there are several features that should be kept in mind about it. Morphologically, it is a kind of pipe running from a cell body to somewhere else. Materials flow from the cell body, or perikaryon, down the pipe, or axon, to nourish it and, some believe, to nourish the structure in which the axon terminates. Going back to the cell body, this has other processes, the dendrites, which together with the axons form the neuropil of the CNS or of ganglia. Material of a nutrient kind flows from the cell body to the dendrites also. Leaving aside the detailed anatomy of nerve cells—which the reader is assumed to know or to be finding in the appropriate place (textbooks of neuroanatomy)—the cell body is in effect a centre of nourishment for the whole cell. It may have another function added to this, that of generator of impulses. But just because billions of cell bodies in the CNS are generators, it must not be thought that all nerve cell bodies have this capacity. Millions of cell bodies that form part of the peripheral sensory mechanisms do not normally exhibit this function. Impulses in sensory fibres arise at receptors and somehow or other simply pass by or through the cell bodies. Even with nerve cells whose bodies *are* generators, it must not be thought that the cell body is the only place where impulses can be generated. An impulse can be originated at any point on a nerve cell—dendrite, cell body or axon—provided an appropriate stimulus is applied. Throughout layer I of the cerebral cortex and all over the outer layer of the cerebellar cortex, impulses are regularly transmitted from axons to dendrites or from axons to axons. One and the same nerve fibre may be activated, at different or the same time, by any of these modes of functional connexion. Very commonly, the connexion is between a terminal filament of an axon and the cell body of another neurone. This is the traditional connexion between nerve cells, forming the synapse (see pp. 10–12) but each of the other forms of connexion have just as much right to be looked upon as synapses.

In diagrams of neuronal pathways and circuits, the synapse is usually represented in some simple fashion as the junction between two neurones. One of the ways to acquire a clearer understanding of the nervous system is to get into the habit of seeing in the mind's eye a whole lot of other neurones which have been deliberately left out of such diagrams. Two statements are worth saying to oneself over and over again until they become firmly bound in the memory:

(1) Every synapse involves more than two neurones.

(2) Every synapse is a region of integration.

After all, there would be no sense in having a join between just two nerve cells. One long cell could function just as well—as happens in the corticospinal tract. Here the cell body is in the cortex and the axon-terminal in the spinal cord may be right down at the sacral end, with no joins on the way. Where shorter neurones occur in chains, each synapse gives the opportunity for a focusing of impulses from several directions. Frequently only one of these directions is under consideration at any time but it is important not to forget the others. The main functional difference between the pyramidal pathway just mentioned and the extrapyramidal mechanisms is that pyramidal impulses get from cortex to peripheral motor neurone without "interference" from other regions, whereas in the extrapyramidal system of neuronal chains there is integration of impulses from many sources before final instructions are sent to the peripheral motor neurone. This type of thing is happening all the time in many parts of the CNS. Where lots of synapses occur in a small region there is a "centre" of large-scale integration—a nucleus such as the red nucleus. Thus, although the anatomical unit of the nervous system is the neurone, the functional unit is the synapse.

One of the additions we could make to our model of the nervous system is to put a small curved arrow in the central region running from the head of the inpointing arrow to the tail of the outpointing arrow. This would represent the existence of spinal reflexes. It will be seen (see p. 99) that spinal reflexes are a good deal more complicated than this, but nevertheless the principle is apparent in our model. For a series of simple, usually evasive reactions the information from the periphery is transferred pretty quickly, at the spinal level, into instructions for the motor neurones. In the intact animal there is integration at one synapse at least in the spinal cord. Here there is a pooling of (a) the stimulatory information that is giving rise to the reflex, (b) information from other, related peripheral receptors, and (c) instructions from higher regions along the descending tracts of the cord. Obviously the spinal mechanisms become less automatic and less predictable as cephalization proceeds, so that in the higher animals spinal reflexes are very much modulated by suprasegmental influences. Indeed, it is the apparatus of the spinal reflex that higher regions use to produce all the manifold peripheral effects that are collectively called behaviour.

Cephalization has resulted in enormous swelling of the anterior end of the neural tube, together with extensive reorganization of neuronal elements and much greater complexity of connexions. But basic principles of function remain. Apart from alterations in morphology, a section of any subcortical region of the brain has the same essential features as a section of the spinal cord. Both sections contain fibre tracts that are carrying impulses upwards and downwards, and both sections contain localized accumulations of nerve cell bodies— collections of synapses, regions of integration, centres, nuclei. Proportionally, of course, there are many more fibres in the cord than in the swollen end of the neural tube, because the increase in size is largely due to the addition of specialized masses of nerve cells, many of them with axons that travel only a short distance to another collection of cell bodies. Nevertheless it is important to recognize that any but the most localized damage to the CNS destroys both nerve cell bodies and nerve fibres; some of the results of the damage may be due to the interruption of impulses from more or less remote regions. Essentially, though, in the intact brain the main difference between the spinal cord and the suprasegmental structures lies in the enormously greater integrating powers of the latter due to the extra synapses.

On the sensory side the thalamus represents the spinal ascending system but with infinitely greater powers of putting together the variety of information streaming in from the receptors, with the object of transmitting (not *transferring*, notice) processed data to still higher regions. These particular higher (cortical) regions possess the wider integrating power of comparing immediate sensory information with the stored experience gained from (a) past sensory experience, and (b) previous cogitation about such experiences.

With regard to motor mechanisms the descending tracts of the spinal cord, though by no means lacking in integrative devices, are thoroughly outdistanced by the integrative potential of the brain stem extrapyramidal foci, fed in their turn by the all-powerful motor regions of cerebral and cerebellar cortex. Over all this supportive type of motor functioning, the pyramidal apparatus exerts a controlling action due to its ability to integrate sensory data with volition in the performance of skilled behaviour.

Thus along with the concept of degrees of integrative power at various levels, arises the concept of levels of dominance. The higher one goes in the CNS, the less are structures dominated by others. True, even the highest regions are *influenced* by other parts of the brain, but the lower the structure the more this influence takes the form of instructions rather than information. Another general principle emerges from all this: *that the degree of dominance is positively correlated with integrative potential, which in its turn is dependent upon the level of synaptic complexity.* Hence one would expect that the details of neuronal interconnexions increase in complexity towards the cortex. This is indeed the case.

A very cursory study of brain function makes it clear that impulses pass from one part of the CNS to others. Closer examination shows that in some cases this is happening all the time, even when nothing seems to come of it. Such "tonic" discharge is a property of very many neurones and quite a few receptors. Even though to the external view a system seems to be activated just when a stimulus is applied, it would be quite erroneous to believe that the system was quite inactive prior to the application of the stimulus. All kinds of internal exchanges of information are taking place continuously. The applied stimulus simply adds a new piece of information of a kind that precipitates action. Very frequently the internal exchanges are of an excitatory nature inasmuch as they make the cells upon which they impinge more ready to discharge. Such tonic excitation is frequently intermingled, in any given neuronal pool, with tonic inhibition. The latter condition arises from the fact that impulses arriving at some synapses render the postsynaptic cell *less* ready to fire. Of course, inhibition does not have to be tonic; it may arise only under certain conditions and then die away as the conditions change. Nor do impulses having an inhibitory effect necessarily originate in cell-bodies that are concerned only with inhibition. Some cell bodies are able to produce excitation at one of their axonal terminals and inhibition at another, at the same time. In this way a cell (which, of course, would belong to a small population all doing much the same thing) is able to increase the chances of some action by (a) exciting supporting mechanisms, and (b) depressing interfering mechanisms. This type of thing happens with both the sensory and the motor aspects of brain function. Thus, the net observable external effect of brain activity represents the algebraic sum of the excitatory and inhibitory processes. The fundamental principle to hold in mind is that *all nerve impulses are of the same nature,* whether producing excitatory or inhibitory effects at their termination. Once again it can be seen that it is the character of the synapse that determines what happens in the nervous system.

The sections that immediately follow deal with various aspects of the brain and its environment in a rather general manner. Nevertheless, it is hoped that the reader will not simply riffle through them before passing on to the topics that interest him more. He should read them carefully and refer back to undergraduate books wherever his recollection of elementary points seems deficient. Such care over these preliminary matters will be well repaid by a better understanding of the rest of the book.

CHAPTER 2

SPECIAL ASPECTS

Electrical Aspects

PHENOMENA AT THE CELL MEMBRANE

Between the surface of a nerve cell and the interior of the cell there is an electrical potential difference. The inside of the cell is negative with respect to the exterior by about 50–100 mV. This so-called resting potential is generally agreed to result from the relative permeability of the resting cell membrane to potassium ions (K) and its relative impermeability to sodium ions (Na). In general, there is about ten times as much Na outside the cell as inside it, whereas the reverse is true of K. Nerve cells examined in a sodium-free solution show no excitability and this property returns when Na is added to the medium. No adequate explanation has yet been put forward to account for these concentration gradients in either nerve cells or other cells. Its effect, though, has been unequivocally demonstrated, viz. a polarization of the cell membrane, with positive poles outside and negative poles inside.

The changes that accompany activation of the nerve cell may be considered under three headings, but they should be looked upon simply as different aspects of the same thing. They are (a) depolarization of the membrane, (b) increased permeability of the membrane to ions and (c) passage of Na into the cell and passage of K out of the cell. With respect to depolarization it may now be said that the term is rather inappropriate. It was once thought that excitation of a nerve cell (i.e. initiation and propagation of an impulse) resulted in a disappearance of the resting potential, but more recent work with refined electronic equipment has shown that a reversal of polarity occurs, the outside becoming negative with respect to the inside, giving an action potential difference about twice the size of the resting potential. The second aspect of nerve cell excitation, membrane permeability, has as yet no generally agreed explanation. One school, led by Hodgkin (1957) considers that permeability changes are the result of physical processes; another school, with Nachmansohn (1959) as its chief exponent, believes that chemical reactions involving acetylcholine are responsible for alterations in membrane permeability.

9

An account of the distribution of acetylcholine and related substances is given by McIlwain (1959). With regard to ion exchange,
the modern use of radioactive materials has established the facts
beyond all doubt and fully confirmed the earlier work in this field.
When a nerve cell is excited there is a sudden ($0 \cdot 1$–$0 \cdot 2$ msec) transfer
of Na into the cell and a much slower (1–2 msec) transfer of K to the
exterior. Entry of Na corresponds to the rising phase of the action
potential and loss of K to the falling phase. Restoration of the resting
potential occurs after about 3–4 msec, due to some unknown oxidative
reactions; activation of a nerve cell in an atmosphere of nitrogen
prevents the return of the resting potential. During the 3–4 msec
that the membrane has a reversed potential it is, of course, not
excitable by any kind or strength of stimulus; this is the absolute
refractory period. When the ionic distribution begins to return to
the resting arrangement, the cell is excitable but only by stimuli
stronger than normally required; this is the relative refractory period.
At the end of this latter period there is again a relative abundance of
K inside and Na outside the cell, and once again the cell is responsive
to stimuli of normal threshold strength because the membrane is
normally polarized. It may be noted that an impulse is not generated
until a sufficient amount of ionic interchange has occurred and then
the impulse (action potential) is always of the same size. This is the
basic reason for the all-or-none law of nervous excitation. Nevertheless, it must be remembered that once an impulse has been generated
the nerve is in an altered ionic state for a brief period and resting
stimulus-impulse relations no longer apply, although the all-or-none
law still does.

PHENOMENA AT THE SYNAPSE

A synapse is the term given to the functional junction of two nerve
cells. It takes the general form shown diagrammatically in Fig. 1. The
presynaptic nerve cell has swellings on its terminations and part of
the surface membrane of such swellings is closely applied to part of
the surface of the postsynaptic cell body (or one of its dendrites).
No special features have been discovered for the parts of the cell
membrane that are in close contact. They are separated by a minute
space, the width of which is constant for any particular type of
synapse. Electron microscopy has shown that granular material occurs
in the synaptic space, but no details of how the space is maintained
have yet been discovered. In the presynaptic swellings many small
spheres are to be seen which have been given the name of synaptic

vesicles. These are from 300 to 500 Å in diameter and occur most densely near the junction of the two membranes. Most authorities seem to be agreed that synaptic vesicles represent quantities of transmitter substances and play a vital part in the transfer of excitation from cell to cell. Both the presynaptic cell and the postsynaptic cell

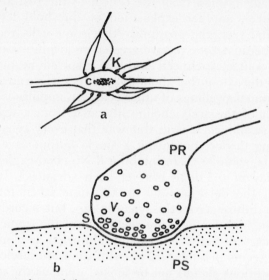

FIG. 1. Diagram to show relations at a synapse. (a) Low-power view illustrating the contact of many terminal knobs (K) from several presynaptic neurones upon the cell body (C) of the postsynaptic neurone. (b) High power view of the region of contact of a single end knob from a presynaptic neurone (PR) onto a postsynaptic neurone (PS). The knob is separated from the cell body by a narrow synaptic space (S) and is charged with many synaptic vesicles (V). The latter disappear on stimulation of the presynaptic neurone and are thought to represent the neurotransmitter which crosses the synaptic space and causes depolarization of the postsynaptic cell body. At excitatory synapses the vesicles are thought to contain acetylcholine.

have resting electrical potentials, and when the presynaptic cell is sufficiently stimulated the action potential is transferred, after a delay of about 0·5 msec, to the postsynaptic cell, the so-called excitatory postsynaptic potential (EPSP). In the case of excitatory synapses it is believed that the synaptic vesicles contain acetylcholine and that this is liberated from the presynaptic swelling at a rate that depends upon the membrane potential. When an action potential occurs, i.e. a nerve impulse arrives, it is said that the rate of liberation is about 1 million times the basal level. Further, it is believed that as acetylcholine is liberated, it passes across the synaptic gap and causes partial depolarization of the surface membrane of the postsynaptic cell body or dendrites. When sufficient acetylcholine has been liberated, the postsynaptic cell membrane is fully depolarized and an impulse is generated. There seems little doubt that some cells need more acetylcholine than others to cause generation of an impulse. Indeed, as a general rule this "threshold" of excitation appears to rise in a steady fashion from the caudal to the rostral parts of the brain. However, another explanation of threshold levels must be borne in mind, viz. the possibility that some cells require greater stimulation because they receive greater tonic inhibition (see p. 282). In fact, of course, each cell body is involved in many synaptic junctions, to the extent that about 80% of its surface area is in contact with the terminal swellings of other cells. An impulse is generated in it as a result of the acetylcholine liberated from a whole series of presynaptic swellings. It is in this way that every synapse serves as an integrating device, producing a single output as a resultant of several inputs, some of them inhibitory. No good explanation of the synaptic delay of 0·5 msec has yet been advanced. It used to be thought that the delay was due to the time taken for transmitter substance to diffuse across the synaptic gap, but according to Nachmansohn "the high temperature coefficient of the latency period and the high energy of activation exclude diffusion as a major factor." However, it seems possible that the diffusion of acetylcholine under synaptic conditions should not be looked upon as the mere crossing of a space—it is the crossing of a space charged with cholinesterase. This latter enzyme has the role of breaking down acetylcholine wherever it occurs, and this undoubtedly happens in the synapse. It may be that synaptic delay is due to the time taken for acetylcholine to reach a concentration sufficiently high for it to cross the gap without being effectively destroyed on the way.

Some synapses are inhibitory. At such junctions the effect of the presynaptic cell upon the postsynaptic cell is to produce hyperpolarization of the latter's cell membrane, the so-called inhibitory postsynaptic potential (IPSP). Argument still rages over the precise mechanism of synaptic inhibition, some workers favouring unknown physical (i.e. ionic) processes and others preferring to postulate an unknown transmitter substance. Micro-electrode recording is reported to have shown that the IPSP is produced by a diffusion of ions across the synaptic membranes and it is believed that the unknown transmitter substance alters the membrane permeability in favour of K and in disfavour of Na. Thus the ionic interchange during inhibition is the reverse of the movements during excitation. The matter is considerably more complicated than that and for interested readers recent reviews are available (McLennan, 1963). For the non-specialist, it is sufficient to know that inhibition at synapses is a fact, that some neurones are always inhibitory while others are excitatory and that inhibition is a most important component of the input to a cell, the output of the latter representing the algebraic sum of the stimulatory and inhibitory effects brought to bear upon it. Not only will this inhibitory mechanism reduce the effect or output from the brain to the periphery, but it can serve to alter the transfer of information and instructions between central structures. It provides an excellent basis for the phenomena of selective dampening of sense modalities in the economy of attention (see p. 62) for the cessation of reverberating circuits, for the action of the hypnogenic centre (see p. 247) and for the central control of receptors. The reader will no doubt be able to think of many more functions in which active inhibition seems to be taking place.

PROPAGATION OF THE IMPULSE

When a point on a nerve fibre is activated, depolarization occurs at that point. Once this has happened, no further activation is required for the excitation process (i.e. the ionic interchange) to continue in both directions along the fibres, for as each region of cell membrane becomes depolarized it automatically affects the polarity of the neighbouring part of the membrane. Thus the action potential travels as a wave of surface negativity towards the axon terminals and towards the cell body. Such a wave is loosely but usefully called the nerve impulse. Those that travel towards the cell body are known as antidromic impulses and in the cell body they produce an antidromic potential, the temporal characteristics of which can be distinguished from those of the spike produced by dromic impulses, i.e. waves of negativity travelling towards the axon terminals. It is not known to what extent antidromic impulses occur under physiological conditions, although it is quite clear that impulses are transmitted at points along some axons to nearby gemmae (see p. 243) and presumably a two-way wave is set up in the receiving fibre. It is unlikely however that the antidromic potential component produces any secondary excitation. Antidromic potentials are, of course, very useful in electrophysiological studies of nervous connexions; they enable the investigator to determine whether a given cell body and a particular fibre are connected by continuity or by a synaptic junction.

Argument continues as to the exact nature of impulse propagation in myelinated fibres. In the unmyelinated fibre, which is morphologically uniform throughout its length, it seems to be agreed that propagation is of the simple wave form described above. But the myelinated fibre has internodes of myelin and nodes where this lipid material is lacking. Micro-electrode measurements leave no doubt that myelin has a much higher resistance than the nerve fibre proper to direct current. The existence of fields of current around the nodes led to the theory of "saltatory conduction" according to which the nerve impulse (i.e. action potential) jumps from one node to another without traversing the intervening internode. Later, more precise, experimentation showed that there is in fact a very weak current in the internode and a fairly large capacitative current in the myelin sheath. Further discussion of this topic and indeed all aspects of impulse conduction may be found in Tasaki's review (1959).

THE NEUROMUSCULAR JUNCTION

Motor neurones of the ventral horns of the spinal cord terminate in a varying number of branches, each of which ends in close approximation to a muscle fibre—the myoneural junction. Just proximal to the junction the nerve fibre loses its myelin sheath and then breaks up into many minute branches that lie flat upon a more or less circular plate, the endplate, which is about 50μ in diameter. Around the endplate the nuclei of the muscle are especially dense, a feature that is interpreted to indicate increased metabolism in that region. Covering the endplate and the nervous terminations is a fairly thick layer of neuroglia having the special name of teloglia. A considerable degree of infolding or invagination occurs at the myoneural junction, so that fingerlike processes intertwine, thus greatly increasing the surface area available for transmission. In much the same way as at a neuro-neural junction (synapse), so at the myoneural junction there is a resting potential on both sides of the gap. Arrival of impulses in the nerve terminal produces an action potential in the cell membrane which is transferred to the muscle fibre. There seems to be no room for any doubt that the transmission of excitation is mediated by acetylcholine that is released from the nerve terminals under the influence of the action potential. This substance crosses the extremely small gap and in some unknown way causes the muscle fibre to contract, probably involving changes in membrane permeability and migration of ions.

Chemical Aspects

Since this text is primarily one of neurophysiology, no great space will be given to the chemical aspects of the brain. Rather the treatment will be of generalities to provide a minimum background knowledge upon which functional matters may be built. This should on no account be taken to imply that the study of brain chemistry is unimportant. On the contrary, there is little doubt that current and future studies in this field will yield much information of great value to our understanding of brain function, and this is especially so with regard to mental phenomena. The reader is earnestly advised to pursue this topic at greater depth in some recent reviews (McIlwain, 1959; Tower, 1960; Sokoloff, 1960) including a study of the influence of hormones upon the brain (Campbell and Eayrs, 1965).

COMPOSITION

As with so many parts of the body, the brain is largely composed of water. If no account is taken of any particular part of the brain, then it may be said that this organ is 80% water. Protein accounts for about 7% of the brain's volume, while the fat content is about 13%. These figures naturally change when the brain's various compartments are considered separately. The most important compartments are (a) the solid matter (23% of total brain volume), (b) intracellular fluid (47%), and (c) extracellular fluid including the cerebrospinal fluid (30%). Cerebrospinal fluid composition is dealt with in a separate section (see p. 23). Protein makes up about 35% of the solid matter, with fats accounting for another 50%; if the brain solids are considered as deriving from grey matter, then protein comes to about 50% and fats to 35%; in white matter there is, of course, a higher fat content (60%) due to the presence of myelin, and the relative lack of nuclei brings the protein content down to about 25%.

With regard to fats no one of the several kinds found in the brain seems to be specific for that organ; they are all found, often in much lower concentration, in other parts of the body. White matter fats are largely composed of cholesterol, cerebrosides and sphingomyelin, whereas the fats in grey matter are mainly phosphatides. Data on the concentrations of various proteins are rather sparse and no clear-cut figures can be given. As with other tissues, it appears that globulins are more abundant than albumins. Somewhat specific for brain tissue are the proteolipids, occurring mainly in the myelinated regions, with such a large fatty portion (50–80%) that many workers consider them as belonging to the fat category.

As can be seen from an examination of the figures above, constituents that are not fats, proteins or water make up only about 4% of total brain volume. This includes the carbohydrates, salts and oxygen. Glycogen is, of course, a predominant component of this fraction, with the di- and tri-phosphates of adenosine coming a close second along with glucose. One should not, however, be misled into believing that substances present in relatively small amounts, such as cytochrome c and pyridoxine are of no importance. Modern careful work is revealing that some of these "trace" materials are essential for the proper working of the brain.

Studies with radioactive substances have shown very clearly that there occurs a considerable turnover of all brain constituents examined, the reason for which is not clear. The highest turnover, as would be expected, occurs with oxygen. At any instant the brain contains just enough oxygen to support metabolism for about 10 sec and so is more dependent than any other organ upon a continuous and adequate blood supply (14% of cardiac output).

METABOLISM

The substances most actively consumed by the brain are oxygen and glucose. Oxygen is utilized at the rate of about 3·3 ml per 100 g of brain tissue every minute, i.e. about 45 ml/min for the average whole brain in the adult. This rate is increased by approximately 40% in children of about 5 years of age. That the oxygen is rapidly taken into combination is indicated by the rate of loss of carbon dioxide, which is numerically so similar to the oxygen uptake that the respiratory quotient is close to unity. So carefully controlled and protected is this metabolic mechanism that it varies hardly at all in even the most severe conditions affecting other aspects of the body's metabolism. Glucose is taken up by the brain at the rate of about 5 mg/min per 100 g, i.e. about 70 mg/min for the average adult brain. This substance provides the source of all the brain's energy requirements and its aerobic metabolism accounts for the major part of the brain's oxygen consumption.

While the process of aerobic utilization of glucose provides the brain with a ready source of energy, other compounds play an important part in directing this energy into suitable channels to serve manifold cerebral functions. Foremost among such substances, perhaps, are the various compounds in which phosphates occur.

There seems little doubt that such materials are utilized at a rate that is proportional to total brain activity, whereas oxygen and glucose consumption are not appreciably altered by such changes in activity as narcosis (raised concentration of phosphates) or epilepsy (lowered concentration of phosphates). Similarly, conditions under which the brain is highly active are accompanied by increased amounts of non-protein nitrogen in the brain, implying an enhanced utilization of protein. It should be noted that while oxygen and glucose utilization of the brain are not markedly changed except by extremely un-physiological states (such as diabetic coma), this is not the case with the peripheral nervous system. The nerves and autonomic ganglia exhibit metabolic rates that are closely related to the degree of electrical activity in these structures. This has led some investigators to hold in mind the possibility that since physiological cerebral activity never involves the whole brain and frequently is associated with excitation in some parts at the same time as other parts are inhibited, then there may be, in whole brain studies, a cancellation of excitatory effects by inhibitory effects as far as oxygen and glucose consumption is concerned.

Vascular Supply

It might be asked why psychiatrists should study the circulation of the brain. At first glance it would seem to be a rather non-clinical topic. But there are many who believe that a psychiatrist (or anyone else) will be able to carry out his duties with greater excellence the more he is aware of the collected data of the basic sciences. Even leaving this homily on one side, the mere fact that mental activity becomes progressively distorted and finally abolished as brain blood flow is decreased should be sufficient grounds for realizing that the present topic has implications that reach to the consulting room couch. A good deal of the gradual deterioration in mental capacity that parallels the expansion of an intracranial space-occupying lesion is due to deficiencies in blood supply to structures involved in cerebration. Similar explanations can be given for disturbances of mental activity and consciousness in myxoedema. The brain, and hence the mind, cannot function properly without a normal blood supply.

ANATOMICAL CONSIDERATIONS

These are adequately dealt with in detail elsewhere. A general picture is given in Fig. 2. Here it is only necessary to draw attention to a few points of special functional significance. In man, nearly all of the blood that reaches the cerebrum gets there via the internal carotid arteries. If these are occluded, unconsciousness occurs in about 5 sec; after 20 sec there is irreparable damage, frequently seen

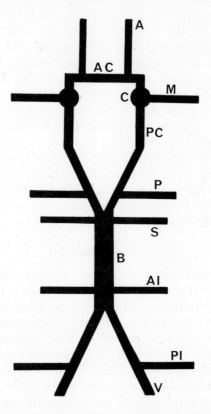

FIG. 2. Diagram of blood supply to the brain. A, Anterior cerebral artery; AC, anterior communicating artery; AI, anterior inferior cerebellar artery; B, basilar artery; C, internal carotid artery; M, middle cerebral artery; P, posterior cerebral artery; PC, posterior communicating artery; PI, posterior inferior cerebellar artery; S, superior cerebellar artery; V, vertebral artery.

as dementia. The vertebral arteries supply significant amounts of blood in man, to the cerebellum, pons and medulla together with a rather small amount to the cerebrum in the region of the pituitary gland. Venous outflow in the human is more complex, comprising four possible routes: (1) internal jugular veins, (2) anastomoses with orbital and pterygoid veins, (3) emissary veins and (4) connexions to the vertebral venous plexus. The last route is of particular importance for it drains a considerable amount of blood from the brain under normal conditions and is also able to accommodate most of the brain's drainage when the internal jugular veins are acutely occluded.

One or two points about the functional vascular anatomy of lower forms is appropriate. These enable a better understanding to be made of some experimental data to be given below. Experiments on monkeys are most suitable for extrapolation to man, for the vascular pattern in this group most closely approaches that of the human. An interesting fact about the cat is that the internal carotid artery is quite rudimentary, often without a lumen. In this species the external carotid artery includes the brain among the many structures it supplies with blood. The vertebral arteries carry most of the blood reaching the brain of the dog; occlusion of these arteries in this species rapidly results in unconsciousness and severe brain damage.

METHODS OF STUDY

These have been devised to determine how much blood passes through the brain in a given time. Compared with almost any other organ, it is more difficult to measure brain blood flow because of the multiple routes of inflow and outflow—especially the latter, for paths of venous drainage are complex in all species. Hence, it is not possible simply to measure the amounts of blood entering or leaving the brain in unit time; indirect methods have to be used. Several such methods were used by earlier workers to give useful approximations of brain blood flow. Such were the techniques of measuring the difference in oxygen concentration in arterial and venous blood, determining displacement of cerebrospinal fluid, observation of retinal circulation and so on. Little reliable information was obtained until Kety (1948) applied his modification of the Fick principle to the problem. Instead of using oxygen or carbon dioxide, the concentrations of which will inevitably alter in passage through the brain, Kety used nitrous oxide. This gas has several advantages. It is inert; it has a partition coefficient close to unity; it reaches equilibrium in a very short time; it can be given to the conscious subject in large enough doses for chemical detection without producing any apparent physiological effect. Kety arranged for the subject, which can be human, to breathe a mixture of oxygen, nitrogen and nitrous oxide. With flexible catheters in the internal carotid and high in the internal jugular veins, serial blood samples are withdrawn. A graph is made of the concentrations of nitrous oxide in these samples and the blood flow is then calculated from the curves by means of the Fick principle (see any textbook of general physiology).

BLOOD FLOW

Figures are available for several species, but we may confine ourselves to man. The above method gives results which when averaged show that 750 ml of blood flows through the brain of a healthy man at rest every minute. This comes to about 54 ml/min for each 100 g of brain tissue. Very little difference is found in the female. An interesting finding was made with hypertensive subjects. In these the total blood flow was 778 ml/min, or 56 ml per 100 g/min. Evidently some kind of compensating mechanism is at work to protect the brain from an abnormally high input of blood. This is most important, for the cranium is rigid and its contents are incompressible. When the volume of one component increases, some other component must be made to decrease or damage must be the inevitable consequence. Such considerations led to the Monro-Kellie principle, which flatly states that the total volume of the cranial contents cannot change. Any tendency towards increase in volume would raise the intracranial pressure, and this automatically results in deterioration of mental activity. The amount of blood in the brain must be kept constant.

MECHANISMS

Mechanisms are available by which this constancy is maintained. One such mechanism involves the cerebrospinal fluid and will be dealt with in detail on page 28. Here we shall simply note that an increase in intracranial volume tends to be offset by the outflow of an equivalent volume of cerebrospinal fluid. Perhaps the most important mechanism for maintaining constant intracranial volume involves reciprocal changes in the diameter of arteries and veins. Under conditions of arteriolar dilatation, the large intracranial veins contract, the total volume of the vascular bed remaining the same. A considerable degree of venous vasoconstriction can occur without negating the desirable effects of the arterial vasodilatation. Of necessity, while brain blood volume remains relatively constant, the flow of blood through the brain must change, under normal as well as pathological conditions.

Factors Controlling Brain Blood Flow

Extrinsic

A proper arterial blood pressure is essential for the adequate interchange of nutritional material between brain tissue and blood. When extracranial conditions result in generalized changes in arterial blood pressure, passive alteration of brain blood vessels occurs to match. Thus the flow of blood through the brain is to some extent under the influence of extrinsic factors. These probably operate under conditions of mild pressure changes.

Intrinsic

However, it frequently happens that large changes occur in peripheral blood pressure, both normally as in muscular exercise, or abnormally as in hypertension or hypotension. It would be wasteful and dangerous to have the cerebral blood flow so severely affected by remote conditions. Some intrinsic mechanism is required to give the brain relative vascular independence. The most obvious mechanism would be change in brain blood vessel calibre, i.e. vasoconstriction and/or vasodilatation. Initially, it was found that adrenaline would cause vasoconstriction and reduced blood flow, but later work showed that this effect was obtained only when the adrenaline was applied directly to the brain or injected into the arteries. The reverse effect of vasodilatation and increased brain blood flow was obtained when adrenaline was injected into the veins. Direct observation of pial vessels in the cat showed that ipsilateral vasoconstriction of these vessels could be produced by electrical stimulation of the cervical sympathetic system. But whereas the stimulation caused an 80% reduction in calibre of skin vessels, it produced a reduction of only 8% in the brain vessels. Also, in cats and humans it is known that blocking of the stellate ganglia does not detectably affect brain blood flow. The overall modern view is that sympathetic vasoconstriction has little part to play in the regulation of brain blood flow. It then becomes necessary to consider vasodilator mechanisms.

There is no doubt, it seems, among those who work in this field that there are vasodilator nerves supplying cerebral vessels in some forms. They originate from the medulla oblongata, reach the greater superficial petrosal nerve via the geniculate ganglion and ramify in the pericarotid plexus. Little more than that is known about them. It is believed that they exert a tonic vasodilator effect upon which other factors can operate. Their role may be highly local and there is no evidence of their existence in man.

The most important factor controlling brain blood flow is the vasodilator effects of the phenomena that accompany brain metabolism. These effects are increase in carbon dioxide tension, decrease in oxygen tension, increase in acidity, increase in temperature. When the *carbon dioxide tension* in systemic vessels rises, the vessels react by constricting. The reverse effect occurs with brain blood vessels. It is likely that normal carbon dioxide tension maintains a tonic tendency towards vasodilatation. When this tension rises so the tendency becomes active, there is vasodilatation and increased blood flow; when the tension falls so the tendency becomes less active and the vessel tends to constrict under the action of its elastic intima. Brain blood flow may rise to a total of 1 300 ml/min (95 ml/min/100 g) with high carbon dioxide tensions, and may fall to 450 ml/min (35 ml/min/100 g) with low carbon dioxide tensions. There is very little doubt that carbon dioxide tension is the overriding factor controlling brain blood flow. *Oxygen tension* in systemic blood vessels has a poor effect in comparison with that of carbon dioxide. But in the brain the tensions of these two gases produce just about equally marked effects. Naturally, the changes accompanying fluctuations in oxygen tension are the reverse of those produced by alterations in carbon dioxide tensions. Low oxygen tension may raise the brain blood flow to 1 000 ml/min (75 ml/min/100 g); high oxygen tension may reduce the flow to 600 ml/min (48 ml/min/100 g). Such figures reflect the brain's urgent need for oxygen. It has been calculated that the normal human male brain will function properly only if it receives 46 ml of oxygen every minute (3·3 ml/min/100 g). Under basal conditions 14% of the cardiac output goes to the brain, carrying 18% of the oxygen absorbed by the lungs. These basal conditions for the brain are comparable to the oxygen requirements of the muscles during heavy work. Small and probably localized effects are produced by the other phenomena of brain metabolism. Increased blood flow due to vasodilatation accompanies acidaemia and rise in temperature. Alkalaemia and lowered temperature produce vasoconstriction and reduced blood flow.

Evidently then, the flow of blood through the brain is varied according to the metabolic needs of the brain itself. While this relationship is not infrequent in the body, it is seldom seen to such a marked extent. The great sensitivity of neural tissue to internal environmental changes, its inability to function properly outside very narrow limits of carbon dioxide and oxygen tensions, its vulnerability to pH and temperature changes, have all combined in the evolution of a mechanism whereby the brain ensures that the vascular system will give it priority of food supply and waste removal.

The above remarks apply equally to local changes in blood flow. These seem undoubtedly correlated with local brain activity. Stimulation of sensory receptors (e.g. retina) results in localized increased blood flow in the corresponding cortical region (e.g. visual area). It is highly likely that the locally increased activity of the brain cells produce a local rise of katabolites and a reduction in anabolites, these in turn affecting the nearby vessels as described above. There is always the possibility that incoming sensory impulses cause the local vasodilatation, but there is no evidence for this. It is puzzling that in man, increased cerebral activity, as with mental arithmetic, is not accompanied by obvious changes in brain blood flow. At the beginning of sleep, an actual increase in brain blood flow has been reported. Hence, no final conclusion can be drawn about the effect on blood flow of the brain's activity.

Any close relationship between brain activity and brain blood flow certainly breaks down under pathological conditions. Administration of drugs, as for example in insulin shock therapy, may reduce the oxygen consumption of the brain by 50% without concomitant change in brain blood flow. In conditions of acidosis the same remarks apply. Naturally, degenerative changes in cerebral vessels frequently disrupt the normal dependence of blood flow upon metabolic activity. Cerebral arteriosclerosis reduces both brain blood flow and brain oxygen consumption, which are no doubt important factors in the genesis of the psychotic behaviour that frequently accompanies this condition. Similar findings accompany senile psychosis. No great changes have been found in epilepsy or schizophrenia.

Cerebrospinal Fluid

COMPOSITION

For a detailed list of constituents and their concentration, see Table I. The main points to remember are that the major solid material is sodium chloride. Next come proteins, glucose, phosphorus and urea. CSF is largely water, and it should look like water; any trace of colour or turbidity is to be regarded as pathological.

The composition at any particular level of the CSF system rarely changes under normal conditions, but during pregnancy and menstruation the glucose content rises and chloride content falls. However,

TABLE I

Constituents of Cerebrospinal Fluid

Constituent	Normal range (mg/100 ml)
Proteins	20–40
Nitrogen	16–22
Amino acids	1·5–2·5
Urea	10–30
Glucose	45–80
Pyruvic acid	0·5–1·25
Lactic acid	11–27
Citric acid	4·5
Histamine	0·2–3·0
Sodium	297–352
Potassium	8–15
Calcium	4–6
Iodine	7–18
Magnesium	1–3
Chloride	410–470
Sulphate	19–27
Iron	23–52 (μg/100 ml)
Aluminium	12·5 (μg/100 ml)

Note: Several constituents in low concentration have been omitted.

the concentration of all constituents varies slightly with place of collection (see p. 27).

It should be noted that all the substances found in CSF are also found in blood, which gives a clue to where it comes from.

ORIGIN

In general terms, CSF comes from the arterial side of the vascular system, enters the ventricles and subarachnoid spaces and goes into the venous side of the vascular system.

Faivre (1854) suggested that CSF arises from the choroid plexus of the lateral ventricles. Cushing (1914), in the course of a legitimate brain operation, exposed the choroid plexus of the lateral ventricle in man and observed the exudation of a colourless, transparent fluid. Dandy (1919) produced experimental internal unilateral hydrocephalus in the dog by blocking one foramen of Monro. This condition did not occur if the choroid plexus had been previously removed.

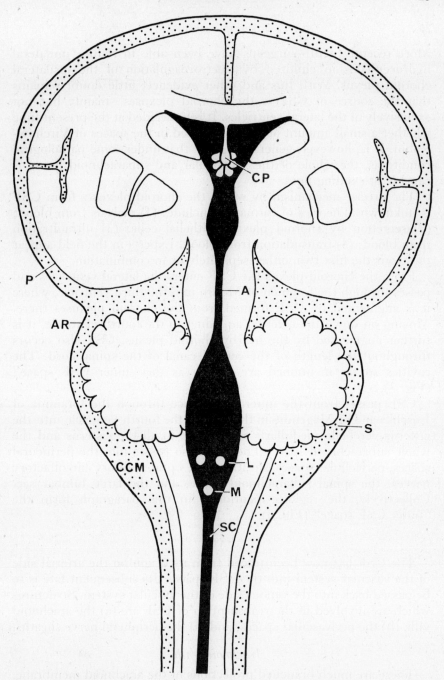

FIG. 3. Oblique section through brain to indicate the internal (solid black) and external (stippled) CSF spaces. A, Aqueduct; AR, arachnoid; CCM, cisterna cerebello-medullaris; CP, choroid plexus; L, foramina of Luschka; M, foramen of Majendie; P, pia mater; S, subarachnoid space; SC, spinal canal.

More recently neuro-surgeons have been able to reduce unilateral hydrocephalus in children by electrocoagulation of the ipsilateral choroid plexus. With this and other evidence, little doubt remains that the source of CSF is the choroid plexuses—mainly but not exclusively of the lateral ventricles. It is undecided at the present time whether a small amount of CSF is formed in the spaces of Virchow-Robin. It is, however, generally agreed that under some pathological conditions, the whole of the ventricular and subarachnoid lining is capable of exuding fluid.

The precise mechanism by which the choroid plexuses form CSF is unknown. Theories of formation include: (1) dialysis from blood; (2) secretion by choroid plexus epithelial cells; (3) ultrafiltration from blood; (4) transudation from blood. Experts in the field appear to favour the first two, either separately or in combination.

From the choroid plexus the CSF enters the lateral ventricles and passes through the foramen of Monro into the third ventricle, where it is augmented by CSF formed from the choroid plexuses there. Moving on down the cerebral aqueduct to the fourth ventricle, it is further augmented by the nearby choroid plexus. CSF also occurs throughout the length of the central canal of the spinal cord. The cavities so far mentioned are known as the "inner CSF space" (Fig. 3).

CSF passes from the inner CSF space through the foramina of Luschka and of Magendie in the roof of the fourth ventricle into the cisterna cerebello-medullaris and thence to all the cisterns and the whole subarachnoid space. The CSF also passes into the perineural spaces, pericellular spaces, sheaths of the optic, auditory and olfactory nerves, the spinal subarachnoid space, and the large lumbar sac. Collectively, the regions mentioned in this paragraph form the "outer CSF space" (Fig. 3).

FATE

The CSF has now been traced from its origin on the arterial side of the vascular system into the CSF spaces. Its subsequent fate is to be passed back into the venous side of the vascular system. Structures which are involved in the reabsorption of CSF are (a) the arachnoid villi, (b) the perivascular spaces, and (c) the peripheral nerve sheaths.

Arachnoid Villi

These are much branched projections of the arachnoid membrane. They push up through the dura into the venous sinuses (Fig. 4), occurring mainly in the central part of the superior sagittal sinus, but also along the sphenoparietal sinus, straight sinus and at the terminations of cerebral veins. They are also found near the roots of the spinal nerves, projecting into the segmental veins. Arachnoid

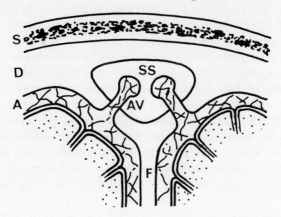

FIG. 4. Diagram to show structures involved in the passage of CSF from the external space into the blood stream. A, Subarachnoid space; AV, arachnoid villi; D, dura; F, falx cerebri; S, skull; SS, sagittal sinus.

villi are formed late in foetal life and their number increases markedly with age. Although these structures are responsible for most of the reabsorption of CSF, they do not account for the amount of re-absorption that occurs in association with the spinal cord.

Perivascular Spaces and Nerve Sheaths

These are of more importance in the spinal cord region because of their much greater number. From these spaces, the CSF passes into the blood stream via the lymphatic system.

In the above description, the implication has been that CSF moves from one place to another in a kind of circulation. The evidence for this is not of the best and for some time there was considerable controversy over the matter. The general opinion now seems to be that CSF does indeed circulate, but very slowly. It is then necessary to inquire what is the driving force.

The strongest evidence for a circulation of CSF is the difference in composition of the fluid in different parts. Near the ventricles, the protein content of CSF is at its minimum (10–16); in the cisterns is found an intermediate value (16–20) and in the lumbar sac the CSF contains its highest concentration of protein (16–24). This increase in protein content is attributed to reabsorption of water along the pathway. But the circulation of CSF should not be visualized as a distinct streaming motion; rather as a continuous mixing and diffusing. The rate of flow seems to be about 130 ml/24 h, which is about equal to the total volume of CSF. One must bear in mind that the fast flow of CSF through a puncture needle is an artifact due to abnormal pressure relationships.

There can be little doubt that the force driving the CSF slowly onward is supplied, very indirectly, by the heart. At each systole a large quantity of blood enters the cranium and a wave of increased pressure sweeps over the brain—seen clearly in the pulsating of the infant fontanelle. Careful exposure of the CSF, avoiding altered pressure relationships, reveals that CSF pressure does indeed fluctuate with the pulse. The absolute pressure varies with posture and is about 60–180 mm H_2O when the patient is horizontal. Although Becht (1920) demonstrated the correlation of CSF pressure with arterial and venous pressures within the cranium, a satisfactory explanation of the mechanism awaited the work of Verjaal (1947). According to this author the CSF pressure is largely determined by the pressure in the vertebral venous plexus, which contains valveless veins so that blood may pass easily in both directions. A model of the CSF system is useful in coming to understand the mechanism involved. This model (Fig. 5) consists of a rigid "cranium" attached to an elastic "spinal sac" enclosed in a rigid "vertebral column" with the elastic "venous plexus" in between. It is obvious that if the pressure of the "CSF" is not equal to the pressure in the "plexus", then one or other must become compressed. Verjaal showed that every change in plexus pressure is reflected by a similar change in CSF pressure. These facts and the model enable an explanation to be given of the various factors which affect CSF pressure.

1. *Changes in intracranial volume.* An increase in volume within the rigid cranium will inevitably cause a displacement of fluid towards the spinal sac, which then expands and compresses the venous plexus. Pressure in the latter rises and becomes reflected in increased CSF pressure. This occurs normally with cardiac pulsations and abnormally with cerebral tumour, oedema or haemorrhage. By manually occluding the jugular veins, the intracranial volume may be experimentally raised. Under these conditions a rise in CSF pressure should be detected; its absence indicates a blockage below the foramen magnum (Queckenstedt test).

2. *Changes in intrathoracic pressure.* Rise or fall of pressure within the chest will be transmitted to the total venous pressure which in turn will be represented in the vertebral venous plexus. Hence, with pressure on the chest wall or abdominal wall there will be a rise in CSF pressure. Such changes are seen to occur in correlation with

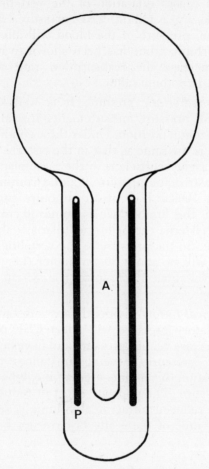

Fig. 5. Model to illustrate the mechanism by which CSF pressure is maintained. The bulbous top represents the rigid cranium. This is attached to (1) an elastic sac representing the subarachnoid space (A) and (2) a rigid outer tube representing the vertebral column. Between the two lies the elastic vertebral venous plexus (P) which is, of course, connected to the rest of the vascular system. A rise in CSF pressure cannot expand the rigid cranium but will result in expansion of the arachnoid sac. This will press against the venous plexus and cause blood to be expelled, thus reducing the CSF pressure to the original level. Converse changes would occur with a drop in CSF pressure.

respiratory rhythm—increased CSF pressure during inspiration, decrease during expiration. When abdominal breathing is occurring, these relations may be reversed.

3. *Changes in amount of CSF.* Obviously, when a CSF puncture is made the drainage reduces the volume of CSF and of the elastic CSF space. This causes dilatation of the vertebral venous plexus which is reflected by a fall in CSF pressure. Also, abnormally, changes in osmotic pressure of the blood will affect CSF pressure. Injection of hypertonic saline has been shown to reduce the rate of formation and increase the reabsorption rate of CSF. Reverse effects occur with hypotonic saline.

4. *Changes in hydrostatic pressure.* It is well known in clinical diagnosis that CSF pressure measurements are valid only when the patient is in a horizontal position. Under these conditions the pressure in the lumbar sac is the same as that in the cisterna cerebello-medullaris, because the right ventricle is in the same plane as the vertebral venous plexus; hydrostatic pressure is not a contingent factor. CSF pressure is about 100 cm H_2O at all puncture sites. In the sitting posture, however, the lumbar sac is some 30 cm below the right ventricle and the cisterna cerebello-medullaris is about 15 cm above the right ventricle. So the pressure in the vertebral venous plexus at the lumbar level will be about 30 cm higher (i.e. 130 cm H_2O) and at the occipital level about 15 cm lower (i.e. 85 cm H_2O) than in the horizontal position.

5. *Pharmacological factors.* Evidently any substance likely to cause changes in circulatory pressure will affect CSF pressure. Pituitrin and adrenaline increase venous pressure and have been shown thereby to increase CSF pressure. Several substances that bring about cerebral vasodilatation (histamine, ergotamine, ether, etc.) are known to raise CSF pressure. The opposite effect of reduced CSF pressure consequent upon reduced intracranial volume is seen when caffeine is administered. Some of these effects have not been demonstrated in the human.

FUNCTION

Among the people who spend their lives working on CSF there seems to be full agreement that this fluid serves an important mechanical function. The whole central nervous system is submerged in CSF; the effect of this is to reduce by *thirty times* the net weight of the CNS. This buoyancy function is a very important matter for a tissue as soft as the living brain. Another aspect of the mechanical function of CSF arises from the fact that water (which is what CSF mainly is) cannot be compressed. The brain is quite loose inside the skull. CSF in the subarachnoid spaces therefore prevents movement of the brain under the effects of light blows to the skull and of rotary movements of the head. The absence of this function is most apparent in patients from whom the CSF has been drained. Until replacement has occurred (24 h) such patients are intensely sensitive to the slightest of head knocks and head movements. Thirdly, still in the mechanical field, the CSF serves to keep the intracranial pressure constant (by the mechanisms we have seen). Any tendency towards a change in pressure inside the skull is immediately transferred to the CSF, which then moves out into the elastic spinal sac thus effecting neutralization of the increase. Fourthly, the final physical function of CSF follows from the two facts that (a) the CNS is the tissue most sensitive to heat, and (b) water has a large latent capacity for heat. Thus by acting as an insulator the CSF in the internal spaces protects the brain from bodily heat and the CSF in the external spaces protects the brain from environmental heat.

So, it seems that the CSF has a buoyancy function, serves as an hydraulic buffer, pressure-equalizer and heat insulator. Even so, the experts believe that the CSF system is too well differentiated, too complex and too well controlled to subserve merely mechanical functions. There is little evidence for any other function, but workers in the field expect future research to show that CSF may (a) remove metabolites from the CNS, and (b) have a biochemical protective role in the removal of foreign substances including bacterial toxins.

Part II

Sensation and Perception

CHAPTER 3

THE PERIPHERY

Somatic Senses

The older view of sensation was that each modality had a special-ized sense organ, an afferent fibre connecting this to the CNS and then a couple of synapses leading to a termination in some specific part of the cerebral cortex. Recent work, especially that utilizing the method of evoked potentials, has shown that this scheme must be modified at every level. It is the business of the present section to examine the modifications required at the peripheral level with regard to the somatic senses in general. The latter are here considered to include the sensations caused by environmental changes that affect the skin and the sensations due to the spatial disposition of the musculoskeletal system.

It is no longer clear that each sense modality has its own specialized ending. This may well be the case with interoceptors and proprio-ceptors, which respond to mechanical distortion. But it is not true, or not entirely true, of the cutaneous receptors. In the older books, and even some of the more recent ones, there are diagrams of several types of encapsulated, highly organized sensory receptors. Weddell (1945, 1961) and his colleagues at Oxford have made a careful search of the skin for such receptors and find that they have a remarkably sparse distribution. Indeed, the specialized cutaneous sense organs are virtually restricted to the regions of skin that are devoid of hair. Not surprisingly, these hairless regions—sole of foot, palm of hand, various mucous membranes—are the highly sensitive areas that were chosen for study by earlier histologists. The Oxford workers found that over the great majority of the skin there were only two types of sensory receptors, if such a term should be applied to such simple structures. In the hairy parts of the skin are found only naked nerve terminals and similar terminals coiled around the bases of hair follicles. Yet common observation tells us that the hairy regions mediate all modalities of cutaneous sensation. Further, although it is agreed that the cornea contains only naked nerve endings, yet Weddell and his co-workers were able to elicit sensations of touch and temperature by careful stimulation of the cornea.

35

So that whatever the specialized endings are doing in the hairless regions, it is evident that they are not the only structures that will transmit information in their alleged modalities. There is some evidence that these complicated, encapsulated endings have been produced by the constant mechanical deformation to which nerve terminals in hairless regions are exposed. In these regions forms of nerve endings are seen which have the appearance of encapsulated organs in the process of development from naked nerve terminals. Again, the conjunctiva in very young people contains only free nerve endings, whereas with increasing age the conjunctiva comes to possess complex terminal swellings. Few external tissues can be subject to such long-term mechanical stimulation (blinking) as the conjunctiva.

From a different point of view, the theory that each modality is only served by its special receptor does not accord with the generally agreed finding that pain can be elicited by intense stimulation of any receptor—including those of the eye and ear. As will be seen later, this is not to be interpreted to mean that there is no specific pain mechanism.

It has to be admitted that there is still some controversy over the matter of specialized nerve endings. However, it would seem safe and reasonably accurate to look upon any given organized sensory terminal as having a particularly low threshold for a given type of stimulus. Other less complicated endings may also be sensitive in that modality but need a stronger stimulus to activate them. There is also the likelihood that a given specialized ending is associated with only one sensory fibre. With the unspecialized endings, on the other hand, this is not so. It has been clearly demonstrated that up to 3 000 naked terminals may be derived from a single afferent, covering not a point but an area of skin. No anastomoses occur between the terminals from different fibres, but there is considerable overlap in the area of skin innervated. As a general principle, each area of skin and each hair follicle is innervated by at least two nerve fibres. Hence, the classical concept of "spots" of sensation must be replaced by one involving overlapping *fields* of sensitivity, varying in size and threshold and serving several modalities.

FUNCTIONAL TYPES OF RECEPTOR

It was once thought that for a receptor to cause impulses in its afferent it had to be stimulated. This is now known to be true only for some receptors. From this point of view receptors may be divided into four classes (Fig. 6). One type is frequently called the "on" receptor; these fit the classical pattern in that they are activated when a stimulus is applied. Another type, the "off" receptor does not react to the application of a stimulus but only to the cessation of a stimulus. A third type of receptor combines both of these properties and reacts both to the onset and to the cessation of a stimulus; these are the

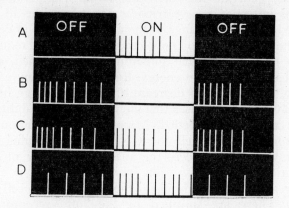

FIG. 6. Responses obtained from the four main types of receptor. A, The "on" receptor that discharges only when a stimulus is applied; B, the "off" receptor that is activated only when a stimulus is withdrawn; C, the "on-off" receptor that fires both when a stimulus is applied and when it is withdrawn; D, the "spontaneous" receptor that fires at a steady state in the absence of a stimulus and responds with increased frequency of discharge to the onset of a stimulus. Note in all four cases the dwindling of the response even though the effective stimulus continues, representing the property of *adaptation*.

"on–off" receptors. Lastly, perhaps the most remarkable class of all, the "spontaneously-discharging" receptors; these, as the name implies, do not require either the onset or the cessation of a stimulus. They fire all the time at a slow steady rate. Earlier workers such as Adrian (1937) with commendable caution felt that these receptors were being activated by very slight stimuli of which the investigators were not aware. Very careful and precise modern work has removed any doubt that spontaneously discharging receptors exist.

Examination of Fig. 6 reveals that in each of the first three classes of receptor impulses cease to be produced after a period of time irrespective of whether the stimulus is still being applied. This illustrates the principle of *adaptation*. It also brings out clearly the nature of receptor sensitivity. The operant condition for activation of receptors is a change in the environment, i.e. *a change in incident energy*. The "on" receptors respond when an increase of incident energy occurs; the "off" receptors respond when there is a decrease in incident energy. Change of incident energy modulates the tonic discharge of "spontaneous" receptors.

It is valid to enquire why these several types of receptor are required by the body. With regard to "on" receptors the reason is clear, for they generate the information that a stimulus has been applied. This information is carried as nerve impulses to the CNS and deposited there as a change in the excitatory state of cell bodies. Now what the CNS needs to know—the information it requires to be deposited in this way—is that something has happened, that there has been a change in incident energy. Removal of a stimulus is such a change. How can news of a decrease in incident energy be brought to the CNS? Only by impulses that alter cellular excitability. This is why "off" receptors are needed. Mere cessation of impulses from "on" receptors does not tell the CNS that a stimulus has been removed for, as we have seen, the adaptive property of receptors causes cessation of impulses even while a stimulus is still being applied. A fresh barrage of impulses, another change in cell threshold is required. These are supplied by the "off" receptors. Teleologically, the purpose of the spontaneous receptors is even more clear. It is apparent from several studies that when the sensory input to the CNS is artificially reduced to very low levels, serious disturbance of brain function occurs, involving both sensory and motor mechanisms. The CNS appears to function properly only when it is constantly receiving impulses. Hence, it is reasonable to believe that the purpose of the spontaneously discharging receptors is to maintain a continuous low-level bombardment of the CNS with "resting" impulses. In this way the central excitatory state, the level of excitability of the appropriate nerve cell bodies is kept at a "standby" level and not allowed to fall to a "stand down" level; the appropriate higher regions are maintained in a state of preparedness for any change in incident energy in the environment. It seems that the most commonly occurring type of receptor is the spontaneously discharging form that responds both to onset and cessation of a stimulus.

THE FREQUENCY CODE

It is appropriate at this point to consider the correspondence between activity of the receptor and activity in the sensory fibres. The essential relationship is that more intense stimuli produce more intense activation of the receptor which results in a higher frequency of impulses in the afferent fibres. Figure 7 shows an experimental demonstration of this relationship. It is becoming more and more clear that the CNS interprets the environment largely in terms of this frequency code, a code in which there is a distinct parallelism between absolute frequency and stimulus intensity. However, it would be too simple a view to consider that the impulse frequency

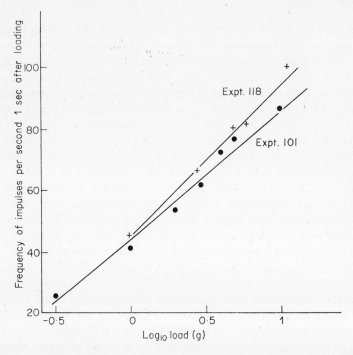

FIG. 7. Responses of a frog muscle spindle to varying loads upon the muscle, i.e. different intensities of stimulation. Note that the impulse frequency is proportional to the logarithm of the stimulus intensity (Fechner's Law). (From Matthews, 1931.)

set up by a receptor reaches all appropriate higher levels unchanged. When dealing with central mechanisms below, it will be seen that the sensory input is subjected to central modification at several levels. Nevertheless, for each level the rule still holds that what the CNS does about the sensory input depends upon the total number of impulses arriving in a given pathway in a given time. Although Fig. 7 may apply to a single fibre, it should be borne in mind that usually a more intense stimulus activates more receptors than a milder stimulus, so that the total number of impulses in a given modality is the sum of the individual frequencies in many fibres. It is this total number of impulses in a given modality that is integrated at various levels (especially in non-specific regions) with the total number of impulses in other modalities so that, in the simplest terms, the dominant stimulus (which may be polymodal) produces the dominant response.

RECEPTIVE FIELDS

It is evident from the previous account of the overlapping and branching of the terminals of sensory fibres that the skin can no longer be considered as made up of sensitive "spots". Current concepts of skin sensitivity demand that the peripheral mechanism of sensation be looked upon as generated by receptive fields. Instructive remarks on this topic are to be found in Ragnar Granit's monograph (1955), from which the following quotation is taken: "In the skin the receptive field is a complex structure of several intermingled modalities, many of which are evoked together by the simplest kind of touch stimulus and many more by pressure. The fields again overlap and the larger ones are punctuated by smaller fields, the smallest of all apparently referring to encapsulated or otherwise organized endings with highly developed specificity. Any one of the modalities may be pictured as a relief map over the skin, in which peaks represent high sensitivity and valleys low sensitivity."

LOCAL SIGN

Common experience soon teaches us that not only do we know that we are being touched but we also know *where* we are being touched— the so-called local sign of sensation. Granit's description of the skin receptive fields makes it rather difficult to see how accurate local sign arises. It was much simpler in the days when it was thought that the skin just had spots of sensitivity corresponding to spots in the cortex. Now we know that any sensory fibre may carry impulses from up to 3 000 terminations the old explanation no longer holds. This should not be taken to mean that topographical sensory representation does not occur in the CNS; several such correspondences will be described in the section on central mechanisms of sensation. But the question must be answered as to how the overlapping, multimodal peripheral organization becomes transformed into the central discrete "maps". Drawing largely upon Granit's (1955) explanation, the mechanism can be considered as twofold. (a) Anatomically, the sensory fibres are collected into bundles in the dorsal roots and more so in the spinal cord, where the modalities are largely separated. Within each modality, i.e. within each sensory tract, there is further grouping according to fibre size and with respect to gross site of origin (lower limb, trunk, etc.). (b) Physiologically, the very existence of skin fields in themselves can be seen to aid spatial discrimination, for a point of touch will inevitably excite several sensory fibres and these have different thresholds and are different distances from the point of stimulation. Hence each fibre sends a different message in the frequency code. Central integration of the messages—a kind of neural triangulation—results in more or less exact localization and modality-discrimination. We may now consider some special points about the various modalities.

PAIN

It was pointed out above that highly intense stimulation in any modality may give rise to a sensation of pain. We should inquire whether this is all that pain is—a high frequency discharge in any sensory fibre. An unequivocal answer can be given. There is no doubt at all that some pain sensations are mediated by specific pathways, at least in the spinal cord. It is a clinical cliché that antero-lateral cordotomy relieves the corresponding somatic region from pain while leaving other kinds of sensations intact. Similarly, properly placed central lesions have been found to have the same effect. More peripherally, the picture is not so clear. It is possible that a given sensory fibre may carry, not necessarily at the same time, impulses that produce a sensation of pain and impulses that produce some other sensation; the two modalities might be separated by differential synaptic resistance within the spinal cord. No final answer can be given on this point, but two pieces of evidence suggest that the pain pathway in peripheral nerves is distinct. (a) Mistreatment of a peripheral nerve by pressure, cooling, chemical anaesthesia, etc., results in graduated loss of sensation from the corresponding somatic region, and very frequently pain remains when all other sensations have been lost. (b) Experimentally, sensations of pain can be pro-duced by very low frequency discharge in single fibres, whereas the same frequency in other fibres does not result in pain; conversely, high frequency discharge in some fibres does not result in pain whereas the same frequency in other fibres does so.

Whether or not pain has its own set of peripheral sensory fibres, there is no doubt that painful stimuli are appreciated by undifferen-tiated, unmyelinated nerve endings. These occur in a network over the whole of the skin at various levels and also in several deeper regions such as the adventitia of arteries, the intermuscular connective tissue, the deep fascia and periosteum. Although no special frequency is required in these fibres to produce pain—anything from 5–100/sec being effective—there arose the concept of double pain, frequently referred to as fast pain and slow pain. The concept was generated by the findings of earlier workers that a painful stimulus such as a pin-prick was reported by the subject to give an immediate sharp feeling of pain, followed within a split second by a different unpleasant sensation. The explanation was that thin fibres carried fast pain and thick ones carried slow pain. However, the concept has been severely criticized recently by workers using highly refined methods of stimulation. By careful *mechanical* application of a pin-prick in several thousand subjects, they were unable to elicit a double effect. It is thought that earlier workers, who used *manual* application of the pin, unwittingly stimulated different pain fibres at two depths in the skin, sensation from the deeper fibres necessarily following a fraction of a second after the sensation from the more superficial fibres.

TOUCH AND KINAESTHESIS

Difficulty has been experienced in defining touch. We shall use the description given by Rose and Mountcastle (1959): tactile stimuli are those which cause displacement of hairs or deformation of skin without injury; by kinaesthetic stimuli we shall mean those which cause displacement or compression of joint capsules.

Touch Receptors

These respond to tactile stimuli. As already mentioned, naked nerve endings can do this, as demonstrated in the cornea. In the course of time, i.e. after much mechanical stimulation, these undifferentiated endings may become modified into some semblance of organization. In addition, the endings associated with hair follicles are exquisitely sensitive to the slightest displacement of the hair. It is a property of all touch receptors that they are fast-adapting, as befits a form of receptor that is subject to such continuous stimulation; in contrast the deep, kinaesthetic receptors are slowly-adapting, corresponding to the relative infrequency with which they are stimulated.

Touch Fibres

These have been a focal point of controversy for some time. For many years it was thought that the large diameter fibres of the peripheral nerves were solely responsible for touch sensibility. More refined methods of investigation, especially the techniques of recording from a single fibre, have shown that touch can be mediated by fibres of all diameters. Not that *all* fibres mediate touch, but a fibre cannot be eliminated from the touch pathway simply on the basis of its diameter. It seems likely that touch fibres of different diameters carry different qualities of touch. Single-fibre recording has shown in the cat that light touch is followed by impulses in fibres of 6–12 μ diameter, whereas sustained pressure is accompanied by activation of fibres with a diameter of 3–5 μ. Hence, as a general rule, the larger the fibre the more sensitive is its receptor.

Kinaesthetic receptors, according to Sherrington were located in the muscles, the spindles or tendon organs of Golgi. Although there is no doubt about the existence or importance of muscle receptors in the reflex control of contraction, it has become apparent that as far as kinaesthesia is concerned, they play very little if any part. Modern work has made it quite clear that the receptors which signal kinaesthetic information—which is in effect joint angle—are located in the joints themselves. Recording electrodes in spindle and Golgi afferents show that the frequency of impulses in these structures bears no clear relation to the angle of the corresponding joint. On the other hand, a definite parallelism has been established between joint angle and the rate of discharge in joint afferents. Two types of receptor are involved: (a) a spray ending type, resembling the Ruffini organs in skin, these occur in the connective tissue capsules of the joints; (b) endings tending to resemble the tendon organ of Golgi in structure and occurring in the ligaments of the joints. Both types adapt very slowly and have a spontaneous discharge, so that information is transmitted while the joint is motionless as well as when it is moving. The disposition of the receptors is in roughly parallel rows and they discharge one after the other along the rows that are in the direction of the movement. Hence as the joint angle increases, receptors further and further from the origin begin to fire. It is obvious that this pattern of discharge up to but not beyond a certain receptor is ideal for indicating the joint angle at any instant.

TEMPERATURE

Within the field of thermal sensation, at least as far as the periphery is concerned, classical notions have stood up well to modern investigations. *Thermal receptors* have always been thought to be of two kinds and recent electrical recording techniques have amply confirmed the existence of receptors especially sensitive to cold and of receptors

especially sensitive to heat. Whether these two receptors are anatomically different is not known. On what the experts in this field consider
to be rather poor evidence, it has been suggested that the Ruffini
organs are sensitive to heat and that cold is appreciated by Krause's
end bulbs. All that is known for certain is that electrodes in one
position pick up discharges when the region is heated but not when
it is cooled, and that regions can be found in which the converse is
true. These experiments also confirmed the classical idea that the
cold receptors are situated more superficially than the warmth
receptors. The absolute depth of the temperature sensitive organs
varies with the site on the body; in general terms the cold receptors
occur at about half the depth of nearby warmth receptors.

It should not be thought however that the role of the temperature
receptors is to signal absolute thermal conditions. For both types of
receptor there is a range of temperature over which they discharge and
these ranges overlap. Under any given set of conditions it is possible
that many units of both types are firing at the same time, though not
necessarily with the same frequency code. As with other receptors,
the thermal organs are really concerned with changes in incident
energy. They signal whether an increase or decrease is occurring,
i.e. whether the temperature in their region is rising or falling. Under
steady temperature conditions there is a steady discharge in the
receptors, the actual frequency being proportional to the temperature.
A change in the steady state is accompanied by a change in frequency
that is proportional to the *rate* of change of the temperature (Fig. 8).

COMPOSITE SENSATIONS

Under natural conditions it must be very rare for a stimulus to
excite only one kind of somatic receptor. With almost any normal
stimulus several modalities are affected. A simple experiment to
demonstrate this is to place a subject's hand in water at about 40° C.
He describes the water as "warm" because (apart from light touch)
only the thermal receptors are activated. If the temperature of the
water is raised a few degrees, the subject describes it as "hot". In
this case the thermal receptors are being stimulated strongly and the
pain receptors mildly. When the water is raised near to boiling point
the subject may well consider it "damned hot" because at this temperature both thermal and pain receptors are being very intensely stimulated. It is this type of composite sensation, this mingling of modalities
that is so important in the transformation of mere sensory input into
affective perception.

Perception, then, is based peripherally upon two patterns of nervous activity: (a) the pattern—frequency of discharge and number of fibres discharging—in each modality, and (b) the pattern of total

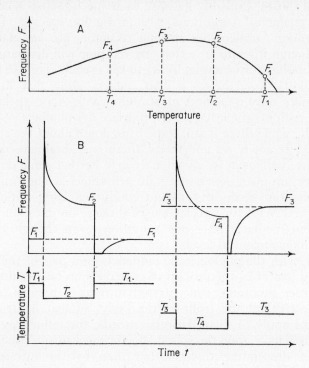

FIG. 8. Graphs of impulse frequency from a single cold fibre plotted against temperature. A, Steady discharge occasioned by gradual temperature changes; B, rapid rate of change of frequency with sudden drop in temperature. Notice in B that the *relative* temperature drop from T_1 to T_2 is the same as for T_3 to T_4 but the *absolute* temperatures are different; nevertheless, the shapes of the frequency curves are similar and the receptor returns, under steady temperature conditions, to a steady discharge at a frequency proportional to the absolute temperature. (After Hensel, 1953.)

number of impulses arriving in the CNS from several modalities. Indeed, for perception there must occur *analysis* of the information in single modalities and *synthesis* of the information in several modalities.

Special Senses

By and large the main differences between the peripheral organization of the somatic and special senses lies in the specificity of the latter, as their name implies. We have seen the great difficulties involved in assigning any histologically demonstrable complex nerve ending to any particular somatic sense. No such problem arises with the special senses. Probably because each special sense is concerned under physiological conditions with a rigidly specific change in incident energy, undeniably specific receptors are associated with them. Although it seems true that any receptor will discharge to any intense stimulus (for example, blows to the eyeball give rise to sensations of light), nevertheless it also appears clear that in natural circumstances only one kind of stimulus will excite special sense receptors, each of which has an appropriate morphology.

Secondly, while there is still some little doubt about the specificity of somatic afferent fibres and tracts, there is general agreement that special sense pathways are distinct. It may be that some dorsal root fibres carry impulses generating pain sensations at one time and at other times (that is, under different conditions) carry impulses of a tactile nature. With the special senses there is no question but that each system mediates only one sensation, even though there are interminglings at central levels.

Thirdly, with the phylogenetic tendency for a part of the body to be directed forwards, the process of cephalization has resulted in the special senses becoming concentrated into small regions (eye, ear, tongue, nostrils) at the front of the body, so that no true spinal mechanisms apply to them. In other words, the influences that the special senses have upon the spinal effector mechanisms are mediated by way of descending tracts rather than by the intrasegmental horizontal connexions found with somatic senses.

VISION

The classical neural pathway for vision contains the usual three neurones and two synapses from periphery to cortex. In order, this section deals with the retina, optic nerve, optic chiasma and optic tract. The lateral geniculate body, optic radiation and visual cortex will be dealt with in the section on central mechanisms (Chapter 4).

The *retina* is a very highly complex structure and its detailed organization is considered in the supplement to this section (p. 90). Here only the broad outline of retinal mechanisms will be considered. The retina contains the first two neurones and the first two synapses of the visual pathway (Fig. 9). Light activates the sense organ—a rod or cone—which excites the first neurone, a bipolar cell. Rods are the sense organs that seem to be concerned largely with non-colour vision and the density of their distribution increases towards the periphery of the retina. The usefulness of rods under monochromatic conditions is indicated by the fact that nocturnal animals frequently possess only rods. Rhodopsin is the pigment found in the rods. This

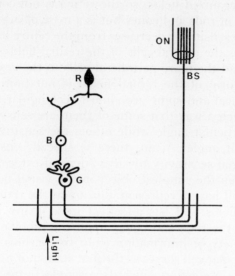

FIG. 9. Highly simplified schematic representation of retinal organization. Light crosses the retina to fall upon and activate the receptor (rod or cone) (R). This excites the bipolar cell (B) which in turn sets up impulses in the ganglion cell (G). Axons from the ganglion cells run along the surface of the retina and turn inwards at the blind spot (BS) where they leave the retina as the optic nerve (ON). (See also Fig. 21.)

is a derivative of vitamin A, deficiency of which leads to night-blindness. Under the action of light rhodopsin is converted to a carotenoid substance, "retinene", which is then changed to vitamin A; in the dark the process is reversed and rhodopsin is re-formed. This pigment is not found in the cones of the retina. These occur most densely in the fovea and the concentration diminishes towards the periphery. Cones, which are outnumbered about 125 : 1 by rods, function best under conditions of bright illumination and are sensitive to colour. They are highly discriminative and, like the rods, send processes to the dendrites of bipolar cells. Actually there is considerable convergence of many light-sensitive organs onto one bipolar cell. As mentioned above some receptors are activated by an absence of stimulus and those in the retina are no exception. Indeed all the four classes of sense organs represented in Fig. 6 are found in the retina, where the distinctions can be demonstrated with great clarity, some receptors discharging when the change in incident energy is towards greater light and others being activated by a reduction in light. Just as skin sensitivity is to be looked upon not as scattered points but as organized fields, so the retina is not composed simply of serried ranks of rods and cones but is a mass of overlapping fields, in each of which sensitivity decreases from the centre to the periphery. In general terms the central cells of the retinal fields respond to the onset of light and the more peripheral cells to the cessation of light. However, the form of the retinal fields is not uniformly circular; many are elliptical and some are almost rectangular. The fields are orientated in such a way that some of them are sensitive to external objects at a particular angle while others are sensitive to objects at quite a different angle. Again, there is special sensitivity towards curves and special sensitivity towards edges of external objects. It is obvious that even the simplest object in the visual field, say a short straight line, will have a representation upon the retina that spreads across several fields and has an effect upon many receptors. The convergence of the rods and cones upon the bipolar cells brings to the latter a variety of information from the various fields affected, and thus the bipolar cell serves as the first station of integration in the visual pathway, projecting onwards a single output which is the resultant of all the impulses reaching it.

These resultant impulses are transmitted from the bipolar cells to the secondary neurone, the "ganglion cell", which sends its axon over the surface of the retina to the blind spot where the axon turns inwards with others to form the optic nerve. Just as the rods and cones converge upon the bipolar cells, so the axons of the latter converge upon the ganglion cells. In man it has been reported that the retina contains about 125 million rods, whereas there are less than 1 million fibres in the optic nerve. Hence the information that passes along the optic nerve has already been considerably compressed and the visual fields have been converted into a more economical representation. Convergence is greatest for the data arising in rods; the human retina contains only about 1 million cones, hence they must have a large share of the optic nerve fibres. Such an arrangement is to be expected when it is remembered that the cones are the most discriminative receptor. Evidently the precision of their response to external objects does not require extensive modification. Indeed it seems as though there is no convergence at all for the cones situated in the fovea region. Each receptor at this location seems to have a separate line through to the thalamus, which would explain the high level of visual acuity of the fovea. As will be seen later, this is partly the explanation of the fact that many aspects of visual phenomena are a direct result of the properties and connexions of the retinal receptors.

In the *optic nerve*, as mentioned above, are the axons of the ganglion cells. Although traditionally considered to be the second cranial nerve, the optic nerve is really a tract that has extended to the brain substance. The reasons are (a) it is enclosed by meninges, (b) it is bathed in cerebrospinal fluid, (c) its fibres lack a neurilemma, and (d) it is composed of secondary fibres that pass directly to the thalamus. Beyond the fovea the axons are myelinated and are of several thicknesses. It is likely that the fibres of largest diameter are concerned with vision proper and that the small-calibre fibres subserve subcortical visual reflexes. Since the receptors in the fovea have a largely one-to-one relation with optic nerve fibres, it is not surprising that a disproportionately large part of the optic nerve is taken up by fibres from this region of visual acuity.

The *optic chiasma* in higher forms is the place where partial decussation of optic nerve fibres takes place. In the lower forms, such as fish, there is complete decussation so that each eye is represented on the opposite half of the brain. With ascent in the phylogenetic scale the percentage decussation becomes less until in man only about half the fibres cross the midline. By and large it is the fibres that are connected with the nasal halves of the retina that cross to the opposite thalamus, corresponding to the temporal half of the visual field. Fibres connected to the temporal regions of the human retina remain on the same side. No entirely satisfactory explanation of the visual decussation has been put forward, but many believe that it has to do with the migration of the eyes from the side to the front of the head.

In the *optic tract* on each side are collected the fibres that correspond to one-half of the visual field and these are simply swept along the base of the brain stem to the region of the thalamus. Most of the optic tract is made up of fibres that subserve the function of vision, but a few fibres, especially those of small diameter are concerned with visuomotor reflexes involving the pupil and the voluntary muscles. These fine fibres leave the tract near the lateral geniculate body and pass upwards to synapse in the pretectal nuclei (Fig. 10). Postsynaptic fibres pass into the tectospinal tract to influence spinal effector mechanisms. In man this system is not well developed; it is more obvious in lower animals which react more predictably and automatically to visual stimuli. Even so, sudden changes in the visual field are still able to evoke automatic head turning in man, due to the visuo-tectospinal activation of neck muscles. Such reactions, although not occurring wholly within the spinal cord, are nevertheless very much of the character of spinal reflexes. Other postsynaptic

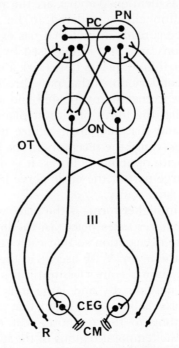

FIG. 10. Pathways involved in the light reflex and ciliary accommodatory changes. Discharges in retinal elements (R) pass along fine fibres in the optic tract (OT) to synapse in the pretectal nuclei (PN) on both sides. These nuclei are interconnected. Postsynaptic fibres run from the pretectal nuclei to the oculomotor nuclei (ON) on both sides. Third-order fibres run in the oculomotor nerve (III) to the ciliary and episcleral ganglia (CEG), from which quaternary fibres pass to the ciliary and pupillary muscle (CM). Missing from the diagram are fibres leaving the pretectal nuclei in the tectospinal and tectobulbar tracts, which subserve automatic motor responses to visual stimuli, e.g. head-turning. PC, Posterior commissure.

fibres pass from the pretectal nuclei to the nucleus of Edinger-Westphal, from which tertiary fibres run in the oculomotor nerve to the ciliary and episcleral ganglia. Fourth order fibres pass from these ganglia to the smooth muscle of the iris. Those from the episcleral ganglion are concerned with accommodatory changes in the pupil; those from the ciliary ganglion are involved in the pupil's response to light (the light reflex). A certain amount of crossing over occurs between fibres in the pretectal nuclei, so that information brought to a pretectal nucleus is passed (after a synapse and hence after integration) across the posterior commissure to the pretectal nucleus of the opposite side. This, plus the fact that the pretectal nuclei receive fibres from several areas of cerebral cortex (occipital and frontal), suggests that, at least in lower animals, visuomotor responses are not as simple as they appear to be at first glance. It is unlikely, however, that much significance should be attached to them in higher primates and man.

AUDITION

Neural pathways involved in hearing are much more complex than those concerned with vision. This section will deal only with the ear and the cochlear nerve. Other important regions are considered in the section on central mechanisms (p. 79).

The *ear* in most mammals is a highly sensitive organ. Changes in incident energy sufficient to produce oscillations of the ear drum as small as the diameter of a hydrogen atom are said to be capable of producing a sensation of sound. Textbooks abound with diagrams and descriptions of the mechanical apparatus of the ear, so no treatment of this topic will be given here. Instead attention will be directed at the receptors. As with vision, there is no doubt about the specific form and function of auditory receptors. These are the hair cells that occur in the organ of Corti (Fig. 11). Unlike most other receptors, the hair cells require an elaborate system of ancillary equipment to enable them to function properly. Vibrations of the air are passed by way of the tympanum, auditory ossicles, oval window and perilymph to the basilar membrane of the cochlea. Distortion of the basilar membrane causes displacement of the hair cells against the tectorial membrane and impulses are discharged into the fibres of the eighth cranial nerve. The hair cells are absent from those animals that are "genetically deaf", such as many Dalmation dogs, albino cats and waltzing guinea-pigs. An enormous amount of experiment and speculation has not yet produced a generally accepted explanation of how the cochlea responds to natural sounds. Details may be found in standard texts of general physiology, where it will be seen that the so-called Wever and Bray theory seems best to fit the experimental results. According to these two workers the cochlea distinguishes the qualities of pitch and intensity by (a) discharging at varying frequencies for tones of low frequency; discharging in particular regions for tones of high pitch; tones of intermediate frequency evoke a combination of frequency discharge and "place discharge", and (b) discharging a varying total number of impulses to correlate with loudness. In this latter regard the mechanism recalls the subject of the frequency

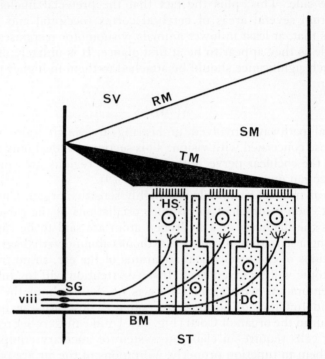

FIG. 11. Diagrammatic representation of the organ of Corti. Vibrations of the tympanum are transferred to the basilar membrane (BM) causing movement of the hair cells (HS) against the tectorial membrane (TM). The hair cell receptors cause impulses to travel down fibres of the auditory nerve (viii) to the spiral ganglion (SG). DC, Distant cells; RM, Reisner's membrane; SM, scala media; ST, scala tympani; SV, scala vestibuli. The whole system must be visualized as a section through a spiral structure.

code described in the section on somatic senses (p. 38). It seems that cochlear appreciation of pitch cannot be brought completely under this scheme, for there is no doubt that sounds of high frequency result in a preferential discharge of impulses from the more ventral regions of the cochlea, whereas low frequency sounds produce most activation in the dorsal part of the cochlea. Nevertheless, there is no point-for-frequency arrangement and in the final analysis the CNS must be presented with information in the frequency code. As with the eye, so with the ear there are discharges in response to the onset of sound and to the cessation of sound. Indeed auditory receptors seem to fall into the above-mentioned four classes, including the class of spontaneously discharging receptors.

Cell bodies of the *auditory nerve* (cochlear branch of eighth cranial nerve) occur in a cluster known as the "spiral ganglion". Distally the dendrites terminate in the hair cell receptors of the organ of Corti described above. Centrally, the axons terminate in the dorsal and ventral cochlear nuclei. The fate of auditory information beyond this point will be taken up in the section on central mechanisms (p. 79). Activity in the auditory nerve is by no means simple. It does not bear an obvious relationship to the stimulus—at least with experimental stimuli such as clicks and pure tones. A single click produces a short sharp volley of impulses in the nerve; with greater intensities the first wave is followed by a second or third wave. With a pure tone of constant intensity the auditory nerve shows a steady train of volleys that by and large reflect the frequency of the tone, though not in any single fibre. Volleys alternate between several fibres in synchrony to produce an overall result that is an accurate representation of the environmental change.

TASTE AND OLFACTION

Receptors for taste are distributed about the oral cavity: tongue, epiglottis, soft palate, fauces and posterior wall of pharynx. They are modified epithelial cells occurring in close contact with ramifying endings of nerve fibres that belong to the seventh, ninth and tenth cranial nerves. Each taste receptor (taste bud) consists of a group of cells forming a small globular mass with a distal pore. From some of the cells fine "hairs" project into the pore. Olfactory sense organs occur in the upper parts of the nasal cavity, as the olfactory mucosa on the superior turbinate, middle turbinate and nasal septum. They take the form of pseudostratified columnar epithelium. At the free end of each cell some 1 000 "hairs" occur; these are finger-like extensions of the protoplasm that serve enormously to increase the exposed surface area of the cell. Electron microscopy of rabbit olfactory mucosa reveals the presence of some 150 000 terminal processes per mm^2. An unusual feature of olfactory receptors is that no synapse occurs between them and the "higher" parts of the CNS. Nerve fibres pass directly from the hair cells, via the olfactory nerve (which is really a tract) to central regions subserving the sense of smell.

Fibres from taste buds are of small calibre and mostly myelinated. Unit recording from these fibres shows that threshold varies among the sensory units, greater concentration of applied solution bringing in more units and hence a greater total number of afferent impulses. Thus the sense of taste follows the usual frequency code system. By and large the tongue may be divided into regions that are particularly sensitive to certain flavours, e.g. the front responds mostly to sweet solutions, the sides to sour and the back to bitter. The midline areas are hardly at all sensitive. Nevertheless there is considerable overlap of sensitivity to give the wide range of flavours that is part of everybody's common experience. At one time it was considered that all taste buds were equal and that selectivity of flavour was brought about by the site of termination of the nerve fibres. This is not now thought to be the case. Application of solutions by micropipette to individual cells within taste buds has demonstrated that the receptor cells exhibit the sensitivity that would be predicted from the site of the taste bud. It is not yet clear whether taste bud specificity is due to specificity of the whole sensory cell or to varying sensitivity of various parts of the cell membrane. There is, however, no doubt that part of the mechanism by which taste information is conveyed to the CNS involves activity in contiguous fibres. It is likely that this mechanism is used to carry information about intensity. A 1% solution of a substance may excite the discharge of, say, 5 impulses in one fibre and 10 impulses in a nearby fibre; a 5% solution of the same substance may still excite only 5 impulses in the first fibre but 30 impulses in the second fibre. The difference in discharge *pattern* thus accounts for part of the mechanism of taste intensity discrimination.

Olfactory nerve (*not* cranial nerve I; see pp. 86–88) fibres run from the sensory hair cells through perforations in the cribriform plate to enter the olfactory bulb. They are extremely fine ($0 \cdot 2\ \mu$ diam.) and numerous (about 10 millions on each side). There is general agreement that each fibre in the olfactory nerve runs to only one hair cell, whereas several taste receptors may be innervated from a single fibre. Probably because of the great difficulty of exposing the olfactory nerve without damage to surrounding structures, very little functional data are available on the kind of electrical activity that goes on in these structures. More work has been done on the olfactory bulb, to be dealt with in the next section.

CHAPTER 4

CENTRAL MECHANISMS

Somatic Senses

SPINAL CORD AND BRAIN STEM

Impulses ascending the peripheral nerves pass the dorsal root ganglion and enter the spinal cord, from which point the mechanisms are considered to be central. Sensory fibres are collected into fairly discrete bundles in the dorsal root, forming the medial and lateral divisions. Within these divisions there occurs a certain degree of topographical distribution of fibres, producing a kind of map of the body region served. On entering the cord, sensory fibres in each modality tend to gather into discrete bundles, the ascending spinal tracts. Anatomical works should be consulted for full details of the disposition of the various sensory pathways. Figure 12 gives schematic representations of the major tracts, with emphasis on the physiological features. It should be noted that (a) all the entering fibres divide into ascending and descending rami, the latter being shorter than the former; (b) at intervals along both rami collaterals are given off which pass round to the ipsilateral ventral horn and engage with motor neurones for spinal reflex purposes (see also Fig. 22); (c) the ascending ramus soon ceases to give off collaterals and continues rostrally to engage, ipsilaterally or contralaterally, with a secondary neurone which in the case of conscious modalities passes to the thalamus from which a tertiary neurone is projected to the cortex; in the case of unconscious modalities (proprioceptive), the secondary neurone passes to the cerebellum. Brief perusal of a modern advanced account of the spinal sensory pathways (e.g. in "Handbook of Physiology. Section 1, Neurophysiology") reveals that Fig. 12 is a gross over-simplification of the situation and that many points are still in dispute such as the intermingling of modalities in various tracts, the exact points of origin, termination and decussation of some sensory pathways, and the presence or absence of minor pathways in man. This account, with its accompanying Figure, is meant to avoid such disputes and to deal only with what is fairly well established.

The spinal cord should not be regarded as merely a kind of rod along which impulses pass from one end to the other. A certain

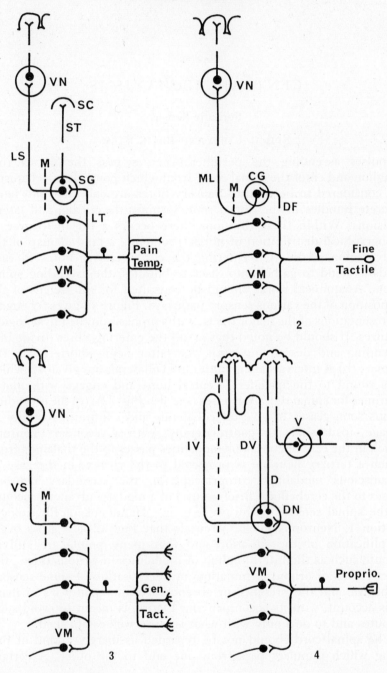

amount of collation and integration of sensory information occurs within it. It seems that many, if not all, dorsal root fibres carry impulses which excite some spinal neurones and inhibit others. Ventral horn motor neurones form a final common path for many inputs, each cell body being in contact with axons from higher regions and from several sensory pathways. A given motor neurone may be excited, for example, by impulses arriving in a proprioceptive fibre but inhibited by impulses flowing in along tactile fibres. Further integration of sensory information occurs as a field effect. Each incoming impulse excites a group of secondary neurone cell bodies. Cells in the centre of the field respond by discharging bursts of impulses at high frequency, whereas cells on the periphery of the field generate one impulse. In between these two extremes of position the cells will discharge a smaller number of bursts of low frequency impulses. Higher regions are thus given more precise information than they would receive if the sensory impulses were simply passed on along the cord in the same form as that in which they enter. This type of modification of incoming information occurs also, of course, when the secondary neurones arise in the medulla.

FIG. 12. Schematized representation of the main sensory pathways of the spinal cord and their higher destinations. VM, Ventral horn motor neurones.

1. The pathway for most pain and temperature information. Fibres travel in Lissauer's tract (LT) for a short distance before synapsing in the substantia gelatinosa (SG), from which secondary neurones pass (a) in the spinotectal tract (ST) on the same and opposite (not shown) sides to the superior colliculus (SC) and (b) across the midline (M) in the ventral white commissure to turn rostralwards in the lateral or dorsal spinothalamic tract (LS) leading to the ventral nuclei (VN) of the dorsal thalamus.

2. The pathway for fine tactile sense. Fibres run in the dorsal funiculi (DF) of the spinal cord to synapse on the same side in the nuclei gracilis and cuneatus (CG). Secondary neurones run as internal arcuate fibres across the midline (M) to join the medial lemniscus (ML) and travel to the ventral nuclei (VN) of the dorsal thalamus. With appropriate change of receptor, this diagram also represents the pathway for the conscious proprioceptive information from tendons and joints.

3. The pathway for coarse or general tactile sensation. Fibres cross the midline (M) almost immediately after entering the cord and ascend in the ventral spinothalamic tract to reach the ventral nuclei (VN) of the dorsal thalamus.

4. The pathway for unconscious proprioception. From the joints and tendons, impulses pass into the spinal cord to a synapse in the dorsal nucleus (DN) of the grey matter, from which secondary neurones (a) ascend on the same side in the dorsal spinocerebellar tract (D) all the way to the cerebellum via the restiform body (inferior cerebellar peduncle), (b) ascend in the ventral spinocerebellar tract on the same side (DV) and on the opposite side (IV) to curve backwards in the region of the pons, reaching the ipsilateral cerebellum via the brachium conjunctivum (superior cerebellar peduncle). The pathway for vestibular information is shown at upper right, where fibres in the vestibular division of the eighth cranial nerve synapse in the vestibular nuclei (V) from which secondary neurones run to the cerebellum.

(Compare these diagrams with those in Fig. 13.)

THE THALAMUS

From the neurophysiological point of view the thalamus is not so much a collection of some thirty distinct nuclei as a structure composed of a more or less unified dorsal region and a differently functioning but still more or less unified ventral region (Fig. 13).

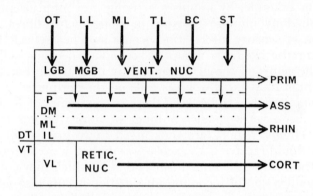

FIG. 13. Physiological organization of the thalamus. Six sensory inputs, from the optic tract (OT), lateral lemniscus (LL), medial lemniscus (ML), trigeminal lemniscus (TL), brachium conjunctivum (BC), and the various spinothalamic tracts (ST), discharge into the lateral geniculate body (LGB), medial geniculate body (MGB) and the ventral nuclei (VENT. NUC) which form the extrinsic nuclei of the dorsal thalamus (DT). Each of these regions (a) projects to its respective primary sensory area of cerebral cortex (PRIM) and (b) sends a small component to the pulvinar (P), dorsomedial nucleus (DM), midline nuclei (ML) and intralaminar nuclei (IL) which form the intrinsic nuclei of the thalamus. The first two of these send fibres to many association areas of the cerebral cortex (ASS); the last two project to rhinencephalic regions (RHIN). In the ventral thalamus (VT) the best known part is the reticular nucleus (RETIC. NUC) which sends fibres to many parts of the cerebral cortex (CORT). The ventral part of the lateral geniculate body (VL) is rudimentary in man. The dorsal thalamus is thus concerned with specific (PRIM) and relatively specific (ASS; RHIN) projections to the cortex, while the ventral thalamus delivers non-specific (CORT) information to the cortex.

The *dorsal thalamus* receives six sensory inputs from the body, two of which are concerned with the special senses and four with somatic senses; these all terminate in the various *extrinsic nuclei* of the thalamus.

(1) Auditory information arrives by the lateral lemniscus and enters the medial geniculate body (both crossed and uncrossed).

(2) Visual information arrives via the optic tract and reaches the (dorsal part of the) lateral geniculate body (both crossed and uncrossed).

(3) Proprioceptive information from the lower body travels via the medial lemniscus to the ventral nuclear region of the thalamus (crossed).

(4) From the head region somatic sensibility is transferred via the trigeminal lemniscus to the ventral nuclear region (crossed and uncrossed).

(5) Proprioceptive information from the dentate nucleus of the cerebellum reaches the ventral nuclear region of the thalamus by way of the brachium conjunctivum (crossed and uncrossed).

(6) Somatic sensory information ascending in the various spino-thalamic tracts adjoins the medial lemniscus and reaches the ventral thalamic nuclear group (crossed).

However, the classical view that sensory tracts send all of their fibres to the thalamus is no longer tenable. Every one of the six sensory inputs to the thalamus sends information elsewhere either by collaterals or directly. What structures the "elsewhere" involves has not yet been fully worked out but we shall be considering some of them later. It must also be accepted on the basis of modern work that the thalamus does not receive information only from the sensory tracts; this aspect of thalamic function will also be taken up later.

Information received by the extrinsic thalamic nuclei is modified to a greater or lesser extent and then projected to the primary sensory area of the cerebral cortex. Thus from the medial geniculate body fibres run to the temporal auditory region; from the lateral geniculate body the optic radiation reaches the occipital visual areas; from the ventral nuclear group fibres spread out to cover the parietal somatic sensory area. Thus, the cortical projections of the extrinsic nuclei represent the *specific* sensory radiations, i.e. each sensory modality follows a strictly localized pathway from the spinal cord to the cerebral cortex.

The other functional division of the dorsal thalamus is composed of the so-called intrinsic nuclei, whose name is derived from the fact that connexions to these nuclei all arise from other parts of the thalamus not from external sources as is the case with the extrinsic nuclei. Major constituents of the intrinsic nuclei are the pulvinar, dorsomedial nucleus, midline nuclei and intralaminar nuclei. Each of these receives sensory information from other regions of the thalamus, modifies and integrates it and then relays it to the cortex in accordance with the following scheme:

(1) The pulvinar and dorsomedial nuclei send fibres to the "association areas" of the neocortex, i.e. not to the specific primary sensory regions.

(2) The midline and intralaminar nuclei send fibres to various parts of the rhinencephalon, i.e. not to the neocortex proper but to the archicortex.

It will be obvious that the intrinsic nuclei of the thalamus are concerned with supplying the cerebral cortex with *non-specific* information, the second group being especially concerned with information of a more primitive kind. Phylogenetically, the nuclei of the second group do indeed become smaller with ascent of the evolutionary scale, whereas the first group of nuclei become progressively larger as specific sensory information plays a larger and larger part in the life of the organism; there is correlative evolution of both the capacity and the neural mechanisms for increasing attention to the specific form of external stimuli and its association with experience, so that the organism comes to rely less and less upon automatic, stimulus-response behaviour.

The *ventral thalamus* is composed of the ventral part of the lateral geniculate body (see above for dorsal part) and the so-called reticular nucleus. In man there is practically nothing to the ventral lateral geniculate body except a small group of cells and it is not known whether it has any function. In lower mammals it seems to be a relay station on the way from the superior colliculus to the tegmentum as part of the tectospinal optic apparatus concerned with automatic motor responses to visual stimuli. Rather more is known about the thalamic reticular nucleus although it has only recently been studied in any detail. Throughout the whole mammalian series there is no striking change in proportional size of the reticular nucleus, suggesting that the functions of this structure are just as important to the human as to the lower orders. We have seen that the dorsal thalamus sends projections to both strictly specific (extrinsic part) and to fairly specific (intrinsic part) regions of the cerebral cortex. This is not the case with the ventral thalamus seen as the reticular nucleus. Projections from this structure pass to very many, probably all, areas of the neocortex with very little specificity at all. In this respect the thalamic reticular nucleus bears resemblance to the midbrain and brain stem reticular formations (see Chapter 14). Because of its very widespread cortical projections the reticular nucleus is often considered to be functionally equivalent to the whole of the dorsal thalamus. Nevertheless some degree of localization is present, for small lesions in the cerebral cortex are followed by degeneration in only a restricted part of the reticular nucleus (as well as in the isotopic region of the dorsal thalamus). This slight localization will later be seen to have some importance.

THALAMO-THALAMIC CONNEXIONS

At this stage we might usefully pause to ask what is the function of the thalamus. Structurally, it is a mass of synapses. The synapse we know to be the unit of integration, so the purpose of the thalamic break in the path from sense organ to cortex must be looked for in terms of integration. Somehow the thalamus must combine several sensory inputs into one output to the cortex, for it is in this that integration consists. Each afferent sensory bundle entering the thalamus sends almost all of its fibres to a fairly localized region, as described above. But in addition each one sends a few fibres to the regions where the fibre-bundles from other tracts terminate. It is this arrangement that gives the opportunity for sense data in various

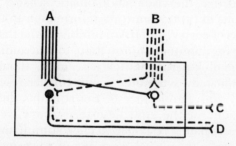

FIG. 14. Diagram to illustrate intrathalamic integration of several sense modalities. Sensory information entering at A is mainly transmitted to region D of the cerebral cortex, but part of the input is able to affect the synapses into which sensory input B is feeding. Thus the modality A is able to influence the information that reaches area C of the cortex, which is a primary area for modality B. In a similar way modality B modifies the information proceeding to area D.

modalities to have an effect on *one* area of cerebral cortex (see Fig. 14). Such connexions have been demonstrated for several modalities and the experts in this field believe that in time all senses will be seen to be so connected within the thalamus.

In addition to the above-mentioned anatomical evidence support for the teleological argument comes from experiments involving

unit-recording from thalamic regions. As would be expected, electrodes placed in the dorsal part of the lateral geniculate body record
the electrical activity of the thalamus evoked by light entering the
eye. When an auditory stimulus (clapping) was added to the experimental situation in the rabbit the magnitude and frequency of the
spikes in the visual thalamus increased. Hence, the auditory pathway
(a) carries information destined for the auditory cortex, and (b) is
able to *facilitate* the thalamic neurones which are carrying information
to the visual cortex. Similar results were obtained in experiments in
which the second stimulus was excitation of a peripheral nerve; that
is, the somatic sensory pathways also have dual functions, one of them
being to facilitate concurrent thalamic visual phenomena. However,
true integration is not simply a matter of facilitation, since the integral
output from a synapse should be the algebraic sum of incoming
facilitatory and inhibitory influences upon the postsynaptic cell body.
Experimental evidence for such intermodal inhibitory effects is also
available. Recording electrodes in the medial geniculate body detect
the thalamic activity due to sounds reaching the ear; this activity is
reduced when concurrent visual or somatic stimuli are given. Hence,
it may be stated that the visual and somatic sensory pathways have
the dual functions of (a) transmitting information to the corresponding sensory areas of cortex, and (b) of inhibiting the thalamic neurones
which are carrying auditory information to the auditory cortex. At
the present stage of experimentation it seems as though the auditory
modality is dominated by the others, but further research may show
that the quality and significance of the stimulus determines modal
dominance. Results of the kind described above were obtained by
recording a cat's thalamic response to click stimuli and then presenting the animal with the visual stimulus of mice in a jar. It is not
surprising that the cat paid more attention to the emotive visual input
than to the neutral auditory input. An experiment of great interest
would be to see whether the thalamic activity produced by a meaningful auditory stimulus (say, squealing of mice) would be inhibited by a
neutral visual stimulus (say, an empty jar).

All this is good evidence that there is interaction between the
sensory modalities at the thalamic level. It is evidence, anatomical
and experimental, that a measure of integration of several modalities
occurs in the thalamus. One might enquire what is the purpose of
this integration. Statements of purpose are guesses, inspired or un-
inspired, and the guess about this particular purpose is that it
generates economy of attention. It seems reasonable to suppose that

a stimulus to the skin requires the co-operation of the eyes rather than the ears. A wastage of neural effort would occur if attention were paid to auditory stimuli under these conditions. Obviously the animal does not stop hearing; it simply tends to ignore what it hears and gives its attention to what is stimulating the skin. Similarly, when the animal's attention is engaged by a more or less neutral visual stimulus, it is reasonable to expect that the visual attention is at a lower level than it will be when a sudden auditory stimulus (even a neutral one) impinges upon the situation. In these circumstances there is inhibition of *inappropriate* and facilitation of *appropriate* modalities. On the other hand, although more or less neutral sense data are continually streaming into the CNS, at times information of considerable meaning enters and it is reasonable to assume that neural effort is conserved by reducing central activity in all sensory modes except the one that corresponds to the stimulus, this one being increased. In these circumstances there is inhibition of modalities receiving *non-significant* stimuli and facilitation of the modality receiving *significant* stimuli. One may presume that appropriate interactions occur when the significant stimulus is plurimodal, i.e. a meaningful object making a meaningful noise.

Thalamic Maps

While the thalamus is under consideration, we may pay some attention to the question of topographical representation or "maps" since there is abundant evidence that such representation occurs.

In the modality of *vision*, the dorsal part of the lateral geniculate body takes the form of a grid reference to the retina. Fibres entering the lateral geniculate body via the optic tract terminate in an orderly sequence, producing a point for point distribution of synapses. Each half of the thalmus (i.e. each lateral geniculate body) carries the representation of the opposite visual field and thus has a grid reference to the temporal half of the ipsilateral retina and to the nasal half of the contralateral retina. In passing we may note that it is the projection from these two representations of retinal halves that produce visual areas I and II in the cerebral cortex (see Special Senses, pp. 71–79), although it should be borne in mind that visual area II has not been demonstrated in primates.

In the modality of *audition* the map in the medial geniculate body forms a topical representation of the spatial distribution of receptors in the cochlea, laid out in correspondence with the frequencies of audible sound. Again there are two representations in the thalamus, projecting to auditory areas I and II of the cerebral cortex (see Special Senses, pp. 79–85).

The *somatic senses* are represented in the thalamus very much in the form of an outline of the body projected upon the ventrobasal nucleus. The arcuate region of this nucleus contains both ipsilateral and contralateral representation of the face, brought by the trigeminal lemniscus. For the lower body, only one map occurs in each thalamus, representing the somatic receptors of the opposite half of the body. Yet on the cerebral cortex there are two somatosensory areas; stimulation of somatic sense organs results in increased activity in areas 1, 2 and 3 of the cortex, the postcentral gyrus, which forms somatosensory area I. However, stimulation of somatic receptors also evokes increased activity in the cortex that is tucked inside the Sylvian fissure between the auditory cortex and the face part of somatosensory area I; this latter region is designated as the second (*not* secondary) somatosensory area or somatosensory area II, a region that has also been demonstrated in the human cortex. Two things may be said of area I that cannot be said of area II: (a) ablation of area I is followed by retrograde degeneration in the ventrobasal nuclei of the thalamus; (b) electrical stimulation of the ventrobasal nuclei evokes electrical activity in area I. There can be little doubt, then, and in fact there is general agreement that the thalamocortical projection of somatic sensory information is from ventrobasal nuclei to area I, a contralateral representation because the sensory pathway has crossed the midline in the spinal cord or medulla.

Somatic sensory area II is still very much a puzzle. Connexions between it and the caudal extension of the ventral posteromedial nucleus of the thalamus have been described. It carries a representation of both halves of the body, not merely the contralateral side. Ablation of the whole area has practically no observable effect. Electrical stimulation of somatosensory area II is accompanied by movements on both sides of the body. In general terms it would seem that this area (and also the second areas of the special senses) represents not a secondary region but a primary one. The marsupials form a primitive mammalian group with what would be expected to be a primitive cerebral cortex. In these creatures the sense modalities are intermingled on the cortex with motor regions in such a way that practically the whole cortex is sensorimotor (Fig. 15). Thus it may be that bilateral representation of sensation and body musculature was the primary condition of the cortex. With increasing specialization and advancing skills, special secondary areas evolved that we now designate as primary (or I) simply because they were discovered first. It is also likely that at this evolutionary distance from the marsupials, the second cortical areas are to a large extent vestigial in higher mammals such as primates.

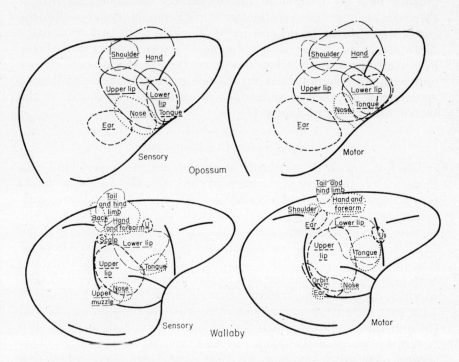

FIG. 15. Organization of the cerebral cortex in Marsupialia, showing how no clear distinction can be drawn between sensory and motor areas. This may represent the more primitive condition that is seen in the "second" sensory and motor areas in higher forms. (From Lende, 1963.)

CORTICO-CORTICAL PROJECTIONS

It is pertinent to inquire what happens to sensory information that has passed through the stages so far described and reached the cerebral cortex. At the outset it has to be admitted that relatively very little is known about this important matter. Obviously a complete answer to the question would carry within itself an excellent explanation of brain function as a whole. However, some information is available. It is known from both anatomical and functional evidence that all sensory areas send fibres to other parts of the cortex. Primary visual area 17 projects to area 18; primary auditory area 22 projects to area 21; somatosensory areas 1, 2 and 3 project to areas 4 and 6. Areas 4 and 6 and, it appears, somatosensory area II send fibres to the cerebellum. Direct interconnexions must not be assumed; it is possible with all or some of the projections mentioned above that there is a synapse between the two cortical points, either within the cortex or below it. In general terms, the role of these non-primary areas (sometimes called association areas) seems to be of importance in converting mere sensation into perception, so that objects are not only seen, heard and touched but also recognized and their significance appreciated. Further consideration of them will be found in the section on learning (Chapter 13).

CORTICO-RETICULAR PROJECTIONS

Much recent work, especially of an electrophysiological kind, has made it clear that very many parts of the cerebral cortex send fibres into the midbrain reticular formation (MRF). This structure, considered as the reticular activating system, is fully dealt with in the section on consciousness. Here it is only necessary to note that the MRF has a place in the consideration of sensory phenomena because it is likely that every cortical manipulation of sensory information, both primary and associational, is treated in two ways: (a) specifically, in which the precise qualities of the stimulus are recognized, compared with past experience and transformed into appropriate action, and (b) non-specifically in which the sensory information is dealt with in terms of its crudest qualities such as intensity and duration. This second mechanism involves the MRF, for it has been shown that neural elements within it can be excited by stimulation of any part of the sensory cortex. The MRF neurones are common to all modalities and do not distinguish between the points of origin of the stimuli, but are concerned with the total magnitude of sensory phenomena at any instant.

SENSO-RETICULAR PROJECTIONS

Earlier in this section it was pointed out that the classical sensory pathways from sense organs to thalamus must not be considered as exclusive. There is now general agreement that the fibres in every sensory mode send collateral branches to the reticular formation of the midbrain. Such collaterals carry immediately to the MRF the largely unmodified sensory messages from the periphery. We have seen that these messages also reach the thalamus, are modified (integrated) there and passed on to the cortex. In the cortex further modification occurs and the final result is, among other things, presented to the MRF. Thus the MRF is kept informed of two things: (a) what is happening to the sense organs, and (b) what the CNS, on the basis of its experience, is doing with the information supplied by the sense organs. These conditions are of course tonic, they go on all the time, even during sleep, and the MRF keeps up a tonic bombardment in what seems to be a non-specific fashion of both cerebral cortex and subcortical structures such as thalamus, hypothalamus and corpus striatum.

RETICULO-CORTICAL PROJECTIONS

Electrical recording techniques have shown that activity in the MRF is projected in a diffuse and non-specific fashion to the cerebral cortex. No matter whether the activation of the MRF is due to stimulation of a sense organ, stimulation of cerebral cortex or (experimental) stimulation of the MRF itself, the result is always a widespread activation of many cortical areas. Thus it may be seen that at least two of the functions of the MRF are: (a) to present many parts of the cortex with non-specific sensory information, while the thalamus is relaying specific messages to localized regions, and (b) to keep many parts of the cortex informed in a non-specific way of what the other parts of the cortex are doing. Since the MRF is a midline structure with neural elements common to both hemispheres, it evidently may serve in the interhemispheric transfer of non-specific information, while such structures as the corpus callosum serve the transfer of specific information from side to side in the cortex.

RETICULO-THALAMIC PROJECTIONS

It has already been pointed out that the reticular nucleus of the thalamus is known to project in a diffuse manner to many parts of the cerebral cortex. Most of the experts in this field, led perhaps by Jasper, now believe that the reticular nucleus of the thalamus should be looked upon as a rostral extension of the midbrain reticular formation, but with somewhat different functions. Anatomical studies have shown that the MRF is composed of some long and many short fibres occurring in chains. Some of these chains of short fibres run forward into the reticular nucleus of the thalamus. As mentioned above, there are differences. These are: (a) whereas the MRF sends tonic information to the cortex, the thalamic reticular region has a phasic discharge to the cortex; (b) when the MRF receives extra stimulation, its discharge to the cortex has low frequency and long duration; information sent to the cortex by the thalamic reticular nucleus has high frequency and short duration; (c) the MRF projects to the cortex with no detectable degree of localization, no points of correspondence between regions in it and regions in the cortex; as we have seen there is some evidence of a slight degree of correspondence between the cortex and the thalamic reticular region, and (d) the effect of the MRF discharge is to raise the central excitatory state of cortical neurones; the thalamic reticular region is able to produce either excitatory or inhibitory effects upon the cortex. Some workers hold the opinion that while the thalamic reticular region projects rather non-specifically to the cortex, yet there is functional localization in that some cortical regions are inhibited at the same time as others are excited. In this way the thalamic reticular region may contribute to the selective dulling and sharpening of senses involved in attention or "set". It is a matter of self-experience that, say, concentration upon the reading of a book is frequently accompanied by an apparent "deafness" to remarks addressed to the reader. Similarly, close attention to some manual task may render the subject temporarily unaware of minor injuries to the skin. There can be no doubt that the auditory or somatic sense organs, respectively, function normally under these conditions and send impulses into the CNS in the usual manner. Some central mechanism must act to reduce the consciousness of relatively unimportant sense data and at the same time heighten the receptivity and hence the consciousness, of the relevent sense data. The thalamic reticular nucleus seems suited for such a purpose.

CORTICO-THALAMIC PROJECTIONS

For very many years it was thought that connexions between the thalamus and the cortex were purely efferent from the thalamus. Recent studies using electrical recording techniques have produced a fundamental change in this view and indeed in sensory physiology as a whole. Functional connexions between the primary sensory areas of cortex and thalamic nuclei have been clearly demonstrated. Since the findings at present are limited to the special senses, consideration of the details are presented in that section(p. 78).

CENTRO-PERIPHERAL CONNEXIONS

Careful work over the last decade has produced irrefutable evidence to support the surprising belief that the brain modifies its own sensory input by direct control of the peripheral receptors. Some earlier anatomical workers had described a few efferent fibres in what were traditionally considered to be wholly afferent nerves and little attention was paid to such reports. But experiments in which record-ing electrodes are placed in or near receptors, with stimulating electrodes in various parts of the brain, have clearly demonstrated the role of such efferent components. As with cortico-thalamic phenomena, most of the research has been concerned with the special senses and is described in that section (p. 71). Here it may be noted that the discharge from muscle spindles in response to a stretch stimulus and the response of touch receptors to mechanical stimulation have been shown to be severely modified by stimulation of various brain areas. Activation of the midbrain reticular formation, motor cortex, anterior lobe of the cerebellum or head of the caudate nucleus produces facilitation of the receptors. That is, with a given constant stimulus the receptors give a higher frequency discharge when these brain areas are being stimulated than under resting conditions (Fig. 16). On the other hand, the reverse effect of inhibition

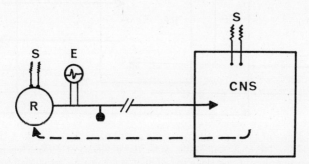

FIG. 16. Method of demonstrating central control of receptors. Stimulating electrodes (S) are inserted into the receptor (R) and into the brain (CNS). When the receptor is stimulated, the recording electrode (E) in the afferent fibre picks up different frequencies depending upon whether the brain is also being stimulated.

of receptors is produced by stimulation of the brain stem reticular formation. In the field of motor physiology it has become apparent that the midbrain reticular formation has a largely facilitatory action upon spinal motor mechanisms, whereas the brain stem reticular formation is largely inhibitory; these roles seem to extend also into the field of sensory physiology. It is apparent that the brain is by no means at the mercy of peripheral receptors. Under normal conditions

the brain exerts a dominance over the type of information being sent
to it as well as being able to process the sense data at several levels
centrally. One could be pardoned for believing that these mechanisms
are all aimed at removing the inevitability of stimulus-response

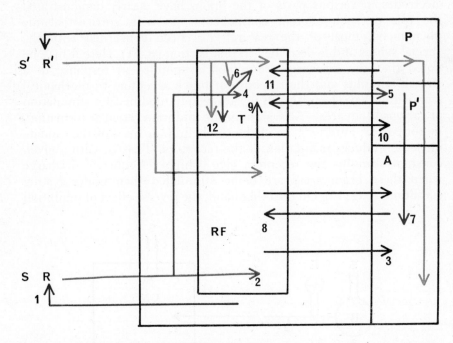

FIG. 17. Schematic diagram to summarize the mechanisms of sensation. A stimulus (S)
activates a receptor (R) that is tonically under the influence of central regions. (1) The
receptor causes impulses to pass along the afferent system to the reticular formation (RF)
and to the thalamus (T). Impulses arriving in the reticular formation (2) are relayed in a
wide and non-specific fashion (3) to association areas (A) of the cerebral cortex. Information
reaching the thalamus (4) is projected to the appropriate primary sensory area (PI) of the
cerebral cortex. At the same time, it is relayed to the regions where other (green) modalities
are supplying information and is itself influenced by the impulses arriving in the other
modality (6) which is projecting to its own primary sensory area (P) of cortex. From the
primary sensory areas, impulses travel by association fibres to the association areas (7).
The activity in the association areas is in part transmitted to the reticular formation (8),
which also projects into the thalamus (9), contributing to the non-specific output of the
thalamus to the cortex (10). Primary sensory areas of the cortex control their own inputs
by cortico-thalamic projections (11). The non-specific output of the thalamus is also
engendered by the collaterals from the extrinsic to the intrinsic nuclei (12). The diagram,
though incomplete and oversimplified, emphasizes that sensation cannot be properly
considered without taking account of (a) stimuli in more than one sensory mode (red and
green arrows), (b) the non-specific projection systems (black arrows), and (c) the "higher-
to-lower" projections (blue arrows).

reactions, giving the organism the opportunity to bring past experience to bear upon the total sensory environment and, once more, to concentrate attention upon what is deemed to be important under any given set of circumstances.

By putting together the pathways and functions mentioned in the preceding paragraphs, all of which apply also to the special senses, it is possible to arrive at a generalized view of sensation as shown schematically in Fig. 17. Such diagrams are suitable only when used to see in one scheme the phenomena of sensation as they appear at present. Figure 17 is undoubtedly incomplete and can only hint at the exciting knowledge that has yet to be acquired. Already recent research has demanded modification of the traditional view of sensation in two respects, (a) the non-rigidity of the effect of external stimuli upon the brain, and (b) the importance of non-specific central sensory mechanisms.

Special Senses

Schematic representation of the pathways for the special senses is given in Fig. 18.

VISION

Lateral Geniculate Body

To begin where the section on peripheral mechanisms ended, we take up the visual pathway where it enters the lateral geniculate body (LGB). This is the thalamic integrative station for the relay of visual information to other regions. Its architecture varies at different phylogenetic levels, but in the higher mammals, including man, a fairly uniform picture is seen that correlates with the development of binocular vision. In the rabbit, which is more or less monocular, no stratification of cells is seen in the LGB. In the cat, which has a fair degree of binocularity, there are three layers of cells. In monkeys and man the LGB is composed of six layers of cells alternating with layers made up of fibres from the optic tracts (Fig. 19). Cell layers numbered 1 and 2 (from the bottom) contain much larger cells than the others. Temporal retinal fibres (uncrossed) terminate in cell layers 2, 3 and 5; nasal retinal fibres (crossed) terminate in layers 1, 4 and 6. Each fibre synapses with several cells in the LGB but in primates there is very little or no overlap. A group of optic tract fibres has a 1 : 1 relationship with a group of LGB cells. The relationships may even be of the form where one fibre synapses with one cell in the region (central cone) of the LGB that represents the macula.

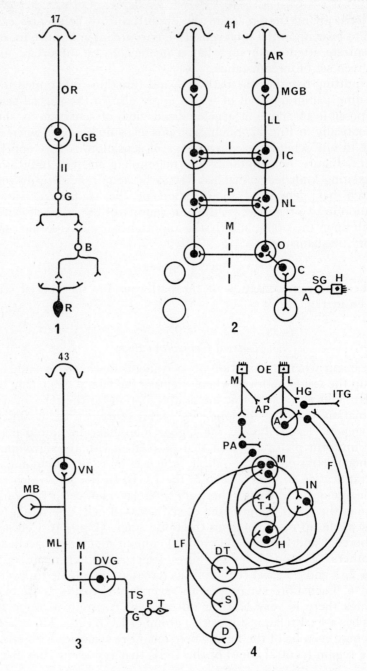

Evidently this non-diffuse transmission system is part of the neuro-logical basis for the highly discriminative powers of the primates. The groups of optic tract fibres that synapse with groups of geniculate cells represent the retinal fields that were described in the last section. Another special primate property is the phenomenon of transneuronal degeneration. If a spot on the retina is damaged in these higher forms, degeneration passes along the corresponding fibres of the optic tract, crosses the synapse in the LGB and continues along the optic radiation to the visual cortex. This is one of the ways in which both the LGB and the visual cortex have been mapped. Incidentally, however small the retinal lesion may be, degeneration is found in all three of the corresponding layers of the LGB. Allowing for this splaying-out of optic tract fibres, there is nevertheless an exact representation upon the LGB of the spatial disposition of the retinal

FIG. 18. Schematized representation of the pathways of special sense.

1. The pathway for vision. Rods or cones (R) converge upon bipolar cells (B) which synapse within the retina with ganglion cells (G). Axons from the latter pass in the optic nerve (II) and optic tract to the lateral geniculate body (LGB), from which tertiary fibres run to the primary visual area of cerebral cortex (17) via the optic radiation (OR).

2. The pathway for audition. Hair cell (H) receptors in the organ of Corti connect with fibres in the acoustic division (A) of the eighth cranial nerve and reach, via the spiral ganglion (SG), the cochlear nuclei (C). Secondary neurones pass to the superior olivary nuclei (O) and synapse with fibres that (a) pass to the superior olivary nucleus of the oppo-site side as trapezoid fibres and (b) ascend to the dorsal nucleus of lateral lemniscus (NL). The latter nuclei are connected across the midline (M) by the commissure of Probst (P), and each nucleus relays fibres to the inferior colliculi (IC) which are interconnected by the inferior collicular commissure (IC). From both inferior colliculi, fibres run in the lateral lemniscus (LL) to the medial geniculate body (MGB) which relays to the primary auditory area of cortex (41) via the auditory radiation (AR).

3. The pathway for taste. Taste buds (T) are connected via the petrosal ganglion (P), with fibres of the glossopharyngeal nerve (G) that enter the tractus solitarius (TS) and synapse in the dorsal visceral grey (DVG) of the medulla. Secondary fibres cross the midline and form the gustatory component of the medial lemniscus, ascending to the posteromedial ventral nucleus (VN) of the dorsal thalamus, from which fibres are relayed to the primary taste area of cortex (43). A small part of the gustatory component of the medial lemniscus (ML) passes to the mammillary body (MB).

4. The pathways involved in the olfactory sense. Receptors in the olfactory epithelium (OE) connect with the mitral cells of the olfactory bulb whose axons run in the lateral (L) and medial (M) olfactory striae of the olfactory tract. Both striae send branches to the anterior perforated substance (AP) and the medial stria sends branches to the para-olfactory area (PA), from which connexions are made with fibres in the fornix passing to the hippo-campal gyrus (HG). The lateral stria sends branches to the hippocampal gyrus and to the amygdaloid nucleus (A), which in turn connects with hippocampal gyrus. From the latter, fibres pass to inferior temporal gyrus (ITG) and by way of fornix (F) to anterior thalamic nuclei (T), the mammillary body (M) and the habenula nuclei (H). The last two structures connect with the interpeduncular nucleus (IN), from which fibres run to the dorsal tegmental nucleus (DT) which also receives fibres from the mammillary body via the dorsal longitudinal fasciculus (LF) as do the salivatory nuclei (S) and the dorsal efferent nucleus (D) of the vagus.

receptors, taking the form of a grid reference system. But it is not just that. In the cat at least, the fibres of the optic tract form two groups as they enter the LGB. One group synapses with cells that

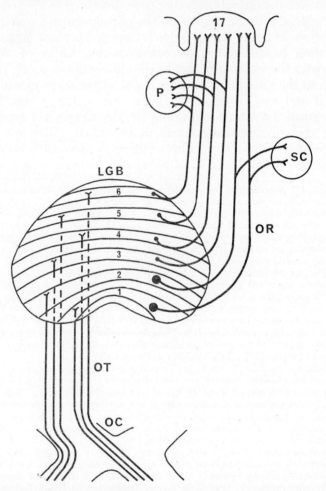

FIG. 19. Diagram of central connexions of the visual pathways. Optic nerve fibres that have crossed in the optic chiasma (OC) travel in the optic tract (OT) to the lateral geniculate body (LGB). This thalamic nucleus has six cell layers (numbered 1–6) which alternate with layers containing fibres from the optic tract. Uncrossed fibres terminate in layers 2, 3 and 5; crossed fibres terminate in layers 1, 4 and 6. Postsynaptic fibres, arising from large cells in layers 1 and 2 and from small cells in the other layers, pass in the optic radiation (OR) mainly to the primary visual cortex (area 17). A few fibres or collaterals pass to the pretectal nuclei (P), to subserve accommodatory and light reflexes, and to the superior colliculus (SC), to give rise to the visuomotor component of the tectospinal tract.

project to the visual cortex and the other group connects with post-synaptic fibres going to the lateral nucleus of the thalamus. Strong stimulation of the optic tract gives rise to two recordable spikes in the LGB, one in the region connecting with the cortex and another, much later, in the region connecting with the lateral thalamic nucleus. The threshold for the latter system is much higher than the first, so one may presume that only strong visual stimuli are relayed to the thalamus. Such intrathalamic connexions seem to apply to all sensory modalities (see p. 58). Optic tract components that innervate tectal regions are dealt with on page 49.

Optic Radiation

The fibres running from the LGB to the visual cortex form the optic radiation or geniculo-calcarine tract. There are many more fibres in it than in the optic tract, due to synaptic diffusion in the LGB. It is generally agreed that the optic radiation contains nothing but fibres running between the LGB and the cortex (perhaps in both directions). Although it is known experimentally that the visual pathway connects with the midbrain reticular formation (see p. 248), no anatomical information is available as to whether the connexion is by collaterals from the optic tract or by postganglionic fibres from the LGB. Stimulation of the optic radiation produces responses in the visual cortex (see below) that are not greatly different from the cortical responses obtained by stimulation of the optic tract or LGB. Hence although the LGB evidently processes information and does not simply relay it, yet the pattern of discharges in the optic radiation is not precisely correlated with the recordable changes in the visual cortex, at least on a statistical basis. It is likely that unit stimulation and recording might yield a closer relationship between geniculate and cortical mechanisms.

Visual Cortex

Although always tending to occur towards the posterior part of the brain, the visual cortex shows great phylogenetic variety in form, position and function. In monkeys almost its whole extent is to be found on the lateral surface, but the evolutionary trend towards expansion of the fronto-parietal association regions has pushed the visual cortex in man almost entirely round to the medial surface, with only a small part visible laterally on the occipital pole. It lies mainly on the dorsal and ventral free surfaces of the post-calcarine fissure, lower free surface of the calcarine fissure and runs deeply into these fissures. It is about 2·2 mm thick. It receives projection fibres from the lateral geniculate body which, for the macular region at the occipital pole, is said to be very nearly a point-for-point relation. Other parts of the lateral geniculate body (and hence of the retina) are represented on the visual cortex in a manner that reflects the organization of retinal elements into receptive fields. The cortical cells seem to be arranged in vertical columns, each column being particularly sensitive to specific visual stimuli, such as the angle of a line at a particular part of the visual field. Adjacent columns, while serving much the same part of the retina, are sensitive to different angles (Fig. 20). According to Hubel (1963) there are two types of cell in the visual cortex, simple and complex. Simple cells respond to lines or slits which have to be precisely placed in the visual field with respect both to angle and to location. Complex cells respond to lines, bars, edges or slits but the exact position is not so important as for the simple cells. Moreover, whereas simple cells cease to show electrical activity when the visual stimulus is even slightly moved, the complex cells continue to fire, even with considerable movement of the object. The behaviour of complex cells in the visual cortex is interpreted to mean that each such cell receives its input not directly from the lateral geniculate body but from a fair number of simple cells that are sensitive to the same type of orientation of the object as the complex cells. Such a concept is consistent with the finding that even the simplest stimulation of the optic nerve results in complex changes in the visual cortex that imply the involvement of three groups of cells. Clare and Bishop (1955) consider that the incoming pulses activate short-axon Golgi cells which in turn sensitize large pyramidal cells, each Golgi cell looking after a group of pyramidals. Recurrent branches from the long axons of the pyramidal cells activate other short-axon cells which then activate another set of pyramidals. It seems likely that the first group of pyramids is concerned with the transmission of primary visual information to nearby visual association areas such as area 18 (p. 204) and that the second group of pyramids leads to more distant secondary association areas such as the supra-sylvian gyrus (where visual and auditory information are associated).

When considering the function of the visual cortex, the phylogenetic level must always be borne in mind together with the fact that some responses to visual stimuli do not involve vision. In the lower animals visuo-tectospinal mechanisms (see p. 49) mediate motor responses to visual stimuli. These are very much of the nature of automatic, involuntary, unconscious spinal reflexes and there is no evidence that the animal actually sees anything until, for example, the head has been automatically rotated towards the object. In addition there is little doubt that even visual perception occurs at subcortical levels

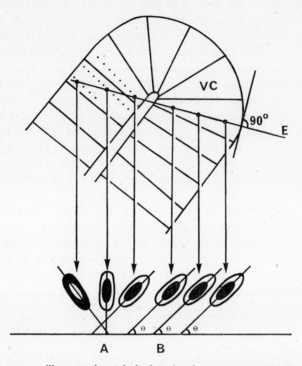

FIG. 20. Diagram to illustrate the orderly functional arrangement of cells in the visual cortex (VC). The line from E represents the track of a recording electrode, inserted perpendicular to the surface of the cortex. On the right-hand side the electrode would record from cells arranged in a vertical column. It would be found that each of the three cells shown responds only to objects in the visual field that are at a certain angle (θ) to the horizontal, as indicated at B. On the left-hand side the electrode would record from three cells that belong to different vertical columns (shown by dots). Each of these three cells would be found to responds to objects in the visual field at three different angles to the horizontal, as indicated at A. The ovals represent the receptive fields of the cells at the tops of the arrows, "off" regions (black) and "on" regions (white). "Off" regions are usually central in the receptive fields, but may be peripheral as at the extreme left. (After Hubel, 1963.)

for all visual phenomena in fish and amphibians. Total removal of visual cortex in, say, the rat, leaves the animal still capable of learning brightness-discrimination tasks. If the visual cortex is removed after such a task has been learned, it is forgotten but can be relearned.

Hence it appears that, in the rat, the visual cortex plays a part in the retention of visual functions that have been acquired by subcortical mechanisms. In man, removal of the visual cortex results in permanent, complete blindness. Evidently, the more primitive subcortical mechanisms, while perhaps still playing a part in the intact human, are unable alone to support the function of vision. Given, then, that the visual cortex receives optic information and converts it to primary sensation, its further connexions as outlined above carry the primary information to non-visual parts of the cortex where it is associated either with past experience or with information in other sensory modes. Stimulation of the visual cortex itself in man causes the subjective impression of flashes of light, washes of colour and so on, but no organized visual scene or memory. Thus it is difficult not to look upon the primary visual cortex in higher forms as an end station of great discriminatory but little elucidatory function. It serves well as the place to which retinal information is sent for subsequent relay to a variety of regions.

As described earlier, there is now no doubt that connexions exist along which impulses are carried from the visual cortex to the thalamus. These have been traced to the posteromedial and ventrobasal parts by electrorecording techniques and seem to represent a kind of servo-mechanism by which the cortex controls the input it receives (Buser *et al.*, 1963; Angel, 1963).

Second Visual Area

In some lower forms, such as cat, rabbit and dog a second visual area (II) has been described, but such an area has not yet been reported in primates. Visual area II occurs adjacent to visual area I and does not seem to receive fibres directly from the thalamus. It contains a mirror-image of the representation found in visual area I and hence is in some way connected to both retinae. Some authorities consider that the second visual area of lower forms is represented by area 18 (see p. 204) in primates. On the other hand, it may well be that the second visual area is phylogenetically prior when the evidence obtained in primitive mammals is considered (see p. 64).

Cerebellar Cortex

Excitation of parts of the cortex of the cerebellum occurs on stimulation of the retina electrically or by light. An area involving the pyramis, folium and simple lobe behaves in this way. The pathway from the retina is not known. Some workers favour relays from the superior colliculus over the known tectocerebellar tract, but more support seems to be given to a pathway in which pontine nuclei receive fibres from the superior colliculus and relay impulses over the pontocerebellar tracts. Stimulation of the occipital visual cortex also causes increased activity in the "visual" areas of the cortex and it is believed that this effect is mediated by occipitopontine pathways.

It is unlikely that the visual connexions to the cerebellum are concerned with vision as such. They are more probably involved in being integrated with the cerebellum's other exteroceptive and proprioceptive inputs in order that the cerebellum may have complete sensory information, so that it may play its part in motor phenomena such as the placing reflexes which depend partly upon visual cues.

AUDITION
Cochlear Nuclei

In the section on Peripheral Mechanisms (p. 51) we left the auditory pathway at the eighth cranial nerve. We now return to this modality where the auditory fibres enter the cochlear nuclei. These occur in the medulla where the auditory nerve enters. On each side there is a dorsal and ventral cochlear nucleus, the dorsal being the larger. Fibres entering the medulla in the acoustic nerve send branches to both nuclei. At least thirteen distinct subdivisions of the dorsal cochlear nucleus have been described and it is said that each entering fibre sends processes to all of these, and in strict order so that the cochlear pattern of excitation is, so to speak, unrolled upon the dorsal cochlear nucleus thirteen times. Some workers believe it is likely that similar connexions occur in the ventral cochlear nucleus. Since each acoustic fibre synapses with 75–100 nuclear cells, and since there are only about three times as many cells in the nucleus as in the spiral ganglion, there must be great convergence of the acoustic fibres upon the nuclear cells. Recordings made from single cells in the dorsal cochlear nucleus show that each cell fires with a characteristic frequency in response to pure tone stimuli of limited frequency range. By and large, the cells in the upper part of the nucleus respond to high-frequency sounds and those in the lower part of the nucleus are activated by sounds of low frequency. The frequency band over which a given nuclear cell responds depends to some extent upon the intensity of the stimulus; as the sound is made louder, so the range of frequencies causing a response becomes wider. It is evident that the degree of complexity of the cochlear nuclei suggests that they are by no means simply relay stations. A good deal of sensory integration must occur within them. As yet, the details of this integration are only poorly known.

Superior Olivary Nuclei

Postsynaptic fibres from the cochlear nuclei pass to (a) the superior olivary nucleus (SON) on the same side, (b) the brain stem reticular formation about the midline, and (c) the SON of the opposite side as the trapezoid fibres. Records made from the SON are similar to those obtained from the cochlear nuclei, but the variety of responsive cells is greater, suggesting that, at least, further frequency analysis of sounds occurs at this level. It is also believed that the SON acts as a relay station mediating auditory reflexes that involve parts of the ear, such as movements of the tensor tympani and stapedius muscles. It has been reported that a small bundle of fibres runs from each SON to the cochlea on the opposite side. This might be one of the pathways by which the central nervous system controls its auditory input.

Nucleus of Lateral Lemniscus

Fibres leaving the SON are collected into the lateral lemniscus and synapse in the nucleus of that bundle. At this point, for no apparent reason, the orderly spatial arrangement seen at lower (and higher) levels of the auditory system is lost. The nucleus of the lateral lemniscus is composed of groups of cells scattered among the lemniscal fibres. Some postsynaptic fibres pass by way of the commissure of Probst to the equivalent contralateral nucleus. No functional data seem to be available for the nucleus of the lateral lemniscus.

Inferior Colliculus

Most of the postsynaptic fibres leaving the nucleus of the lateral lemniscus pass to the inferior colliculus on the same side. This colliculus also seems to receive some fibres that come without synapse from the cochlear nuclei and from the SON. Hence, the type of auditory information reaching the colliculus varies from the unmodified cochlear output, through the altered character of the SON discharge to whatever type of messages are relayed by the nucleus of the medial lemniscus. Each inferior colliculus is connected to the equivalent contralateral structure by the inferior collicular commissure and by strands of intercollicular grey matter. The chief nucleus of the inferior colliculus shows no lamination, but in the more superficial, subsidiary nucleus the cells are arranged in orderly layers. Many workers believe that because of the complexity of its structure and connexions, the inferior colliculus should be looked upon as a "higher" region, not merely as a brain stem nucleus.

Recording from this nucleus again shows that single cells are selectively responsive to particular frequencies, and again the effective band is narrow with low intensities of sound and widens somewhat as the intensity is increased. There is little doubt that in lower vertebrates the inferior colliculus is the main region for such little auditory integration as occurs in these forms. Such creatures require simply a mechanism by which a sound signifying danger or prey shall activate the motor apparatus for escape or attack. The inferior colliculus, by means of its tectobulbar and tectospinal connexions, is ideally suited as the central integrative relay station for such responses. With the development of a nervous system capable of attaching symbolic meaning to sounds, i.e. of relating a given sound with a particular object or event rather than with non-specific danger, it became necessary that the auditory input should be correlated on a wider scale with other inputs and with past experience. Thus, in the higher forms the integrative and analytic properties of the thalamus and cortex have been added to the auditory system. However, it is likely that in "startle responses" the inferior colliculus still plays a considerable role, even in man. In the field of vision, of course, much the same remarks apply to the superior colliculus.

Medial Geniculate Body (MGB)

Postsynaptic fibres from the inferior colliculi run in the lateral lemniscus (and then the inferior quadrigeminal brachium) to synapse in this, the main thalamic end station for auditory information. Each MGB is composed of a so-called principle part, made up of small, densely packed cells arranged in a curving layer, and a smaller magnocellular region containing, as would be expected from the name, large cells. Considerable doubt has been expressed that the magnocellular part has anything to do with audition, though some workers claim that it projects to auditory area II of the cortex (see below).

The principal part of the MGB, when used as a basis for single-cell recording, shows a spiral pattern of tonal responsivity which corresponds to that of the cochlea, although there is no such complexity of cellular organization as found in, say, the dorsal cochlear nucleus.

However, it is also found that some cells do not respond to pure tones but are activated by such stimuli as clicks and general noise. The tone-responsive cells again show a widening of the effective frequency range with increase in intensity of sound. It is not yet known with any degree of clarity just what the MGB does with the auditory (and other) information it receives, but all workers are agreed that it cannot be looked upon as simply a relay station. There is evidence that some degree of conscious appreciation of pitch occurs at the MGB level even in man, and many lower animals exhibit the capacity of the MGB to discriminate between sounds of different frequency.

It must be remembered that, as with the lateral geniculate body and all other extrinsic thalamic nuclei, some of the postsynaptic fibres of the MGB pass to other parts of the thalamus, both extrinsic and intrinsic. In this way the thalamus aids in the matter of multimodal sensory integration (see p. 61).

Also, there is no doubt now that cells in the auditory cortex send axons to the MGB, thus controlling and modifying the output over the auditory radiation (see below). One puzzling aspect, not only of MGB function but of the auditory mechanism as a whole, is that some MGB responses to sound are very long-delayed. Recording electrodes in the MGB pick up activation in many cells about 6 msec after the application of a sound, but some impulses do not arrive there until after the neurological eon of 125 msec. There seems to be no explanation at the moment of what has been happening to the auditory information during all of that time, though it is apparent from the complexity of the pathway that much dispersion and reverberation must occur.

Auditory Cortex

The great majority of fibres leaving the MGB travel as the auditory radiation to the primary auditory area on the superior temporal gyrus (area 41). This is often now called auditory area I because of the subsequent discovery of a second auditory area (see below). Area 41 has a rather thick (3 mm) layer of cells, the main bulk being taken up by the granular layers; the pyramidal cells are unusually small. The MGB seems to project to the cortex in an essentially point-to-point fashion, so that a pattern of excitation in the organ of Corti is exactly represented on the cortex. This has been demonstrated quite clearly in animals where the auditory cortex is superficial (cat, monkey) and there is no reason to suppose that it does not apply to the human auditory area, which is largely within the sylvian fissure. Each cochlea is fully represented in both hemispheres, due to the multiple cross-over points mentioned above. Thus unilateral loss of the primary auditory area has little detectable effect on hearing.

Single-cell recording from the auditory cortex shows, as with the MGB, some units that respond to pure tones and others that will respond only to more complex sounds such as clicks and general noise. Once again the effective frequency band of tone-sensitive cells widens as the intensity of the sound is increased. It is likely that although there is a *proportional* decrease in tone-sensitive cells from the lower to higher regions, yet there is an *absolute* increase in them because of divergence at every level. It is thought that whereas the tone-sensitive cells are connected to a restricted part of the cochlea (or one of its replicas), the non-tone-sensitive cells receive a few fibres from all parts of the cochlea (or one of its replicas) and so respond to multifrequency sounds at any level of pitch-range. Another trend from the lower to higher regions is the appearance of cells that do not seem to respond to any kind of sound; in the primary auditory area, 40% of the cells are of this type. It is not, perhaps, unreasonable to look upon such "deaf" cells as being concerned with the integration of information from several "non-deaf" cells, with a view to carrying the resulting summary of auditory information to association areas. On this view of the function of "deaf" cells, there is obviously little need for them in lower regions.

Lest it seem a clear and simple concept that the presence of tone-sensitive, frequency-specific cells indicates that frequency is the basic parameter in auditory sensation, it should, perhaps, be pointed out that frequency specificity is only clearly demonstrable when the intensity of the stimulus is at or just above threshold level for the particular cell being studied. At higher intensities, indeed, the electrically recorded relationship between frequency of sound and discharge of central cell is not so well correlated as the subjective estimation of pitch. Quite evidently, the intensity of sound as well as its frequency is analysed by the CNS. Unfortunately relatively little work has been done in this field.

The exact functions of the primary auditory area remain obscure. Certainly it receives information that could be called mere sound. What it does with this information is unknown. Loss of a primary auditory area on one side in man is not followed by any detectable deficit. Bilateral loss, in the few cases in which it is known to have occurred, causes a slight (and possibly more apparent than real) defect in localization of sound source but nothing else that can be attributed to the lesion. In monkeys, removal of the auditory cortices seems to produce a slight loss in acuity of hearing; cats and dogs can still learn sound-based conditioned responses after this operation provided that the sound is simple. In these forms the auditory cortex is necessary for learning that involves a two-tone or three-tone sequence and thus plays a part in the synthesis of stimuli (p. 219). Stimulation of the primary auditory area in man gives rise to the subjective impression of elementary sounds such as clicks, buzzes, roaring noises. If the same spot is re-stimulated after a very short interval, then the same sensation is experienced, but after a longer interval a totally different "sound" occurs. It would seem, then, that the precise nature of the subjective phenomenon is not simply a property of the actual cells stimulated.

As mentioned below, the auditory cortex sends fibres to the medial geniculate body to control its own input. Other efferent paths link the primary auditory cortex with the auditory association areas (22 and 37, see p. 203) and also with visual association areas (18 and 19, see p. 204). It is likely that a number of other intercortical connexions occur and the total of these probably represents the real function of the primary area—as an integrative focus from which classified information is radiated to cortical regions that subserve unimodal and multimodal association, as with the visual cortex (see p. 75).

Second Auditory Area

In lower animals (cat, dog) another auditory area has been found; this abuts onto the primary area and contains a mirror-image of the cochlear representation found in auditory area I. Unlike visual area II, auditory area II has been found in monkeys and in the chimpanzee. Some workers believe that area II is connected with the magnocellular part of the medial geniculate body; others report a connexion with the posterior region of the principal part of the medial geniculate body, and there is little doubt that there are interconnexions between auditory areas I and II. Auditory area II may represent the primitive condition of the cortex, on the basis of observations made in Marsupialia (see p. 64).

Cerebellar Cortex

Electrical recording from the vermis of the cerebellum shows that sound stimuli are followed by excitation in that region. Degeneration of cells in the basal part of the dorsal cochlear nucleus occurs after lesions in the vermis. The pathway from the cochlear nucleus is not known but most authorities believe that the tectopontine tract from the inferior colliculus to the pons, followed by the pontocerebellar pathway, represents the most probable route. Also as in the field of vision, stimulation of cerebral cortical areas results in excitation in the cerebellum and conversely.

It is considered improbable that these pathways have any significance in the sensation of hearing, but simply serve to add more sensory information to the cerebellum's input from other sources, so that it has a more complete picture of the external situation to aid its control of the muscles.

TASTE AND OLFACTION

Although the central pathways mediating the gustatory sense are complicated and ill-understood, yet there is general agreement that at all levels there is an extremely close anatomical association between taste elements and somatosensory elements. In the medulla, for example, electrodes in parts of the tractus solitarius respond equally whether the tongue is stimulated by touch or by flavoured solutions. This is not single unit recording, so there is little doubt that different but close-together neurones are responding. Similarly in the thalamus, excitation produced by flavoured solutions is picked up in the region that is also excited by touch stimuli to the face (arcuate nucleus). Again, in the cortex, taste stimuli evoke action potentials in the region of somatosensory cortex that responds to electrical stimulation of the structures involved in chewing. Hence, the overall picture is that taste differs from the other special senses in that no part of the central nervous system is exclusively or even mainly devoted to its mediation. Moreover, no known part of the taste pathway seems to have a very decisive role to play in this sensory mode. Lesions in the taste region of the thalamus or cortex usually do little more than raise the threshold for discrimination. Stronger solutions are needed in a choice-testing situation, but unpleasant materials such as quinine are rejected at the same concentrations as by normal animals. In man, lesions of the inferior part of the postcentral gyrus may or may not result in (among other things) small deficits in tongue sensibility. Stimulation of the face and tongue area of cortex in the human is accompanied by hallucinations of taste sensations. Most workers seem to believe that consciousness of mere flavour can occur at the thalamic level, even in man, whereas the cortex is necessary for the identification of substances and the affective tone that accompanies this. Such beliefs are tentative and speculative but useful nevertheless.

Olfaction is perhaps the oldest and, in higher forms at least, most degenerate of the special senses. There appears to be in the modern animal brain a vast and complex system that once was present for

olfactory purposes only but is now gradually acquiring other functions. It is small wonder that the neurophysiology of the sense of
smell is highly intricate. No great service would be done to the
reader by an expansive survey here; the Bibliography (p. 301)
will take those interested to better sources. There follows a general
account only.

Olfactory Bulb

The receptors in the olfactory epithelium send fibres through the
cribriform plate of the ethmoid bone to synapse in the olfactory bulb.
These fibres are extremely thin, are unmyelinated and have the
slowest conduction rate of all nerve fibres. It is these small fibres
that represent the true olfactory nerve, comparable with, say, the
oculomotor or the vagus. By common consent, however, the historical
designation of cranial nerve I to the olfactory tract is still used.
The olfactory bulb, a swelling on the end of the olfactory tract, lies
over the cribriform plate and contains large, so-called "mitral" cells,
frequently arranged in a layer central to molecular and granular
layers. Fibres from the receptor cells synapse with the mitral cells
and with nearby "tufted" cells. It has been reported that each group
of mitral (25) and tufted (70) cells obtains information from about
25 000 receptors.

Olfactory Tract

This is frequently called the olfactory nerve or cranial nerve I.
It contains the axons of some 50 000 mitral cells. Most of these pass
backwards as the lateral and medial olfactory striae, but a few very
thin fibres pass into the anterior limb of the anterior commissure
and extend into the olfactory tract of the opposite side. It seems
from both animal and human data that destruction of both olfactory
tracts permanently and completely abolishes the sense of smell.

Higher Regions

Studies involving degeneration after ablation of the olfactory
tracts and those concerned with recordable activity after stimulation of
the olfactory tracts have implicated the following regions in olfaction:
prepyriform cortex, amygdaloid nuclei, nucleus of the stria terminalis,
septum, hippocampal formation, midline thalamic nuclei, mammillary body, habenula nucleus and, rather oddly, the globus pallidus.
The precise role, or any kind of role, in olfaction of these structures
is still highly obscure. In many of them there is a very long latency
of response (up to 38 msec) that as yet has no explanation except in

anatomical terms of chains of neurones. Lesions in one or other of these higher regions do not abolish or greatly impair olfaction. Destruction of the prepyriform and amygdaloid regions severely interferes with olfactory conditioning, so these areas may be concerned with olfactory associations and odour-memory.

Supplement on Sensation
SOMATIC SENSES
Receptors

Despite some concentrated research upon receptors, it is still not understood how they initiate impulses in the afferent nerve fibres. Two main schools of thought are extant. One considers that at least some receptors produce a change in the potential of the afferent when they are subjected to mechanical distortion (Loewenstein, 1961). On this view, the size of the potential generated in the afferent will be proportional to the area of receptor that is distorted, giving a physical basis for intensity discrimination. It has been suggested that distortion of the receptor membrane in some way alters the ionic permeability of the membrane and that this in turn affects the afferent resting potential (see p. 9). Another view is propounded by Hunt and Takeuchi (1962) on the basis of experiments in which they recorded from different points along a Pacinian corpuscle. They believe that the receptor acts as an electrical sink for the potential in the nearby afferent. Stimulation of the receptor by mechanical means or stimulation of the afferent (giving antidromic impulses to the receptor) resulted in the appearance of negativity in the receptor, with a latent period that was dependent upon the distance of the recording electrode from the nerve terminal.

With regard to muscle spindle receptors, it has become apparent that these are much more complex structures than was at first thought. At least two types of fibre are present in the spindle (Boyd, 1962). A few very long fibres with "nuclear bags" (densely packed nuclei) in the middle region are supplied by large-diameter ($2 \cdot 5-6 \, \mu$) fibres terminating in end-plates. More numerous are the shorter fibres with a "nuclear-chain" in the middle region, supplied by small-diameter ($1-2 \, \mu$) fibres that terminate in a network of very fine endings. From both of these types of intrafusal fibre, one large afferent originates; in addition a number of small afferents arise from the nuclear-chain fibres. No knowledge is yet available about any separate roles of these two types of fibre but speculations and further details of current research in this field are given by Perl (1963).

D

Although, as mentioned on page 35, there is a strong school of thought that specialized receptors must be looked upon with considerable caution, yet some evidence has been produced (Iggo, 1962) that hairy parts of the skin contain organized neurovascular domes with disk-like nerve terminals that initiate impulses in the afferent when stimulated by very light touch or by cooling. Specialized epithelial cells closely associated with the neural disks are thought to be the actual receptors.

The sense of vibration in man has never been understood. Some help comes from the studies of Hunt (1961) in which he was able to demonstrate that at least some Pacinian corpuscles in the cat generated action potentials in their afferents when subjected to vibrations of 50–800 c/s, whereas other types of receptor did not.

Thalamus

It has been stated (p. 59) that spinothalamic pathways terminate in an intermingling fashion in the ventrobasal nucleus of the thalamus. This is only one of possibly four thalamic sites of termination of fibres in these pathways, although the physiological significance of the others is not yet known. In addition to the ventrobasal nucleus, spinothalamic fibres are also said to end in (a) a part of the magnocellular region of the medial geniculate body, (b) the midline intralaminar nuclei, and (c) the reticular nucleus of the thalamus. Possible functional roles in perception of these various thalamic terminations are considered by Mountcastle (1961). The existence of the intralaminar synapses has raised again the matter of fast and slow pain. It has been reported that, in the cat, noxious stimuli to any part of the body cause evoked potentials in the intralaminar nuclei, one very quickly and the other half a second later (Albe-Fessard and Kruger, 1962). Since the medial region of the thalamus has been implicated in human pain perception, these findings may form a basis for the two types of pain sensation. Before leaving the question of pain, the clinically minded reader might be directed to an interesting account of complete congenital indifference to pain in an individual whose brain showed no obvious abnormality (Magee, 1963). This topic is reviewed at length by Critchley (1956).

The impression has deliberately been given in the earlier sections that in the sensory modalities a synapse always occurs between the receptor and the thalamus. This view is a simplified one and needs to be modified. Although the occurrence of a synapse in this location is the rule in lower animals and is true for the majority of ascending fibres in the higher animals, yet there is good evidence that some fibres pass directly to the thalamus. Mehler (1957) has made a phylogenetic study in this field which shows that the number of these parallel pathways increases with ascent of the evolutionary scale. This has been interpreted by Bishop (1961) to represent the increasing degree of specific central control of motor activity that is seen in the higher animals.

Cerebral Cortex

It has now become apparent that just as the skin is made up of receptive fields, so the somatosensory cortex carries representations of these fields. Moreover, within each of the overlapping fields on the cortex there are neurones that respond to only one kind of somatic stimulus, e.g. hair-bending or light touch (Brooks *et al.*, 1961). Some of the fields on the cortex were not constant in location but varied with continuing stimuli to the skin. Very frequently the cells in the variable fields started by exhibiting unimodal sensitivity and then, as the boundaries of the field shifted, began to respond to other types of stimuli. It is considered that alterations in synaptic interchanges at lower levels might account for varying types of bombardment of given cortical neurones.

Somatic sensory area II has not yet been demonstrated in the primate. Studies made by the evoked-potential technique have shown that this area in the cat overlaps considerably with auditory area II, i.e. in some regions of cortex stimulation by sound or by exciting a peripheral nerve evokes an action potential in the same neurones. With successive stimuli the particular result obtained depended upon which stimulus came first and how long after it the second one was applied (Berman, 1961). In view of these results, one may cogitate as to what part is played in them by the terminations, mentioned above, of spinothalamic pathways in the medial geniculate body. Representation of the body upon somatic sensory area II is by no means as precise as in the corresponding area I. This has been carefully examined by Celesia (1963), who finds a particularly vague and overlapping representation of arm and leg areas and confirms that both sides of the body are represented on area II and that the latency of evoked potentials is much shorter than for area I.

On several occasions in earlier parts of this section mention has been made of the central control of sensory input. It has been said that the CNS affects the receptors and the thalamus (see p. 69) but no details of central regions or centrifugal pathways were given.

Practically nothing is known from this anatomical point of view. However, it has recently become apparent that the sensorimotor cortex, at least in the cat, is able to influence the activity of the ascending systems of the spinal cord. Lundberg *et al.* (1963) have shown that electrical stimulation of the sensorimotor cortex causes a stimulatory effect upon the ventral spinobulbar tract and an inhibitory effect upon the ventral spinocerebellar tract. The authors believe that the centrifugal effects are mediated by the pyramidal tract.

SPECIAL SENSES

Vision

The organization of the retina as given previously was tremendously simplified, as can be seen from an examination of Fig. 21 which is taken from the excellent book by Polyak (1941). A text covering the work of several investigators using more modern techniques has been presented by Smelser (1961). An excellent short review of both retinal structure and visual pigments is available (Dartnall and Tansley, 1963). One factor that has emerged from studies with the electron microscope is that the retinal receptors have a lamellar structure which seems to result from the orderly arrangement of molecules of visual pigments. Such stratifications might explain the specific sensitivity of various cells to the angle of objects in the visual field (see p. 76). It is also possible that part of this mechanism is the special gross morphology of the receptor, for it has been shown that some cones at least have localized thickenings on them.

It has already been pointed out that all receptors, including visual ones, exhibit the property of adaptation. This is seen very clearly with respect to retinal receptors under special conditions. The eyes are never at rest. Even under the most immobile of natural conditions there is a slight continuous nystagmus (Ditchburn and Ginsborg, 1953) which, of course, means that no natural image is ever still for very long on the retina. If by experimental devices, either the eye is fixed or the object is moved in synchrony with the small eye movements, then the image does indeed fall upon one set of receptors. Under these conditions the image disappears after a short time, leaving a grey background. A very slight movement of either object or eye is sufficient to bring the image in view again, as is a slight increase or decrease in the intensity of the visual stimulus. Such phenomena can be explained on the basis of receptor adaptation and on the view that receptors signal *changes* in incident energy.

However, it should be noted that some workers (Clarke and Belcher, 1962) believe that the disappearance of fixated images is due to some mechanism further along the visual pathway but distal to the cortex, with the lateral geniculate body as a favourite site. Along similar lines it has recently been shown that the firing frequency of retinal ganglion cells depends not so much on the intensity level of a light

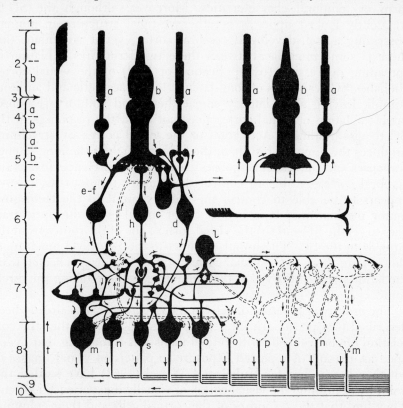

FIG. 21. Schematized impression of retinal organization. It is assumed that light is falling upon the left hand group of receptors (a, b, a). Excitation is transferred from the receptors to (i) horizontal cells (c) which raise the excitatory state of adjacent receptors (i.e. the right-hand group, a, b, a), and (ii) bipolar cells (d, e–f, h) of the centripetal variety which transfer the excitation to the ganglion cells (m, n, o, p, s) whose axons collectively form the optic nerve. The bipolars serve as analysers of the optic information. Centrifugal bipolar cells (i, dotted outline) receive impulses from three sources— ganglion cells, centripetal bipolar cells and from fibres (f) of unknown but central origin by which the brain controls its visual input because the centrifugal bipolar cell transmits impulses to the receptors. Excitation is spread horizontally to nearby ganglion cells by the amacrine cells (1). Note the convergence of receptors upon bipolars and of bipolars upon ganglion cells. (From Polyak, 1941.)

stimulus, as upon the rate of change of intensity, both towards increase and towards decrease (Enroth-Cugell and Jones, 1963).

Investigations on the *superior colliculus* (SC) have shown that at least in the cat this structure is a complex multimodal integrating region. Electrical recording from the SC reveals that visual, auditory and somaesthetic stimuli all evoke potentials but not identical in form or temporal characteristics. Moreover, although the SC is frequently looked upon as a rather vestigial structure in animals possessing a well-developed cerebral cortex, yet it is evident that there is some interplay between these two structures. Ablation or spreading depression (by application of KCl) of the visual cortex abolishes SC responses of long-latency to somaesthetic and auditory stimuli, leaving short-latency somaesthetic and auditory responses intact; ablation of visual cortex does not affect the responses in the SC to visual stimuli. Activation of the visual cortex by strychnine produces the opposite results in the SC inasmuch as the long-latency responses and the visual responses are augmented. Hence, just as the cerebral cortex is able to control the sensory input to itself, so it appears to be able to control the sensory input to the tectospinal motor mechanisms. It is believed that impulses in the optic tract pass to (a) the SC and (b) the visual cortex; one of the routes from the latter is to the SC. The impulses direct to the SC travel much more slowly than those to the visual cortex, so that impulses reflected from the latter arrive at the SC at the same time as those taking the direct route.

The orderly orientation of cells in the *visual cortex* has already been described (see p. 76). An interesting question was whether the correlation of cortical cells with retinal fields was something that developed as a result of repeated exposure to patterned visual images or whether it was innate. Hubel and Wiesel (1963) have settled this point by examining the visual cortex of visually inexperienced kittens. They find that the responses of the cortical cells and their columnar organization is essentially the same as in the adult. Hence, it seems reasonable to believe that in higher mammals at least the visual system develops in such a way that even before light has ever entered the eye the arrangement of components takes a form that is especially sensitive to specific orientation of objects in the visual fields.

Audition

A considerable amount of research has been carried out recently upon the *organ of Corti*. Electron microscope studies have shown that the hair cells in this structure have varying numbers of lamellae at their outer edges which are continuous with the cell membrane. Some workers (e.g. Hawkins, 1964) believe that these lamellae are "involved in the conduction of the excitatory process from the apical, transducer end of the hair cell to the basal, transmitter end, where the cluster of nerve endings surrounds it." However, there is a school of thought which believes that the hairs of the receptor cells are in contact with the basal body of the cell and that this latter structure is the one that generates excitation. There remains little doubt that the hair cells are activated by movements of the tectorial membrane, but it is possible that actual bending does not have to occur. It seems as though the hairs of the inner cells do not touch the tectorial membrane if it is not vibrating under the influence of sound (Engstrom *et al.*, 1962); perhaps hair cells in such locations are specifically so placed to signal variations in intensity of sound.

Recordings made simultaneously from several regions of the *cochlea* have shown that excitation travels along this structure in a wave form. Thus the cochlea should not be looked upon as being excited only in a certain place by a sound of particular pitch, although there may well be a place-specific component involved that serves in pitch discrimination. One still-puzzling aspect of the cochlea is its relatively abundant efferent nerve supply. Several workers have shown that about 500 efferent nerves terminate in granular endings upon the hair cells of each cochlea (see, for example, Smith and Rasmussen, 1963). Despite careful and experienced attempts to demonstrate a function for these fibres (Galambos, 1960), many of which arise from the ipsilateral and contralateral olive, the only useful information about them is that cochlear potentials are enhanced and the auditory nerve potentials reduced when they are stimulated (Fex, 1959). It is reasonable to suppose that they are part of the mechanism by which central structures control the sensory input.

Similar central control is found in the *cochlear nucleus*. Cells in this structure are well known to exhibit spontaneous firing. If one ear is destroyed and the other ear stimulated by sound, the spontaneous firing in the ventral cochlear nucleus on the side of the damaged ear is inhibited (Pfalz, 1962). For particular neurones the inhibition is often frequency-specific, so that, according to Pfalz, one of the roles of central control of sensation in audition may be to focus the system for various frequency bands.

Records made from single neurones in the *medial geniculate body* have revealed rather interesting temporal properties. Nelson and Erulkar (1963) have shown that under the influence of a steady tone, the thalamic auditory cells take several seconds to reach a state of maximal excitation and then take several seconds to return to the resting state when the sound is stopped.

Studies on the *auditory cortex* have been very numerous of late, being largely concerned with topographical relations (Woolsey, 1961) and behavioural studies following ablations (Neff, 1961). As with the visual and somatosensory areas of cortex, there seems to be good evidence that the cells of the auditory cortex are arranged in vertical columns, each column being composed of cells with similar sensitivity characteristics. Unfortunately it has not been possible to delineate on the auditory cortex anything like a precise frequency map, or indeed any kind of map, but it behaves like other areas in having regions that respond to the onset of a sound and other regions that respond to the cessation of a sound. It is thought that during a sound stimulus active inhibition of some cortical regions occurs which then disappears when the sound stops. Though it is not possible to state precisely what the auditory cortex does, it is clear that this structure is not necessary in the cat for discrimination of intensity or pitch. However, cats with ablated auditory areas cannot distinguish between two-tone or two-duration patterns. This latter function of the auditory cortex appears to be acquired by experience, for ablation of the auditory cortex in 7–9-day-old cats did not abolish their ability to discriminate tone and duration patterns (Scharlock *et al.*, 1963).

Perception

Very little can be said about the manner in which sensation is transformed into perception (i.e. subjective impression), except that a great many factors seem to be involved including psychological ones, whatever they are. This latter point is shown clearly in a combined study of sensory estimation and personality type (Petrie *et al.*, 1963). It was found that certain types, called "augmenters" exhibit both intolerance to pain and a tendency perceptually to increase the size of objects (under blindfolded conditions) held in the hands. Others, called "reducers" show considerable tolerance to pain and tend perceptually to decrease object size. The remainder of the subjects formed a group called "moderates" who have a normal tolerance to pain and who do not make perceptual changes in object size. In clinically normal augmenters and reducers the perceptual distortion disappeared or was considerably reduced after a 15 min rest from testing. When schizophrenics were examined, however, it was found that (a) they shifted from extreme augmentation to extreme reduction, and (b) the perceptual distortion persisted after the rest interval. Whether perceptual distortion might serve as a diagnostic aid in mental disease is a point that should perhaps be looked into more closely.

An excellent long review on various aspects of perception has been prepared by Teuber (1960).

Part III

Movement and Posture

CHAPTER 5

BASIC MECHANISMS

In the higher animals the spinal cord has two main functions: (1) it serves as a line of communication between the brain and the body, by means of its ascending and descending fibre tracts, and (2) it behaves as a correlating and reflecting structure by which information from the periphery is organized and returned to the periphery. It is with the second of these functions that this section deals. It should be remembered that in the intact animal the two main functions of the spinal cord do not operate separately. The mere fact that in order to examine spinal reflexes properly, the cord must be separated from the brain, indicates the dominant modifying role of higher regions.

Figure 22a shows the more common type of diagram used to illustrate the simple spinal reflex. However, this leaves a great deal out of the picture. Also, if the neuronal connexions shown in the diagram really existed, it is far too complex. The diagram suggests that an impulse travelling in the dotted fibre results merely in the passage of an impulse down the efferent fibre to the muscle it supplies. Such a system does not need a central mechanism at all. A loop at the periphery between the sense organ and the muscle would suffice.

A more accurate and informative type of diagram is based on the illustrations published by Ramon y Cajal in 1909. Figure 22 shows the two basic forms of the improved diagram. In Fig. 22b, the afferent fibre enters the cord through the dorsal horn and then bifurcates into ascending and descending branches, *as all spinal afferent fibres do*. The ascending branch passes to supraspinal regions, frequently with synapses at spinal levels. Collateral branches leave both the ascending and descending rami, sweep around the grey matter to the ventral horn and there synapse with motor neurones. Note that each afferent fibre gives origin to several collaterals and thereby influences several motor neurones. Nevertheless, only a few motor neurones in a short segment of cord are stimulated; it is an example of the *circumscribed* type of spinal reflex, which is always monosynaptic. The other main type of spinal reflex is seen in Fig. 22c. Here the afferent fibre, after bifurcating as usual, sends collaterals into the dorsal horn, where they synapse with interneurones. Each afferent fibre synapses with several interneurones. The

99

interneurones also bifurcate and send collaterals to the ventral horn motor neurones. In this form many motor neurones over a fairly wide segment of cord above and below the level of entry of the afferent fibre are stimulated. This is an example of the *diffuse* type of spinal

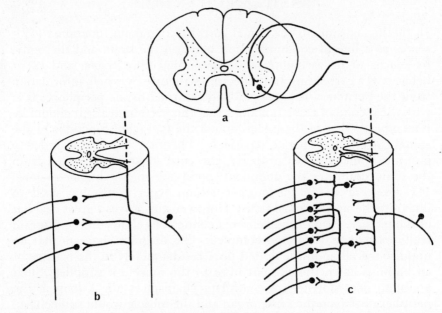

FIG. 22. Diagrams to illustrate the basic patterns of spinal reflex. (a) A common but inaccurate representation of the reflex arc. (b) Apparatus of the arc involved in mono-synaptic or circumscribed reflexes. The dorsal root afferent fibre divides into ascending and descending branches, each of which gives off collaterals along its length; the ascending branch passes up to suprasegmental levels. Several collaterals from one afferent pass around the central grey matter to synapse directly with a group of ventral horn motor neurones. (c) Apparatus of the arc involved in polysynaptic or diffuse reflexes. Organization of the afferent is similar to that for monosynaptic reflexes, but here the collaterals synapse with interneurones. The latter send branches for short distances up and down the cord, each branch giving off a number of collaterals which synapse with ventral horn motor neurones. Since the collaterals from one afferent synapse with several interneurones it is clear that with this apparatus a narrow input to cord can be transformed into a wide output to the muscles.

reflex, which is always polysynaptic. These two types of neural connexions, originating in the anatomical studies of Cajal, have been amply confirmed by more recent experimental findings. Common observation also distinguishes between the circumscribed (plantar, cremasteric, epigastric) form of reflex and the diffuse, often body-wide kind seen when a noxious stimulus is applied. In the diffuse reflexes impulses enter the cord over very few dorsal root fibres, but the effector impulses are radiated out over many ventral roots, throwing both pairs of limbs into action.

Characteristics

Spinal reflexes have certain features which are invariable. Such characteristics are seen only in the spinal preparation or in very low forms, such as fish. Spinal reflexes are as follows.

(1) *Involuntary*. They are not activated by any kind of willing. This is understandable, since the will is in some way connected with higher regions.

(2) *Unlearned*. The pattern of response to a stimulus that activates the spinal effector mechanisms seems to be a property of the arrangement of the spinal neurones. No experience is needed to bring them into operation; and no amount of experience alters the pattern. Again, no doubt because experience is a process involving the higher regions.

(3) *Predictable*. Because experience is ineffective in altering spinal reflexes, they are inevitably predictable. Given the normal arrangement of spinal neurones, then a given stimulus is unvaryingly followed by a corresponding response. Such repeatability occurs from before birth until the death of the mature animal.

(4) *Not dependent upon consciousness*. It will be seen later that consciousness is very much attached to higher regions. Since these are not concerned in purely spinal reflexes, it follows that such reflexes can be elicited in the absence of consciousness. Indeed, in the intact animal, spinal reflexes can be more easily demonstrated when the supraspinal regions have been anaesthetized.

(5) *Immediate*. The monosynaptic type of reflex has a very short latent period; the polysynaptic response occurs a little later. But both types are the fastest reflexes known. The relatively short path from peripheral affector through the cord to peripheral effector is responsible for the immediacy of the reactions. Since a given stimulus inevitably produces a given response, there is no need for time-wasting circulation of information through large circuits.

(6) *Serve adjustive and protective purposes*. This characteristic is indeed the function of the spinal reflexes. In the very low forms this is just about all the spinal effector mechanisms are used for—to adjust a limb in relation to another limb, or to move the whole or

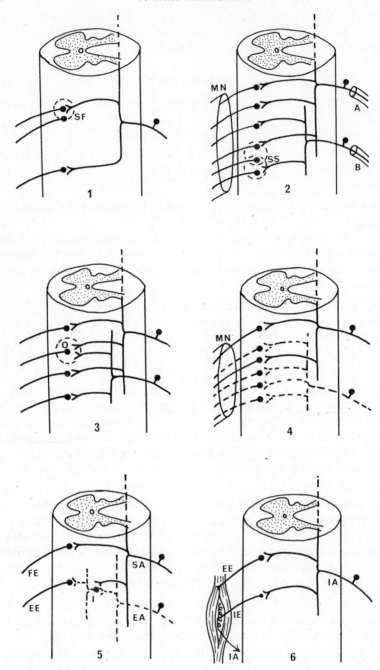

part of the body away from a source of discomfort. As phylogenetic development proceeds, this automatic function needs more and more to be modified in the light of the total sensory input and in the light of experience. Gradually the purely spinal reflexes become merely the basic equipment upon which higher regions bring more complex influences to bear. Even so, the spinal reflexes, even in the primates, retain their ancient purposes. It should perhaps be reiterated that the afferent fibres which ascend the cord to more dominant regions, are the same fibres which are sending collateral branches to the ventral root motor neurones.

Properties

Arising out of the spatial arrangement of the neural elements involved in spinal reflexes, certain patterns of neural activity are derived from a stimulus input, irrespective of the actual stimulus or response. These non-specific properties are as follows.

(1) *Temporal summation*. Repetitive equal stimuli applied to pre-synaptic fibres produce a postsynaptic discharge of gradually increasing magnitude and frequency. This is due to the *recruitment* of surrounding neurones in a subliminal fringe. An impulse arriving at a synapse produces some kind of change (rise in central excitatory state) in the nearby nerve cell. With a single impulse, this change is not sufficient to cause that neurone to discharge. But the change persists in time (hence *temporal* summation), for a few more impulses arriving at the synapse are sufficient to raise the neighbouring

---

FIG. 23. Basic mechanisms that illustrate the properties of spinal reflexes.

1. Temporal summation. Repetitive impulses in the topmost afferent collateral cause the immediate discharge of the topmost motor neurone and gradually raises the excitability of the middle motor neurone which is in the subliminal fringe (SF) and which eventually discharges.

2. Spatial summation. When the two afferent nerves (A, B) are stimulated together, extra neurones in their overlapping subliminal fringes also immediately discharge because of the spatial summation (SS) of the fringes to threshold level.

3. Occlusion. The response obtained when the two nerve fibres are stimulated together is less than the sum of the responses obtained on separate stimulation because some neurones are occluded (O) by common innervation.

4. Fractionation. When the motor nerve (MN) is stimulated, both solid and dotted fibres discharge. Only one group discharges when one of the afferent nerves is stimulated.

5. Reciprocal inhibition. Impulses in the sensory afferent (SA) fibre cause discharge in the flexor efferent (FE) motor neurone and, via an interneurone, cause inhibition of the extensor efferent (EE) motor neurone. EA, Extensor afferent.

6. The stretch reflex. Impulses in the intrafusal afferent (IA) cause discharge in the extrafusal efferent (EE) *large* motor neurone and also by a collateral cause discharge in the intrafusal efferent (IE) *small* motor neurone.

neurones to a discharging state, thus giving an efferent output greater than the afferent input (Fig. 23.1).

This kind of input, repetitive equal-sized impulses, is characteristic of the activity of stretch reflex fibres; and temporal summation is characteristic of such reflexes. On the other hand, the type of sensory input in a flexion reflex is not repetitive, and temporal summation is not characteristic of flexion reflexes.

(2) *Spatial summation.* If two afferent *nerves* (i.e. bundles of nerve fibres) from a muscle are stimulated separately, the individual responses of the muscle are not so great as when the two nerves are stimulated together.

This phenomenon also involves a subliminal fringe. Each afferent fibre connects with a group of neurones that supply a corresponding group of muscle fibres. When the two afferents are stimulated simultaneously, there is a summation of the excitatory state supplied by each afferent, so that the region in between the two groups of neurones reaches threshold level. Neurones lying in this region and supplying a third group of muscle fibres (Fig. 23.2) will discharge under these conditions, and the resultant tension will be that much increased.

Symbolically, if A and B are two afferent nerves producing tension x and y respectively, then:

$$A \to x$$

$$B \to y$$

$$\text{but } A + B > x \text{ or } y$$

(3) *Occlusion.* The response obtained on simultaneous stimulation of two afferent nerves is never as great as the sum of the responses obtained when the two nerves are stimulated separately (Fig. 23.3).

Symbolically, symbols as before and c being the common efferent component:

$$A \to x + c$$

$$B \to y + c$$

$$\text{but } A + B < x + y + c \quad (\text{not } A + B \to x + y + 2c)$$

(4) *Fractionation.* Stimulation of the motor nerve to a muscle always gives a bigger response than stimulation of an afferent nerve which activates that muscle (Fig. 23.4).

This phenomenon represents the very important principle of *convergence*. Any afferent nerve synapses with a group of neurones whose axons travel in the efferent ventral root nerve to the muscles. But several peripheral nerves will activate a given muscle. Thus the motor root is made up of fibres arising postsynaptically from several afferents; the afferents *converge* upon the motor root. Stimulation of the motor root is hence equivalent to the stimulation of several afferent nerves.

Symbolically, $A \rightarrow x$

$$M \text{ (motor)} \rightarrow > x$$

(5) *Reciprocal inhibition*. When a flexor is made to contract, there is inhibition of the opposing extensor muscle, and vice versa. Linking the flexor and extensor inputs is an interneurone (Fig. 23.5). The function of the interneurone, it seems, is to produce inhibition at the synapses of the opposing muscle.

In the intact animal, reciprocal inhibition does not occur automatically. Information from the higher integrative regions may cancel the purely spinal reflex, as, for example, in the simple matter of standing in which both extensors and flexors are contracted. Similarly, the form that reciprocal inhibition takes depends upon the overall situation. It may be semi-automatic as in walking, running, swimming, where it produces the alternation of action in antagonistic limb muscles without continuous volitional attention.

The Stretch Reflex

At this point it is convenient to summarize the details of muscle innervation. Muscle consists of *extrafusal* fibres, which do the contractile work of the muscle, and of *intrafusal* fibres which form the muscle spindle. From here the annulospiral ending sends group I fibres to the dorsal roots of the spinal cord, in which they synapse with ventral root motor neurones. In addition, the afferent fibre also engages with the cell body of a motor neurone which supplies the intrafusal fibres. These are the small motor neurones or γ-efferents. In modern terminology, this forms a feedback system (Fig. 23.6).

When the annulospiral receptor is activated by stretch, the extrafusal fibres are reflexly caused to contract. If no other changes occurred this contraction would cancel the stretch stimulus, the receptor would cease to discharge and the contraction would come to a premature end. Under normal conditions, when impulses flow in the muscle afferents, both large and small motor neurones are discharged.

The impulses passing down the small motor neurone, cause contraction of the intrafusal fibres, so maintaining deformation of the annulospiral receptor, which continues to issue impulses to the afferent and so the contraction of the muscle is prolonged.

The stretch or myotatic reflex plays its greatest role when tensions are very high, when the pull on the muscle is considerable. However, should the tension rise to dangerous levels, a safety reflex comes into operation.

The Inverse Stretch Reflex

In the decerebrate preparation, the limbs are extended. Attempts to flex such a limb meet with strong resistance, but if the force applied is increased sufficiently, the extensor muscles quite suddenly relax. This is the inverse stretch reflex causing a *lengthening reaction*, in which the tendon organ of Golgi is involved.

Figure 24 shows the layout of fibres in muscle innervation as in Fig. 23.6, but with the addition of the tendon sensory organ of Golgi. This sends fibres of type I-B to the dorsal root of the spinal cord, in which synapses occur with both large and small motor

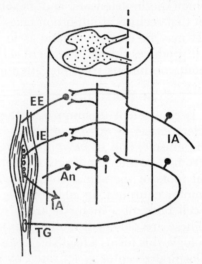

Fig. 24. Mechanism of the inverse myotatic reflex. Moderate stretch causes impulses to flow in the intrafusal afferent (IA) which activate both the large motor neurones forming the extrafusal efferent (EE) and the small motor neurones which control the intrafusal efferents (IE). With immoderate stretch, impulses in the afferent from the tendon organ of Golgi (TG) cause discharges in the interneurone (I) which (a) inhibit the two efferents and (b) excite the motor supply of antagonist muscles (An).

neurones, supplying the muscle to which the tendon is attached. Tendon organs of Golgi react to mechanical deformation, produced either by passive stretching of the muscle or by active contraction of the muscle. Initially, as the muscle begins to shorten, the contraction is sustained by the myotatic reflex. As the tension increases, the tendon organs begin to discharge and the inverse myotatic reflex starts to operate, acting as a brake or damper on the direct myotatic reflex. In addition, the tendon organs activate the opposing muscles. Thus the synergism of direct and indirect stretch reflexes enables a smooth, controlled contraction to take place. Under conditions of excessive tension, the tendon organ discharge becomes great enough to cancel the discharge from the annulospiral receptor. It should be clear that while the neural elements of the stretch reflex form the basic mechanism of movement and posture, they would be of little use to a higher mammal without the controlling influence of supraspinal regions.

CHAPTER 6

PYRAMIDAL AND EXTRAPYRAMIDAL CONTROL

Under the heading of basic mechanisms we examined the spinal equipment available to the body. In the present section we envisage these basic mechanisms as being at the disposal of higher regions, and we look into the means whereby suprasegmental regions utilize and dominate the spinal effector apparatus.

Motor Neurones

Starting from below and working upwards, there are a few points to remember about the ventral horn motor neurones.

(1) There are large and small (γ-efferent) neurones in the ventral horn and both of these kinds are influenced by higher regions.

(2) The ventral horn cell is a final common path that can be affected by impulses arriving along several pathways—not only the one under discussion at any time. Indeed, 80–90% of the surface area of the ventral horn cell body is covered by synaptic knobs from axon-terminations of influencing cells.

(3) Motor nerve cells that supply slowly contracting *red* muscle have a higher excitatory postsynaptic potential than the motor nerve cells supplying fast contracting *pink* muscle. Which of these forms a muscle actually takes is determined by the type of nerve supplying it. Buller *et al.* (1958) have shown that if, in the young kitten, the nerve supplying a muscle which would normally become red, is sectioned and cross-united with the distal end of a similarly sectioned nerve to a genetically pink muscle, then the latter develops as a red muscle.

(4) It is rare for ventral horn cells to be in direct synaptic connexion with fibres from the cell bodies of suprasegmental regions. According to Hoff and Hoff (1934), about 80–90% of ventral horn cell bodies are in synaptic connexion with internuncial neurones.

INTERNUNCIAL NEURONES

A good deal of work has been done on these neural elements over the last decade as a result of improvement in refined methods of electrophysiology. A detailed review is available (Hunt and Perl,

1960). It has been found that internuncial neurones differ in several ways from the motor neurones, and it seems that the ability to carry out smooth movements owes a good deal to these special properties.

(1) Internuncial neurones tend to respond to a *single* afferent volley by a *repetitive* discharge at high frequency.

(2) However, a cell which usually responds in this way, often reacts to a weaker stimulus by a single discharge.

(3) A very common feature of many internuncial neurones is the presence of a continuous, subliminal, background discharge.

(4) Arising out of (3) it seems that *under natural conditions* the response of an internuncial neurone is a modulation of the tonic discharge.

(5) Nearly all, and possibly all, internuncial neurones have extensive peripheral receptive fields. Thus, these elements may be looked upon as semifinal *common* paths.

From these properties, interposed so to speak between the thinking regions and the unthinking spinal reflex apparatus, a series of functions emerges.

(1) *Integration.* The internuncial neurone serves as a place where several afferent routes may converge and the total information transformed into a resultant before being passed on to the ventral horn cell.

(2) *Amplification.* By responding to a single input with a multiple output, the internuncial neurone is able to increase the importance of descending instructions.

(3) *Temporal control.* By the same property, the response passed on to the motor neurone may last longer than the incoming instructions, so the internuncial neurone is utilized as a controlling influence in the dimension of time.

(4) *Regulation.* It has been shown that during the course of motor phenomena generated by higher regions, the pattern of excitability of the spinal interneurones is continually changing. In this way, the interneurones are able to regulate the possible interfering effect of plain spinal reflexes, which unhindered might render the voluntary movement less effective.

Upper Motor Neurone

These are the neuromotor components whose cell-bodies occur in regions other than the spinal cord. They fall broadly into two groups, (a) the long fibres of the "pyramidal system" and (b) the chains of shorter fibres in the "extrapyramidal system". In the supplement to this section (p. 143) evidence is presented to support the view that these two systems should no longer be considered separately.

Pyramidal System

An alternative name is corticospinal tract, but both terms possess more tradition than accuracy. The pyramids are the elevations on the ventral surface of the medulla which were considered to compose the great descending motor system. But it has been shown that whereas the motor cortex contains about 68 000 cells (in man) yet there are 1 000 000 fibres in the pyramidal tract. Similarly, the term cortico-spinal is not entirely satisfactory because some fibres in the tract do not originate in the cortex and some of them do not enter the spinal cord (e.g. cranial outflow). However, these terms though vague may be retained with mental reservations.

Leaving out obscuring detail, the pyramidal system can be repre-sented as in Fig. 25. Structures involved are the cortex, internal capsule, basis pedunculi, pons, medulla and spinal cord. Fibres from the larynx and face regions of the motor cortex pass to the medial part of the internal capsule and down to the pons. Here they synapse in the nuclei of cranial nerves III, V, VII, IX, X, XI and XII. Postsynaptic fibres leave the CNS in these nerves, forming the *corticobulbar* branch of the pyramidal system. From other regions of the motor cortex the fibres pass onwards to the medulla where, just below the olive, there is a partial decussation. About 80% of the fibres cross to the other side and descend as the crossed (or indirect) corticospinal tract. The other 20% remain ipsilateral and descend into the cord as the uncrossed (or direct) corticospinal tract.

The functions of this tract may be examined in several ways. One of them is to section the pyramids, and this was done by Tower (1935). In the monkey, Tower cut the pyramid on one side just above the decussation level. The results were (a) a loss of initiation of movement and a generally reduced usage of the contralateral extremities; (b) a considerably diminished threshold of spinal reflexes; (c) the positive supporting reactions were depressed, and (d) there was a marked lack of phasic movements.

On the side contralateral to the lesion, the loss of initiative was severe, but not complete. The limbs would generate movements if restraint was applied to the unaffected limbs and a strong stimulus given. Within 4–5 months, disuse atrophy appeared in the affected limbs.

With bilateral section of the pyramids there occurred the expected

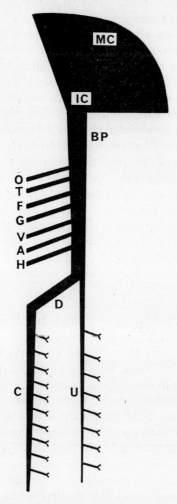

FIG. 25. Schematic representation of the pyramidal system. From cell bodies in motor areas of the cerebral cortex (MC) axons sweep down through the internal capsule (IC) and on through the brachium conjunctivum (BP). In the bulbar region fibres pass out to the oculomotor (O), trigeminal (T), facial (F), glossopharyngeal (G), vagus (V), spinal accessory (A) and hypoglossal (H) cranial nerves. In the lower medulla there is an inter-digitating decussation (D) to give a large crossed (C) and a small uncrossed (U) cortico-spinal tract. (See also Figs. 29 and 41.)

duplication of the effects of unilateral lesions. Under these conditions, however, the paralysis was considerably more incapacitating, since there was no unaffected side to compensate. In addition the axial musculature also exhibited hypotonia. Improvement occurred over a few weeks. The animals became able to sit, then to stand and then to effect a disturbed but useful locomotion.

Two clear conclusions could be drawn from these experiments: (a) the pyramidal system as here defined is not the effective pathway for the tonic inhibition of spinal reflexes that is known to be a constant feature in the waking animal, since there were no symptoms of release (i.e. spasticity) on section of the pyramids, and (b) the pyramidal system is essentially concerned with the *least stereotyped* muscular activities. In its absence there is a virtual loss of fine digitation and very few postural corrective movements.

The "highest" part of the pyramidal system is the motor cortex. Until 1870 it was believed that the cerebral cortex functioned as a unitary organ, but in that year Fritsch and Hitzig made the observation that stimulation of the frontal part of the dog cerebral cortex was accompanied by movements of the contralateral muscles. Stimulation of other parts of the cortex did not have this effect, and so was born the concept of localization of function in the cortex. This topic will be discussed at greater length in the section devoted to this part of the CNS. For the moment only the motor aspect of localization will be dealt with.

Since the original observation of Fritsch and Hitzig, many workers have studied the cortical motor mechanisms: Ferrier, Horsely, Schaeffer and Sherrington in animals; Foerster, Penfield, Erickson and Rasmussen in man. These workers prepared maps depicting the site of motor functions in the cortex, frequently following the outlines of the histologists' cytoarchitectonic maps. A map given by Sherrington is shown in Fig. 26. Such maps are incomplete and inaccurate, but this is no criticism of the workers who produced them. Only with the spurious wisdom of hindsight are we able to see the reasons why early motor maps are unacceptable. These reasons are (a) no systematic comparative studies were made; (b) the early workers did not explore the relevant sulci and the medial surfaces; (c) there was failure to eliminate the interfering effects of afferent systems; (d) it was not known to the earlier workers that the neural threshold rises in the rostral direction, so that strength of stimuli must be correspondingly increased, and (e) they did not have the advantage of microelectrodes.

With the benefit of this knowledge, more recent workers, e.g. Woolsey and his colleagues (see Woolsey *et al.*, 1950), have produced maps of greater accuracy and completeness. These investigations were made with single small electrodes (punctate stimulation) in a

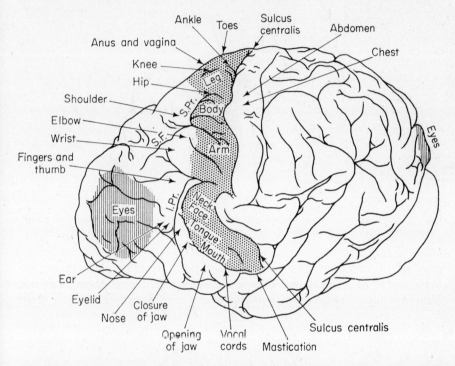

FIG. 26. One of the earliest maps of functional localization in the cortex, redrawn from Sherrington (1906). While of great value when first published, it has subsequently been shown as inaccurate and incomplete.

comparative series with exploration of sulci and the medial surfaces and with increasing strength of stimulus as the electrode was moved more rostrally. Interference from activity in other regions was avoided (or minimized) by working with animals under deep pentobarbital anaesthesia.

Application of this experimental procedure to the rat, which has few sulci, showed that a large part of the frontal cortex had motor functions. It was also apparent that the old maps were wrong in their interpolation of the arm area between the head and the trunk. Complete continuity of epaxial musculature was found to be the case.

Much clearer results were seen when similar methods were applied to the cat. The more detailed maps were obtained by study of the monkey brain. Careful punctate stimulation of the frontal surface of the brain gave the overall picture shown in Fig. 27. Considerable

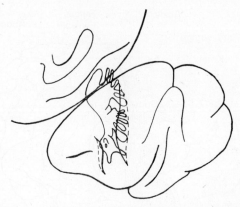

FIG. 27. Representation upon the brain of the monkey of motor area I as determined by punctate stimulation in the deeply anaesthetized animal. (After Woolsey *et al.*, 1950.)

overlap occurred at each stimulation point (see original paper of Woolsey *et al.*, 1950) but it was clearly evident that there was no interruption of epaxial muscle representation. It was also clear that

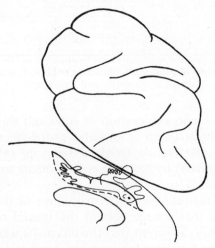

FIG. 28. Representation upon the brain of the monkey of motor area II as determined by punctate stimulation in the deeply anaesthetized animal. (After Woolsey *et al.*, 1950.)

the main part of the forelimb digits is represented on the anterior wall of the central sulcus; the main part of hindlimb digits, together with the tail, is represented on the medial surface of the hemisphere.

Further exploration with punctate electrodes revealed a *supplementary motor area* on the medial surface, with another complete representation of the contralateral body musculature (Fig. 28). In man, vocalization and contralateral movements have been reported to follow stimulation of the medial surface so it is likely that a supplementary area is also present in the human.

Extrapyramidal System

It is obvious from Tower's (1935) experiments on pyramidal section that the corticospinal system does not account for the whole of motor phenomena. It is well known that removal of cortical motor areas or section of the brain stem results in hypertonia and much more serious paralysis than was found on section of the medullary pyramids. The regions and pathways involved in this discrepancy are designated as the extrapyramidal system.

Anatomically, the system has not yet been clearly delineated (Fig. 29) and most knowledge of its connexions has been derived from physiological experiments and from clinical observations. There is general agreement that no extrapyramidal elements connect the cerebral cortex directly (i.e. without synapse) to the spinal cord.

Revealing experiments have been carried out in cats with sectioned pyramids. With electrical stimulation of the cortex in such animals, ipsilateral movements occur. These are slow to appear, build up slowly and tend to outlast the stimulus. Under light anaesthesia the movements show some degree of integration, frequently take on a rhythmic character and sometimes are of a postural nature. In general, the movements so produced differ from those initiated by pyramidal stimulation in that the former are ipsilateral, slow and non-phasic. Nevertheless, it is clear that regions of cortex are able to *excite* movements in the absence of the pyramidal system.

Destruction of extrapyramidal regions of the cortex shows that this system as here defined includes inhibitory mechanisms. The results of such destruction are hypertonia, contracture, exaggerated tendon reflexes and clonus. The overall picture is that the extrapyramidal system is concerned with the organized use of muscle *en masse*, whereas the pyramidal system is involved under conditions of discrete muscular activity. Since these two forms of movement occur together in normal circumstances, it is likely that the pyramidal and

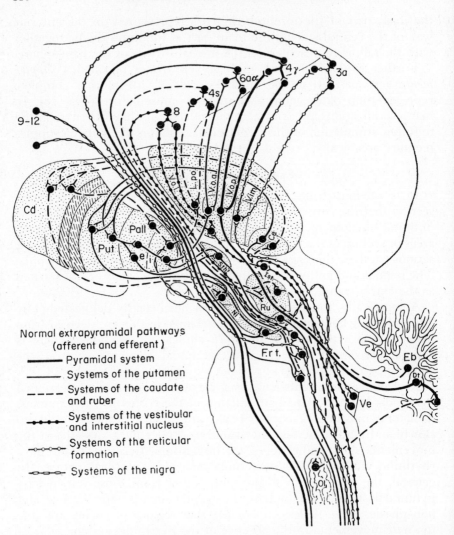

FIG. 29. Connexions of the extrapyramidal system projected onto the sagittal plane, with pyramidal pathways superimposed. Afferent connexions to the striatum pass from the emboliform nucleus (Eb), through the centrum medianum (CE) to the caudate nucleus (CD) and the putamen (Put). From the caudate nucleus efferents pass to (1) the substantia nigra (Ni) and (2) through the two parts of the globus pallidus (Pall, e, i) to the latero-polaris (L.po) nucleus of the thalamus. A two-way connexion occurs between the latter and the suppressor area of cortex (4s). From 4s fibres run to the red nucleus (Ru) and reticular formation (F.rt.), giving off collaterals on the way to the caudate nucleus. Two pathways emerge from the putamen, (1) to the substantia nigra, (2) to the ventro-oral

Continued at foot of page 117.

extrapyramidal systems operate simultaneously, in synergism, and that the extrapyramidal system exerts the tonic inhibition on spinal effector mechanisms.

CINGULATE GYRUS

Recent work indicates that the cingulate gyrus is to be considered as a part of the extrapyramidal system, in view of its anatomical connexions with striatal regions and in view of physiological studies. Showers (1959) has applied electrical stimulation to this region in the monkey and observed the effects on motor mechanisms. Two more complete representations of body musculature were found. Changes in facial expression were obtained by stimulation of all parts of the cingulate gyrus. Stimulation of the anterior region and back towards the middle section elicited movements, in order, from head to tail; similar sequential effects were found on stimulation of the posterior region and forwards to the middle section. Thus, the cingulate gyrus contains two tail-to-tail representations of the muscles. When the monkey cingulate gyrus is lesioned, muscle responses are heightened but there is no sign of paralysis.

The involvement of the cingulate gyrus in motor phenomena has been seen from time to time in the human. Chemical lesions of this region have been accompanied by epileptic seizures in man, cat and monkey. Andy and McChinn (1957) have shown that epileptic seizures can be propagated to the opposite hemispheres by concurrent stimulation of the cingulate gyrus.

Although the physiological role of this region has not been fully clarified, it would seem that the cingulate gyrus was the first cortical overseer controlling the activities of the older subcortical structures. The progress of phylogeny has now produced a larger bulk of cortex with a wider range of overseeing powers and, in places, a more precise localization of body parts.

Continued from previous page.

thalamic nucleus (V.o.a.). From the substantia nigra fibres descend in the nigroreticular tract and ascend, via a relay in the globus pallidus, to the subthalamic nucleus (S. th.). The latter is connected with the globus pallidus and probably also the red nucleus. From the globus pallidus fibres pass to the red nucleus and the reticular formation. The red nucleus gives rise to the rubrospinal tract and the reticular formation gives rise to the reticulospinal tract. Areas 9–12 of the cerebral cortex connect in the substantia nigra with the caudatonigral and nigropallidal pathways. Area 4γ and $6a\alpha$ of the cerebral cortex connect in the substantia nigra with the putamenonigral pathway. Area $6a\beta$ also sends collaterals to the putamen and reticular formation. From the vestibular nuclei (Ve) fibres pass via the interstitial nucleus (Ist), and also directly to thalamic nuclei (V.o.i. and V.i.m.) to take part in statokinetic responses. (From Jung and Hassler, 1960.)

SUPPRESSOR AREAS

In 1936, Hines described a narrow strip of cerebral cortex in the rostral region of area 4—between 4 and 6—removal of which in the monkey resulted in spasticity. This is now designated as area 4s; it corresponds to the pericruciate cortex (see section on posture, p. 137) in carnivores. The application of a chemical excitant (strychnine) to area 4s has been found to depress the electrical activity normally present in area 4, the motor area. According to McCullogh (1947) excitation of area 4s results in a stimulatory discharge to the caudal part of the head of the caudate nucleus. Discharges from this structure produce inhibition in the thalamic region which projects to the somatosensory cortex (area 3). In this way, sensory information from area 3 to area 4 is cut off and hence there is a reduction in the electrical phenomena in the latter (Fig. 30). Using the strychnine method, McCullogh's group have reported the existence of similar suppressor effects in areas 2, 8, 19 and 24.

The physiological significance—indeed, the actual existence—of suppressor areas is still a matter of disagreement. Meyers (1953), for example, claims that no evidence exists for cortical suppressor mechanisms in cat or man.

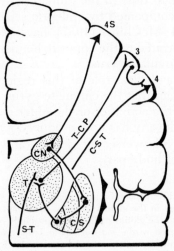

FIG. 30. Diagram of the mechanism of cortical suppression of motor pathways. Impulses arising in suppressor strip 4s pass to the caudate nucleus (CN) and are relayed to the corpus striatum (CS) from which fibres enter the thalamus (T) and inhibit the activity of spinothalamic (S-T) pathways. Hence, excitation in the thalamocortical pathway (T-CP) is reduced and the sensory cortex (3) does not issue instructions to the motor cortex (4), thus reducing the activity in the corticospinal tract (C-ST).

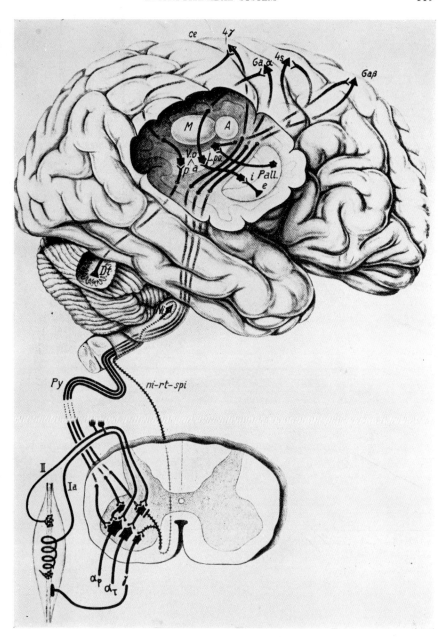

Fig. 31. Some connexions of the basal ganglia, with special emphasis upon the mechanisms of Parkinsonism (see p. 145). (From Hassler, 1962.)

BASAL GANGLIA

Since, according to McCullogh, suppressor areas involve parts of the basal ganglia, it will be convenient to deal with them at this point. The term is used rather loosely to include various combinations of the following structures: caudate nucleus, putamen, globus pallidus, subthalamic body, red nucleus, substantia nigra, some hypothalamic nuclei and parts of the reticular formation. Interconnexions, as shown in Fig. 31, have been described, but there is not yet firm agreement on the details. It is generally conceded that the chief efferent component is the globus pallidus and that the main afferent supply is from the cerebral cortex and thalamus.

Functionally, the basal ganglia form a highly obscure system. Some recent views are presented in the supplement to this section (p. 145). It seems clear from animal experiments that in the absence of the cerebral cortex the basal ganglia play no essential part in the organization of movement for locomotion or postural adaptations. Stimulation of the putamen, caudate nucleus and claustrum inhibits phasic movements induced by stimulation of the motor cortex. Stimulation of the globus pallidus alone has no effect on motor phenomena. When stimulated during a cortically induced phasic movement, the latter is inhibited and the limb enters a state of plastic tone, passively movable and retentive of the new position.

Clinical observations in man implicate the basal ganglia in Parkinsonism, athetosis and chorea. The first of these seems to be closely associated with the substantia nigra and the globus pallidus. Destruction of the globus pallidus region electrically or chemically sometimes produces dramatic abolition of chronic Parkinsonian tremor. Thus, it is possible that the nigropallidal pathway normally inhibits the globus pallidus. Spontaneous lesions in the nigra would then release the globus, which would produce Parkinsonian tremor, the latter being relieved by destruction of the globus. On the other hand, most experimental evidence suggests that the globus pallidus discharges inhibitory information. Athetosis and chorea are usually associated with damage to the caudate nucleus and putamen and only rarely with the globus pallidus. Motor effects in these conditions have been diminished by section of the ventral fasciculus of the spinal cord. Bucy and Keplinger (1961) suggest that lesions in the basal ganglia remove inhibitory influences that normally play on the cerebral cortex, thus allowing an abnormal discharge over extrapyramidal pathways.

CHAPTER 7

CEREBELLAR MECHANISMS

Sessile animals do not possess identifiable balancing organs. Nor do the Protozoa. But all other free-living groups, from medusoid coelenterates up to man, have acquired some specialized structure whose function is to preserve an appropriate disposition of the parts of the body, relative to each other and with due regard to changes in the environment. In the more simply organized animals a balancing organ is required largely for the maintenance of a level trim. As the body becomes phylogenetically more differentiated so there is greater need for balancing (motor co-ordination) of its parts. The development of a muscular system and limbs brings speedy movement. Fast moving animals or rapidly acting limbs are at the mercy of momentum unless an overall controlling mechanism develops at the same time. In the vertebrate this controlling mechanism is the cerebellum.

Cerebellar apparatus is present in the lowest animals with a true backbone, the lampreys. It takes the form of a simple commissure at the anterior end of the hindbrain. Enlargement of the cerebellum occurs to some extent in the cartilaginous and bony fishes, but a distinct bulbose structure does not appear until the Amphibia are reached and even in this group and the Reptilia, the cerebellum is anatomically insignificant in comparison with that of birds. Similarly, the avian cerebellum never approximates in complexity to the mammalian organ. These phylogenetic differences correlate well with the known functional roles of the cerebellar divisions. The *archicerebellum*, found in fish, is connected almost entirely with the vestibular apparatus. Its function was and is to aid in the maintenance of whole-body equilibrium. The *palaeocerebellum*, characteristic of amphibians, reptiles and birds, is connected largely to the proprioceptor pathways from the muscles, tendons and joints. The correlation of symetrical limb movements for postural and progressional purposes is the business of the palaeocerebellum. Mammalian forms are distinguished by the possession, among other things, of a well-developed cerebrum. The *neocerebellum* is predominantly connected with the cerebrum and officiates in the performance of limbs acting independently and in the execution of skilled movements.

E
121

Variations in form of the cerebellum are found even within each of the major animal phyla, in association with specific modes of progression or especially well-developed groups of muscles. Among mammals, for example, the great limb agility of the cat is correlated with a highly developed tonsil; a large simple lobule is characteristic of animals which exhibit great head mobility, such as the deer; the cerebellar "hemispheres" are most highly developed in those animals, primates and man, which have adopted the upright posture.

Probably no other part of the body has been such a happy playground for nomenclature-minded anatomists as the cerebellum. Several distinct and overlapping systems are available for those with a taste for scientific lexicography. But since the main purpose of

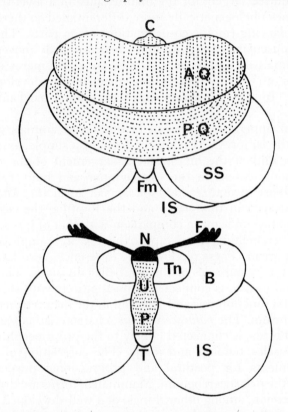

FIG. 32. Main divisions of the cerebellum. Above, dorsal view; below, ventral view. AQ, Anterior part of quadrangular lobe; B, biventral lobule; C, central lobule; F, flocculus; Fm, folium; IS, inferior semilunar lobule; N, nodule; P, pyramis; PQ, posterior part of quadrangular lobe; SS, superior semilunar lobule; T, tuber; Tn, tonsil; U, uvula.

naming parts is to identify them, we shall choose the system that identifies most parts. It is as arbitrary as any other system. Figure 32 shows, diagrammatically the main subdivisions in dorsal and ventral view, modified from Ranson.

The flocculus on each side is continuous with the nodule, forming the flocculonodular lobe, which is very small in man; with part of the uvula it represents the archicerebellum, shown black in the diagrams. The palaeocerebellum consists of the central lobule, the quadrangular lobule, most of the uvula and the pyramis, as shown in the stippled parts of the diagrams. The neocerebellum comprises the rest of the cerebellum but it also encroaches to some extent on the uvula (archicerebellum) and the posterior part of the quadrangular lobe (palaeocerebellum). It should be noted that the cerebellar "hemispheres" are not separate as in the cerebrum, but are everywhere continuous with each other.

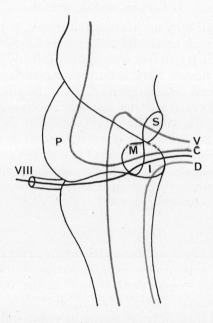

FIG. 33. Input pathways to the cerebellum. The dorsal spinocerebellar tract (D) enters via the restiform body (inferior cerebellar peduncle, I). The ventral spinocerebellar tract (V) continues upwards and then curves back to enter via the brachium conjunctivum (superior cerebellar peduncle, S). Corticocerebellar pathways (C) relay in the pons (P) and enter via the brachium pontis (middle cerebellar peduncle, M), through which also pass the fibres derived from the vestibular nerve (VIII).

The cerebellum consists of a great cortical surface (containing cell bodies) covering white matter that is produced into thin transverse folds, the folia. Buried in the central white matter are the internal nuclei (dentate, fastigial, globose and emboliform), all of which are bilateral.

The cerebellum is connected to the rest of the nervous system by the bundles of nerve fibres, afferent and efferent, forming the superior, middle and inferior cerebellar peduncles. Figure 33 shows their relations.

Connexions

The pathways into and out of the cerebellum may be conveniently considered in relation to the phylogenetic divisions. In this way some functional ideas are more clearly seen.

ARCHICEREBELLUM
(*Flocculus, nodule, uvula*)

Afferent fibres arise in the vestibular division of the eighth cranial nerve (auditory) and enter the cerebellum by way of the inferior cerebellar peduncle (restiform body) either directly or after a synapse in the vestibular nuclei. Very little decussation occurs. Cells of the archicerebellar cortex send *efferent* fibres mainly to the fastigial nucleus. Some fibres reach the fastigial nucleus directly from the vestibular nuclei. As with the other cerebellar internal nuclei, the fastigial nucleus is an efferent relay station. It sends fibres, in the fastigio-bulbar tract, back to the vestibular nuclei and to the descending reticular formation. Thus, via the vestibulospinal and reticulospinal tracts, the archicerebellum is able to influence the final common path motor neurones (Fig. 34).

PALAEOCEREBELLUM
(*Central lobule, quadrangular lobule, uvula and pyramis*)

Afferent fibres arise from several sources. (a) One is from the proprioceptive and somaesthetic fibres in the dorsal and ventral spinocerebellar tracts. Dorsal tract fibres enter via the inferior peduncle; ventral tract fibres continue upwards and then sweep back through the superior peduncle (brachium conjunctivum). (b) Fibres arising in parts of the extrapyramidal system, mainly from the red nucleus, pass via the contralateral inferior olive and inferior peduncle into the cerebellum. (c) A very few fibres, whose function is not yet

known, arise in the lateral reticulate nucleus. (d) Tactile and proprioceptive fibres from the nucleus of the fifth cranial nerve (trigeminal)
pass into the cerebellum via the inferior peduncle. Efferent fibres
associated with the palaeocerebellum synapse mainly in the dentate

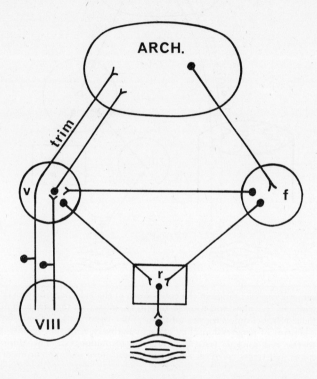

FIG. 34. Schematic representation of the connexions of the archicerebellum (ARCH).
The input arises in the vestibular nerve (VIII) and passes either directly or by a synapse
in the vestibular nucleus (V) to the archicerebellum, carrying information on body trim.
The efferent pathway is to the fastigial nucleus (f) which relays directly to the reticular
formation (r) and also to this same region via a synapse in the vestibular nucleus. Fibres
in the reticulospinal tract synapse with ventral horn motor neurones.

nucleus, but also in the globose and emboliform nuclei. From these
nuclei postsynaptic fibres sweep out of the cerebellum through the
superior peduncle to terminate in the red nucleus and descending
reticular formation. The palaeocerebellum is thus able to bring an
influence to bear on the ventral horn motor neurones through the
reticulospinal and rubrospinal tracts (Fig. 35).

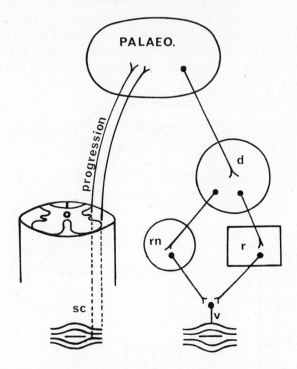

Fig. 35. Schematic representation of the connexions of the palaeocerebellum (PALAEO.). The input arises in the joint and muscle receptors, passes in the spinocerebellar tracts (sc) to the palaeocerebellum, carrying proprioceptive information about limb position to aid in the control of progression. The efferent pathway is to the dentate nucleus (d) and relays to the red nucleus (rn) and reticular formation (r). The rubrospinal and reticulospinal tracts converge upon the ventral horn motor neurones (v).

NEOCEREBELLUM

(Superior and inferior semilunar lobules, biventral lobule, tonsil, tuber)

Afferent fibres have been found to arise from all four lobes of the cerebral cortex, and probably from all or nearly all areas of these lobes. They reach the cerebellum by way of relays among the pontine nuclei, from which the decussated postsynaptic fibres pass through the middle peduncle (brachium pontis) to the cerebellum. *Efferent* fibres from the neocerebellar cortex terminate chiefly in the dentate nucleus. Postsynaptic fibres from the dentate nucleus pass by way of the superior peduncle mainly to the thalamus (ventrolateral nucleus), with some collaterals to the reticular formation and red nucleus. From the thalamus, fibres are relayed to the motor regions of the cerebral cortex (precentral gyrus, areas 4 and 6) (Fig. 36).

With the material in the last three paragraphs at our disposal we can see quite clearly the essential differences in the function of the phylogenetically distinct parts of the cerebellum. The archicerebellum

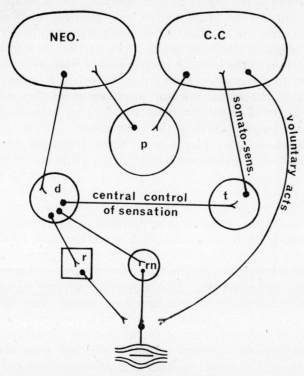

FIG. 36. Schematic representation of the connexions of the neocerebellum. The input is derived from somatosensory pathways to the cerebral cortex (C.C) which sends information via relays in the pons (p) to the neocerebellum (NEO.). The efferent pathway is to the dentate nucleus (d) from which relays pass to the reticular formation (r) and red nucleus (rn). The reticulospinal and rubrospinal tracts converge upon the ventral horn motor neurones. From the dentate nucleus, fibres pass to the thalamus (t) to serve in the central control of the sensory input. Hence the neocerebellum is able to control movements that support the voluntary acts produced by the cerebral cortex.

and the palaeocerebellum resemble each other in standing at the highest point of reflex pathways. Although the neocerebellum is able to function in this way by means of its rubrospinal and reticulospinal connexions, yet the overwhelming majority of its afferent and efferent fibres are centrally placed; it has little to do with the periphery directly. The archicerebellum considers the information presented to it by the continuous (tonic) stream of impulses arising in the vestibular apparatus. This information "describes" the position of the body with reference to the earth's centre of gravity and also reveals the state of motion of the body. Strictly speaking, the information refers accurately only to the head, but in rigid animals, such as the fish, head movements are in effect whole-body movements. Even in the non-rigid animals, the head tends to be carried in a more or less definite relation to the body. A change in this relation is immediately transmitted to the archicerebellum. Appropriate messages are then dispatched to the spinal effector mechanisms so that whole-body equilibrium, trim, may be maintained. The archicerebellum is primarily the balance organ of the vertebrates.

Animals whose limbs play a more active role than those of fish, have in addition a palaeocerebellum. This gives attention to tonic information arising in the great proprioceptive and tactile systems—information that "describes" changes in the relative positions of the parts of the body, especially the limbs. Once again, the cerebellar apparatus is able to reflect back appropriate information to the body musculature through the spinal effector mechanisms. In this way is established a proper co-ordination of the muscle groups involved in locomotion and posture. At the same time of course, there is integration of the archicerebellar mechanisms. Now, the neocerebellum receives information in a secondary way. Sensory data of all forms continuously reach the cerebral cortex and become incorporated into the totality of response. Part of the mechanism of integration is the presentation by the cerebral cortex of selected sense data to the neocerebellum. The latter, working in conjunction with the other two cerebellar divisions, compares these data with its own primary proprioceptive and tactile information and reports back, so to speak, to the cerebral motor cortex. It is as though the neocerebellum, in its proprioceptive wisdom, revises the cerebral plan of action—derived from limited data—into a course appropriate to the given state of the whole body. In this way the three cerebellar divisions blend into a unity, not only among themselves, but with the whole motor system, so that, for example, there may occur the complex and highly discriminative muscular pattern of violin-playing. While the cerebral mechanisms are controlling the intricate movements of the fingers, the cerebellar mechanisms are instigating the appropriate control of the less spectacular but equally necessary movements of lower limbs, trunk and head. The physical basis for this unification of cerebellar activity is beautifully revealed in the histology of the organ.

Histology

In no part of the cerebellum is the histological picture different from any other part. Such uniformity of structure parallels the uniformity of function described above, and this is even more definitely suggested by the cell connexions (Fig. 37). As with the

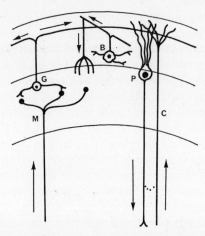

FIG. 37. Histology of the cerebellum. Input is either by mossy fibres (M) whose cell bodies lie outside the cerebellum or by climbing fibres (C) whose cell bodies lie in the internal cerebellar nuclei. Terminals of the mossy fibres connect with dendrites of granular cells (G). These send bifurcating axons for some distance parallel to the long axes of the cerebellar folia. Climbing fibre terminals and granular cell axons interdigitate with the dendrites of Purkinje cells (P) that form the efferent component of cerebellar equipment. Axons from Purkinje cells pass out of the cerebellum to connect with extrapyramidal motor systems; they also send recurrent collaterals back to the cerebellar cortex (dots) in a form not readily distinguishable from climbing fibres (hence, reverberating circuits). Basket cells (B) occur in the upper layers and send bifurcating axons at right angles to the axes of the cerebellar folia. Where a basket cell axon contacts a granular cell axon, excitation passes from the latter to the former and thence to basket cell terminations around Purkinje cell bodies. Basket cells and granular cells are thus able to spread excitation in both directions over the cerebellar cortex.

cerebrum, the cerebellum consists of fibrous white matter and cellular grey matter. The white matter contains afferent and efferent nerve fibres.

Afferent fibres are of two types. (a) *Climbing fibres* which, it is said without universal agreement, arise from cell bodies in the internal nuclei of the cerebellum or as recurrent collateral branches of efferent

fibres. They are of small diameter and pass up to the highest regions
of the grey matter in a manner which has been likened to a climbing
vine. They branch repeatedly. We shall meet them again later.
(b) *Mossy fibres* are not a bit mossy in themselves. They are of large
diameter and pass with much branching into the lower regions of the
cerebellar cortex. The endings of the branches are expanded into
structures that look to some eyes like moss leaves. Mossy fibres are
believed to originate in cell bodies outside the cerebellum—pons,
olive, vestibular nuclei.

The cortex of grey matter containing the cell bodies is very distinctly
composed of two layers. These are an outer *molecular layer* and an
inner *granular layer*. At the junction of these two layers occur the
most conspicuous cellular elements. These are the flask-shaped
Purkinje cell bodies. There are rows of them side by side throughout
the entire cerebellar cortex. At the top end of the Purkinje cell bodies
a dense bush of dendrites extends upwards through the molecular
layer to terminate at the very edge of the cortex. The dendritic bush
is a flat one, the branches all lying in a plane at right angles to the axis
of the folium. From the rounded bottom of the Purkinje flasks, root-
like axons drop vertically down through the white matter *en route*
to the internal nuclei. The Purkinje cells form the efferent elements
of the cerebellar cortex.

We have now to connect the afferent inflow with the efferent
outflow. The simplest connexion is effected by the climbing fibres.
Each of these, when it reaches the molecular layer, becomes associated
with a particular Purkinje cell. The climbing fibre divides branch for
branch (more or less) with the branches of the Purkinje cell's dendritic
bush and so becomes just about as closely applied to its favoured
Purkinje cell as one neurone can be to another. This one-to-one
relation of climbing fibre to Purkinje cell lends support to the belief
that the climbing fibre is a recurrent collateral or—much the same
thing—originates in one of the internal nuclei. The climbing fibres
would then serve to establish reverberating (i.e. temporally extended)
circuits.

With the other type of afferent fibre (the mossy fibre described
above), the final branches terminate as flattened expansions in the
granular layer of the cortex. The granular layer is so named because
it contains *granule cells*. These are small, closely packed, heavily
granulated cells with three to five quite short dendrites ending in
structures like claws. A close association exists between these claw-
like dendrites of the granule cells and the flattened expansions of the

mossy fibres. In this way, each mossy fibre establishes connexions with many granule cells, and each granule cell synapses with three to five mossy fibres. Each granule cell sends a thin axon up into the molecular layer where it divides into two long branches that stream parallel to the axis of the folium running through and synapsing with the dendritic bushes of many Purkinje cells. Hence any one mossy fibre eventually connects with many Purkinje cells and any one Purkinje cell is connected with many mossy fibres. Now, the arrangements described above allow for the activation of Purkinje cells in rows *parallel* to the axis of the folium. In the molecular layer are *basket cells*, each of which gives off a single, long, characteristic axon that runs at right angles to the axis of the folium. As the basket cell axons run across the parallel axons of the granule cells, synapses occur and impulses in the granule cells are transferred to the basket cells. The basket cell axons give off branches as they pass near Purkinje cells. In this way rows of Purkinje cells *at right angles* to the folium are activated. Hence, a single mossy fibre is able to influence an *area* of Purkinje cells which may in turn influence a *group* of muscles.

Cells of Golgi Type II are distributed throughout the two layers of the cerebellar cortex. It appears that these cells serve to set up reverberating circuits among the granule cells and among the basket cells.

The overall histological picture, then, is one of widespread and temporally prolonged activity—the kind that would be expected in an organ concerned with body-wide muscular co-ordination. It should not be assumed that an impulse in a mossy fibre will necessarily *discharge* all the Purkinje cells to which it is connected. But it may be safely believed that such an impulse will raise the central excitatory state (c.e.s.) of the Purkinje cells. With each succeeding impulse-arrival, not always from the same afferent fibre, the Purkinje cell c.e.s. will rise nearer to threshold until discharge occurs. Presumably the "wiring diagram" is arranged in such a way that a new input from, say, the cerebral cortex impinges upon a series of Purkinje cells which are at a particular c.e.s. due to the proprioceptive information reaching the cerebellum from other sources. Some of the Purkinje cells will be discharged by the extra c.e.s. induced by the cerebro-fugal impulses. These will be the cells that connect, via the internal nuclei, with the appropriate pathways of the great descending motor systems to sensitize them in such a way as to result in effective muscular activity. It should be borne in mind that efferent impulses from the cerebellar cortex pass across several synapses (in internal nuclei, red nucleus, thalamus, reticular formation) before reaching spinal effector neurones. Since every synapse is an integrating region, it is obvious that this arrangement allows for (a) non-cerebellar influences to join and modify the pattern of efferent discharge at each synapse, and (b) multiplication of efferent routes at each synapse, so affecting a larger section of the musculature.

Experimental

SPONTANEOUS ELECTRICAL ACTIVITY

The term "spontaneous" in this context may be interpreted in two ways. It may be held to mean the electrical activity occurring in the absence of experimental interference, and it can be considered to imply electrical activity arising within the structure under investigation (as opposed to such activity due to afferent impulses). In both

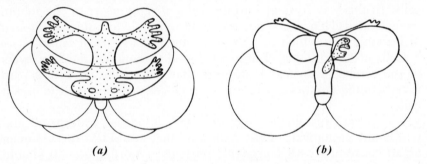

(a)   *(b)*

Fig. 38. Representation on the dorsal (a) and ventral (b) surfaces of the cerebellum of motor areas that correspond to parts of the cerebral motor cortex.

senses, the cerebellum can be said to exhibit spontaneous electrical activity. Snider and Eldred (1949) were able to record electrical changes in the cerebellum even when all of the peduncles had been sectioned, i.e. with the cerebellum isolated from the rest of the nervous system. According to Swank and Brendler (1951) sinusoidal waves of low voltage and a frequency of 100–300/sec can be picked up from the cerebellar surface. Brookhart and his colleagues (1951) declare that these slow waves originate at the level of the Purkinje and granular cells. Fast waves of 1 000–2 000/sec are detectable at the cortex, but their origin is not known. Opinion seems to favour the idea that the fast waves represent the afferent input to the cerebellum and the slow waves correspond to the efferent discharges. Localized changes in electrical activity in the monkey cerebellum corresponding

to localized changes in limb muscle activity were recorded as long
ago as 1943 by Adrian, who also showed that such local changes
spread after a while to neighbouring areas. This is experimental
evidence for the presumption of stimulus-spread derived from the
histological picture. Similarly, stimulation of the cerebral cortex,
electrically or by strychnine, is accompanied by discharges in the
contralateral cerebellar cortex. In this way, and in others, localization
of function is demonstrated.

LOCALIZATION

Figure 38 shows Adrian's (1943) classical diagram of cerebellar
areas corresponding to parts of the cerebral motor cortex. Since then
more refined experimental methods have resulted in more precise
maps involving homunculi.

CHAPTER 8

POSTURAL REACTIONS

From what has been described so far we may tabulate the following basic neural elements as those concerned with postural reactions in the higher mammals (Table II).

This is a formidable list and covers a good deal of the nervous system, suggesting that postural reactions play a much more important part in an animal's life than is generally realized. Perhaps the all-pervading presence and automaticity of posture, together with its role in the play of life as a supporting actor rather than as a dramatic lead, account for the widespread lack of interest in postural matters among students of neurophysiology. A glance at Table II should convince the most disinterested reader that the great bulk of neural activity going on over any waking period is concerned with postural mechanisms and deserves serious consideration. No doubt the processes of thinking and the procedures of discrete voluntary motor activity may be ranked higher on the homocentric scale, but a short acquaintance with patients possessing postural deficits shows that these "higher" activities depend very greatly upon a background of normal postural adjustments.

In the absence of voluntary instructions the normal nervous system arranges that the body and its parts adopt spatial relations which are appropriate to the environmental conditions at any given time. This gives a resting posture. In the presence of voluntary instructions—i.e. during the performance of a corticospinal act— the normal nervous system arranges for a disposition of the "unused" parts in a manner appropriate to the act being carried out. This gives an active posture. Both of these adjustments are effected by contraction of the striped muscles of the trunk and limbs. There is no difference between a voluntary contraction and a postural contraction with respect to the mechanics of the muscle *fibre*, the chemistry and physics of contraction, the nerve impulse or the final motor pathway. But the activity of the muscle as a whole is very different in these two situations. Postural contractions involve continuous, low-frequency discharges down the motor nerve fibres to small groups of muscle fibres. The frequency of arrival of impulses to any one group of fibres is sub-tetanic and the arrival of impulses to different groups

TABLE II

Basic Neural Elements Concerned with Postural Reactions in Higher Mammals

1. Afferent structures

A. Receptors

   (a) Muscle spindles and tendon organs of Golgi
   (b) Joint receptors
   (c) Mesenteric enteroceptors
   (d) Vestibular hair cells
   (e) Retinal receptors

B. Peripheral fibres

   (a) Somatic afferent component of spinal nerves, dorsal root ganglion and dorsal roots
   (b) Vestibular branch of eighth cranial nerve

2. Central structures

   (a) Dorsal funiculi of spinal cord ⎫
   (b) Nuclei gracilis and cuneatus of medulla ⎪
   (c) Medial lemniscus of medulla   ⎬ Conscious proprioception
   (d) Posterolateral ventral nucleus of thalamus ⎭
   (e) Dorsal and ventral spinocerebellar tracts   ⎱ Unconscious
   (f) Restiform body and superior cerebellar penduncle ⎰ proprioception
   (g) Superior, lateral and medial vestibular nuclei
   (h) Medial longitudinal fasciculus
   (i) Abducens and oculomotor nuclei
   (j) Brain stem and midbrain reticular formation
   (k) Cerebellum
   (l) Cerebral cortex

3. Efferent structures

   (a) Cerebello-reticular, -rubral and -spinal bundles
   (b) Rubrospinal tract
   (c) Reticulospinal tract
   (d) Vestibulospinal tract
   (e) Ventral motor neurones (large and small), ventral roots and somatic efferent component of spinal nerves

of fibres is asynchronous, so that the contractions are out of phase and tend to produce a continuous pull rather than a tremorous reaction. By variation of the total input to a given muscle, the continuous pull can be varied in intensity to meet the overall conditions. All that has been described in this paragraph utilizes the basic spinal effector mechanism, the apparatus of the stretch reflex (see p. 105), as will be seen more clearly later.

Brain Stem Sections

Stretch reflex mechanisms, while essential for postural reactions, are by no means sufficient. This is seen clearly after section of the spinal cord. Initially there is loss of postural adaptations and of spinal reflexes below the section. Later, when spinal shock has worn off, it becomes possible to elicit stretch reflexes but the loss of postural adaptations is permanent. Hence there can be no doubt that higher regions of the CNS are necessary. Section of the brain stem at the midcollicular level (i.e. between the inferior and superior colliculi) is the classical means of demonstrating the defect of posture known as decerebrate rigidity. Under these conditions all antigravity muscles stay strongly contracted, so that the animal's limbs are stiffly extended. Evidently then, the section has cut off an inhibitory influence emanating from higher regions. It will be seen shortly that this is by no means the full explanation of decerebrate rigidity. The abnormal postural tone remains in force even when the animal is turned onto its side or back. That the response is not simply extensor rigidity but is a true antigravity phenomenon is shown by the form decerebrate rigidity takes in the three-toed sloth. In this species interruption of higher influences upon the segmental mechanisms results in contraction of the flexor muscles, since these are the muscles used by the sloth to preserve its upside-down habit.

Sections above the midcollicular level have much the same effect as described above, as do cuts below the level until the plane of section occurs at the point of entry of the eighth cranial nerve, as reported by Sherrington in 1906. Decerebrate rigidity changes immediately to the flaccidity typical of ventral root section when the brain stem is cut at the level of the vestibular nerve. Thus decerebrate rigidity cannot simply be due to the removal of inhibitory influences but is partly a result of unopposed facilitatory activity originating in lower regions. The most important structure involved is Deiter's nucleus (lateral vestibular nucleus). If this nucleus is destroyed on one side, then subsequent midcollicular section is followed by decerebrate rigidity of the opposite side only. Similar results are obtained by section of the ventral funiculi of the spinal cord. Degeneration studies show that under these conditions the vestibulospinal tracts suffer serious damage. Evidently then, the vestibulospinal tracts exert a major postural influence upon the apparatus of the stretch reflex. The vestibulospinal facilitatory influence is reflex in nature, with afferents arising in the vestibule and in the muscles and joints (Fig. 39). Decerebrate rigidity occasioned by a midcollicular section is abolished from the hindlimbs if the dorsal roots from the limb muscles are cut. In the case of the forelimbs it is necessary also to cut the vestibular nerve.

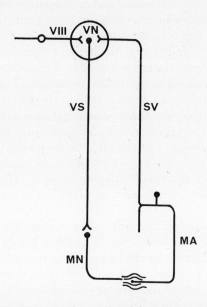

FIG. 39. Diagram to illustrate the reflex nature of decerebrate rigidity. Impulses in joint and muscle afferents (MA) pass in the spinovestibular tract (SV) to the vestibular nucleus (VN) which reflects instructions back along the vestibulospinal tract (VS) to the ventral horn motor neurones (MN). Information in the vestibular nerve (VIII) plays its main part in regard to the forelimbs.

It should be clear by now that the facilitatory mechanisms of Fig. 39 are the ones upon which higher regions exert an inhibitory action. It is the cutting off of these inhibitory influences that allows full play to the vestibulospinal mechanisms causing strong extensor contraction. No clear picture can be given of the origin of inhibitory impulses. There is evidence that area 4s of the cerebral cortex (pericruciate cortex of carnivores), parts of the caudate nucleus and the anterior lobe of the cerebellum are involved. If these regions are destroyed, then a pronounced antigravity posture is assumed, but such destruction is not equivalent to a midcollicular section even though the end effect appears to be the same. Decerebrate rigidity caused by destruction of the sites named is *not* relieved by lesions in Deiter's nucleus.

But a preparation in which area 4s and the anterior lobe of the cerebellum have been removed and the vestibular nuclei destroyed, can be converted to a flaccid state by midcollicular section. Although it may occasion surprise that a midcollicular section can result in flaccidity, a pause for reflection makes the situation clear. In such a preparation the midcollicular section is not cutting off inhibitory impulses because these have already been removed. It is evidently abolishing another facilitatory mechanism that is additional to the vestibulospinal effects described above. The additional facilitatory structure is the brain stem reticular formation. Tonic sensory input to the midbrain and brain stem reticular formation generates a discharge in the reticulospinal tracts which has an excitatory action upon the apparatus of the stretch reflex. Midcollicular section cuts off all or most of this discharge, but the effect is seen only in the preparation described immediately above, otherwise it is masked by the strong excitatory effects of the vestibulospinal system. It is also likely that the red nucleus plays some part in a similar way by means of the rubrospinal tract.

Hence in the intact animal inhibitory regions such as the anterior lobe of the cerebellum and area 4s exert a tonic depressing effect upon the two facilitatory mechanisms of the brain stem. The postural state at any time is thus determined by the algebraic sum of the inhibitory and excitatory discharges (Fig. 40).

Postural Adjustments

This long analysis of the mechanisms of decerebrate rigidity is intended to clarify the basic apparatus concerned with postural adjustments. At the outset it must be emphasized again that posture can only be sensibly considered in terms of adjustments. Postural equipment is in operation all the time and is changing all the time. Sometimes, when a particularly striking change occurs, it is described as a particular kind of postural reflex. But the neural apparatus of posture has not suddenly become active when the reflex is observed; it has been active all along and has now altered its activity under the new conditions in order to go on doing what it has been doing all along—adjusting the body and its parts to the best mechanical advantage.

With the above neural mechanisms in mind, the reader is recommended to analyse the descriptions given in textbooks of general physiology of tonic neck reflexes, tonic labyrinthine reflexes, righting reflexes and supporting reactions.

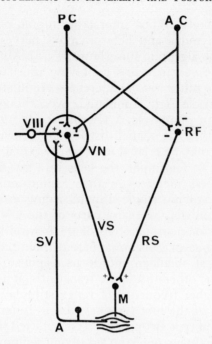

Fig. 40. Overall picture of the mechanisms involved in postural reactions. Muscle afferents (A), via the spinovestibular tract (SV), and fibres in the vestibular nerve (VIII) carry information to the vestibular nucleus (VN). This is not free to make its own decisions but receives inhibitory inputs from the pericruciate cortex (area 4s in primates, PC) and from the anterior lobe of the cerebellum (AC). These regions also send inhibitory impulses to the reticular formation (RF). The instructions carried via the vestibulospinal (VS) and reticulospinal (RS) tracts to the motor neurones (M) is thus an algebraic sum of their excitatory and inhibitory inputs.

Supplement on Movement and Posture

BASIC MECHANISMS

Motor Neurone

The impression has been given in earlier parts of this section that the ventral horn motor neurone discharges as a result of the algebraic sum of excitatory and inhibitory impulses reaching it from a variety of paths. This is the view which is generally agreed upon and which has the largest amount of experimental support. However, it is possible that a dual mechanism operates. It may be that the ventral horn motor neurone sometimes discharges according to the number of impulses arriving in the synaptic knobs that cover its surface, and sometimes discharges when fewer impulses arrive at some special part of the cell body. When interacting inputs of varying size are given via homonymous and heteronymous nerves, the response is frequently not the algebraic sum (Hunt, 1955). Moreover, the EPSP (see p. 11) of a motor neurone supplying muscle A is sometimes larger when some other muscle afferent is stimulated than when the afferent from muscle A is stimulated, even though only the latter causes contraction of muscle A (Eccles *et al.*, 1957). Hence some workers believe that the spatial distribution of synaptic connexions on the cell body may be related to areas of special sensitivity.

It is tempting to look upon the cells in a given neurone pool as being more or less identical in their connexions and properties. Modern work involving single unit recording is making this seem more and more unlikely in many parts of the CNS. Certainly with regard to the motor neurone pools of the ventral horns clear differences between adjacent cells are apparent. Some cells discharge for a fairly long time at small amplitude in response to low frequency reflex stimulation; others fire quite transiently at a higher amplitude and require a higher frequency of reflex stimulation (Granit *et al.*, 1956). Neurones of the first type have been designated "tonic" and those of the second type as "phasic". It is believed that the differences between them are due to one kind supplying red muscle and the other kind supplying pale muscle. There is also no doubt now that the cells in a given neurone pool differ in their thresholds, each cell having what has come to be called a firing index. Some cells fire every time they are subjected to excitatory stimuli and are said to have a firing index of 100; others fire with varying numbers of stimulations and have intermediate firing indices. Another group of cells has, for any given form of stimulus, a firing index of zero, inasmuch as they never discharge, however many times a particular stimulation is made (Hunt, 1955). It seems reasonable to suppose that the cells in a given pool that have a firing index of 100 are the ones that need little or nothing more than the impulses arriving in the dorsal roots to cause them to effect spinal reflexes. Cells with intermediate firing indices are likely to be much more dependent upon simultaneous bombardment by several routes and those that have zero firing indices may well be mostly concerned with the synergism of groups of muscle and therefore would receive their most effective afferents from higher regions.

Those women who have suffered the "quickenings" of pregnancy would probably exhibit no surprise to learn that reflex activity begins before birth. Only recently, however, has there been scientific evidence available to confirm the young wives' tales. In the guinea-pig (gestation period 68 days) spontaneous electrical activity begins in a discontinuous fashion as shown by the EEG at 40 days and becomes continuous at 48 days; reflexogenic responses occur around the 54th day (Bergstrom, 1962). Human spontaneous activity seems to begin in the pontine region at about 70 days, but reflexogenic responses do not occur until about the 84th day; the stretch reflex clearly appeared at the 98th day (Bergstrom and Bergstrom, 1963). Summarizing the appearance of various avoidance reflexes in the human foetus in terms of weeks of menstrual age, Humphrey (1964) gives the perioral as being the first to develop (at 7·5), then, in order, the eyelid (10–10·5), the lip (14·5) and the inside of the nostrils (24). In other words the foetus responds at those ages with avoidance movements in response to manipulation of those areas.

Pyramidal System

In the earlier part of this section devoted to the pyramidal system and in Fig. 25 a rather simplified working view was given. It is necessary to point out that there are some dissentient opinions with regard to the origin and composition of the corticospinal tract. There seems to be general agreement on at least one point—that all the cell bodies of this system are in the cerebral cortex, in lower animals and in man (Lassek and Evans, 1945). But views are still divided about which parts of the cortex are involved. The earliest workers believed that the cells of origin occurred in many parts of the cortex. Then more critical work gradually narrowed down the area until it became limited to what is now called the motor area, the precentral gyrus or the Betz cell region. More modern work has swung the pendulum again and it now appears that pyramidal fibres originate in parts of the cortex other than the precentral gyrus. Indeed, counts of the Betz cells show that they correspond to only about 3% of the fibres in the human pyramids. A summary of the findings reported in recent literature is given by Crevel and Verhaart (1963) who, from their own and others' work, conclude that while some pyramidal fibres originate in the frontal, precentral and postcentral regions, only very few or none arise in occipital or temporal regions. Further, they maintain that there is no evidence for the belief that 50% of pyramidal fibres originate outside the pre- and postcentral cortex; practically all of the cortocospinal tract originates in the anterior two-thirds of the cortex.

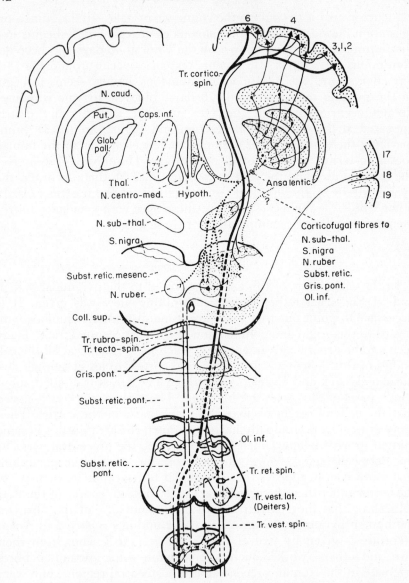

FIG. 41. Descending motor pathways that argue against a separation of pyramidal and
extrapyramidal systems. (From Brodal, 1963.)

KEY. Ansa lentic., Ansa lenticularis; Caps. inf., internal capsule; Coll. sup., superior colliculus; Glob. pall.;
globus pallidus; Gris. pont., pontine grey matter; Hypoth., hypothalamus; N. caud., caudate nucleus;
N. centro-med., centro-medial nucleus; N. ruber, red nucleus; N. sub-thal., subthalamic nuclei; Ol. inf.
inferior olive; Put., putamen; S. nigra, substantia nigra; Subst. retic. mesenc., midbrain reticular substance;
Subst. retic. pont., pontine reticular substance; Thal., thalamus; Tr. cortico-spin., corticospinal tract;
Tr. ret. spin., reticulospinal tract; Tr. rubrospin., rubrospinal tract; Tr. tecto-spin., tectospinal tract;
Tr. vest. lat. (Deiter's), lateral vestibular tract; Tr. vest. spin., vestibulospinal tract.

Extrapyramidal System

An impressive body of argument has been assembled by some workers, based upon both anatomical and functional evidence, to support the view that no useful purpose is served in maintaining the traditional separation of the pyramidal and extrapyramidal systems. Indeed it is proposed in some quarters (Meyers, 1953; Brodal, 1963) that a removal of this distinction results in a truer understanding of motor phenomena. Historically, the pyramidal system consists of the cortical Betz cells of the precentral gyrus (area 4) and the axons of these cells down to their synapse with cell bodies in the spinal cord. All other motor apparatus is assigned to the extrapyramidal system, which thus includes motor cortex other than precentral gyrus, subcortical motor nuclei such as the corpus striatum, red nucleus, substantia nigra, subthalamic nuclei, caudate nucleus, superior and inferior colliculi, olivary nucleus and pontine nuclei. The anatomical argument (Fig. 41) against a separation of the two systems is that fibres in the medullary pyramids (a) arise from areas of cortex traditionally looked upon as extrapyramidal (areas 1, 2, 3 and 6), (b) give off branches to at least several and possibly all of the subcortical nuclei mentioned above, and (c) these subcortical "extrapyramidal nuclei" receive fibres from area 4 of the cerebral cortex (Brodal, 1963). In addition, most of these subcortical nuclei receive afferents that can only be sensibly regarded as components of the sensory part of the sensorimotor apparatus (Fig. 42).

Functionally, it is claimed that there are no pressing reasons why the pyramidal system should be considered to have the exclusive right to the control of discrete movement with the extrapyramidal equipment playing a merely supportive role. Discrete movements are said to result from stimulation of cortical areas other than precentral gyrus (Penfield and Rasmussen, 1950). Moreover, section of corticospinal fibres in the cerebral peduncles does not lead to very marked deficits in discrete movements in man or monkey (Bucy and Keplinger, 1961). This recalls the work of Tower on section of medullary pyramids mentioned on page 110. An excellent and full review of "extra-pyramidal" participation in discrete movements in man, with extensive coverage of the literature, is given by Jung and Hassler (1960) from which Fig. 20 is taken.

Basal Ganglia

Although the basal ganglia are normally included in the extrapyramidal system, they deserve (and have been given) considerable

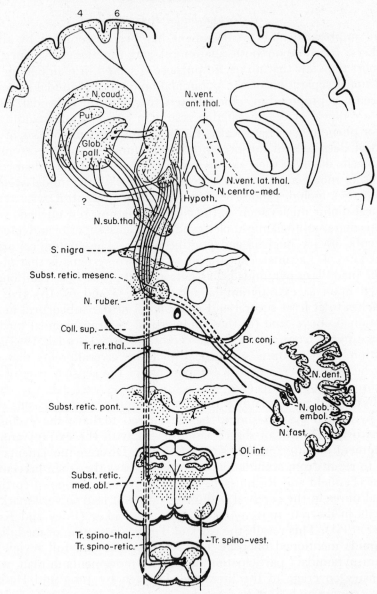

FIG. 42. Ascending pathways that affect the motor system and suggest that no real distinction may be drawn between pyramidal and extrapyramidal systems. (From Brodal, 1963.)

KEY. Br. conj., Brachium conjunctivum; Coll. sup., superior colliculus; Glob. pall., globus pallidus; Hypoth., hypothalamus; N. caud., caudate nucleus; N. centro-med., centro-medial nucleus; N. dent.,

Continued at foot of page 145.

attention in their own right, partly because of their large relative size and partly because they seem to be inevitably implicated in human motor pathology. It has recently been shown that the globus pallidus and possibly also the putamen and substantia nigra contain representations of the body in the form of an homunculus rather like that on the motor cortex (Hassler, 1961). Whether these are sensory or motor is not clear and it is entirely possible that they are sensorimotor. For many years it was thought that the globus pallidus was the seat of trouble in Parkinson's disease, but more recent work locates the lesion in the substantia nigra with the possible but not essential involvement of the globus pallidus. Hassler (1962) has developed an argument (see Fig. 31) regarding the intricate neuromuscular mechanism of Parkinsonism which leads to the conclusion that the nigral and pyramidal systems are antagonistic. If this is so then destruction of the basal part of the ventrolateral thalamic nucleus should relieve Parkinsonian tremor in the same way that ablation of the motor cortex does but without the paralysis that follows the latter operation. Destruction of the ventrolateral nucleus of the thalamus in over 500 patients has indeed resulted in complete relief of both tremor and rigidity. Hence there seems little doubt that the pyramidal system normally facilitates the basic motor system (globus pallidus, dentate nucleus) responsible for semi-automatic movements and that the nigral system (which is invariably destroyed in all Parkinsonian patients) normally exerts an inhibition upon this system.

Another interesting aspect of pallidal function that has only recently become apparent is its possible role in attention and arousal. Stimulation of the globus pallidus in patients under general anaesthesia causes them to "waken" while the stimulus is on, inasmuch as they open their eyes, look around the theatre, move about and attempt to make conversation. Frequently the patient, whether anaesthetized or not, cannot prevent himself from laughing in a quite natural fashion when the globus pallidus is stimulated. It appears therefore that the globus pallidus, and possibly other basal ganglia, must be looked upon as functionally connected with the midbrain reticular formation (see p. 248) that serves to alert the organism in response to non-specific stimuli. In view of the somatotopic representation on

Continued from previous page.

dentate nucleus; N. fast., fastigial nucleus; N. glob.-embol., globose-embolliform nuclei; N. ruber., red nucleus; N. sub thal., subthalamic nuclei; N. vent. ant. thal., ventro-anterior nucleus of thalamus; N. vent. lat. thal., ventro-lateral nucleus of thalamus; Ol. inf., inferior olive; Put., putamen; S. nigra, substantia nigra; Subst. retic. med. obl., reticular substance of medulla oblongata; Subst. retic. mesenc., midbrain reticular substance; Subst. retic. pont., pontine reticular substance; Tr. ret. thal., reticulothalamic tract; Tr. spino-retic., spinoreticular tract; Tr. spino-thal., spinothalamic tract; Tr. spino-vest., spinovestibular tract.

the globus pallidus, it is possible that this structure serves, perhaps with other basal ganglia, to alert the organism in a more specific manner. Put in other words, the globus pallidus may be a region that is worthy of further attention not so much as an extrapyramidal motor structure but as a psychomotor centre of considerable importance.

Cerebellum

Perhaps the most interesting of recently investigated problems of cerebellar physiology involve its role in sensory mechanisms. It was thought for many years that the cerebellum received only proprioceptive information until Dow (1939) showed that potentials were evoked in the cerebellum when a cutaneous nerve was stimulated. The special senses became included when Snider and Stowell (1942) demonstrated that the optic system is connected with the cerebellum and later (1944) showed that this was also true for the auditory system. Neurosurgeons have disagreed about the effects of cerebellar lesions on sensory abilities in the human, some (e.g. Holmes, 1939) reporting no effect and some claiming tactile, auditory and visual deficits. Animal experimentation has produced reports that cerebellar lesions result in a great reduction in startle responses to loud noises (Chambers and Sprague, 1955). Although it is tempting, and some have succumbed to the temptation, to believe that the cerebellum has a role to play in conscious sensation, there is as yet no evidence that this is so. All the data so far accumulated can be explained in the same way as can the proprioceptive input to the cerebellum. In this view, the cerebellum is supplied with information from all the sense modalities so that it may better utilize its centrifugal connexions to exert its supportive role in muscular activity. All the alleged sensory deficits mentioned above may be explained on the basis of slightly deranged muscular powers, either in the limbs, the orbit or the ear. It is to be hoped that future research will clarify some of these points.

There is fairly good evidence, reviewed by Dow (1961) from which this account is largely taken, that various parts of the cerebellum are able to exert effects upon autonomic mechanisms. Stimulation of the cerebellum has been reported to result in cardiovascular changes, sham rage, respiratory inhibition and alterations of pupil size. In the section on the autonomic system (p. 156) it will be seen that the cerebral cortex is similarly implicated in visceral responses. It is likely that both the cerebral cortex and the cerebellum are able to influence the autonomic changes that are appropriate to the particular type of muscular activity that is being generated by the former and modulated by the latter.

Part IV

Visceral Functions

CHAPTER 9

AUTONOMIC MECHANISMS

General

In comparison with the somatic nervous system, two main differences are seen in the disposition of the autonomic system (Fig. 43).

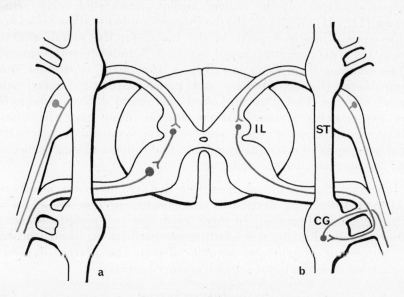

FIG. 43. Comparison of somatic (a) and autonomic (b) neural connexions. CG, Collateral ganglion; IL, intermediolateral column; ST, sympathetic trunk. The green fibres are common to both somatic and autonomic systems. Blue and red fibres in each system are homologous with each other, the blue somatic fibre being an interneurone and the blue autonomic fibre being a preganglionic sympathetic fibre. The collateral ganglion is homologous with the ventral horn neurone pool and has indeed migrated from that site during development, so that the red postganglionic sympathetic fibre represents the red somatic motor neurone.

(1) The postganglionic fibre of the somatic system has its cell body within the spinal cord (ventral horn cell), whereas the cell body of the postganglionic autonomic fibre occurs in an outlying ganglion. Embryologically, the autonomic postganglionic cell is somewhat

homologous with the ventral horn cell, the former having migrated from the spinal cord in the course of development. Reference to texts of neuroanatomy will show the arrangement of the paravertebral chain of ganglia—with fusion in the upper regions to give compound cervical and stellate ganglia—and the collateral or prevertebral ganglia further removed from the spinal cord (solar plexus and inferior mesenteric).

(2) Whereas the peripheral somatic nerves leave the spinal cord in an unbroken series, autonomic nerves arise in three distinctly separate groups: (a) the *cranial* outflow, associated with cranial nerves III, VII, IX and X; (b) the thoraco-lumbar outflow associated with widely dispersed parts of the body; (c) the sacral outflow, associated with peripheral sacral nerves 2, 3 and 4 (genito-urinary). This anatomical division parallels a functional separation into sympathetic (thoraco-lumbar) and parasympathetic (cranial and sacral) systems. The other important anatomical difference between the two systems is that parasympathetic fibres have their final synapse in the effector organ, whereas in the sympathetic system the final synapse is in a remote ganglion. The functional significance of this arrangement will be seen later.

It is important not to look upon these two systems (parasympathetic and sympathetic) as necessarily antagonistic in function. This is often, but not always so. In many cases the two systems function synergistically. Finally, it is worth remembering that, by convention, the autonomic systems are entirely *efferent;* the afferent impulses are carried over the usual somatic sensory pathways.

SYMPATHETIC SYSTEM

The anatomical arrangement of the fibres in this system (Fig. 44) provides a key to its function. Points to note are that (1) fibres in any ventral root run to more than one lateral ganglion; (2) any single fibre sends collaterals to more than one lateral ganglion.

Indeed, the postganglionic fibres outnumber the preganglionic fibres by about 20 : 1. The ratio varies with species and with different ganglia. Thus, we are concerned with a diffusely acting system. Activation at A (Fig. 44) may produce responses in organs supplied by nerves from 1, 2 and 3. Activation at B may result in responses in organs supplied by 3, 4, 5 and 6. Since sympathetic innervation is extensive and diffuse, activation of this system may produce widespread, general effects on the body as a whole. This does not mean

that sympathetic effects are *necessarily* widespread. It will be seen
below that sympathetic functions can be quite discrete. Nevertheless,
this system has a tendency to act diffusely. In other words, the
sympathetic system tends to co-ordinate several activities throughout

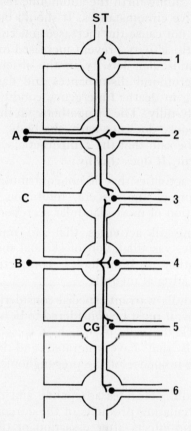

FIG. 44. Schematic representation of fibre connexions in the collateral ganglia. Note
that if the cell bodies at A discharge, excitation is transmitted to fibres 1, 2 and 3. When
the cell body at B generates an impulse, excitation occurs in fibres 3, 4, 5 and 6. C, Spinal
cord; CG, collateral ganglion; ST, sympathetic trunk.

the body to a given end. What is the end? Cannon (1939) in his great
work on this system, gave the general rule that activation of the
sympathetic system *prepares the body for increased activity under
emergency conditions.* The sympathetic system is not alone in responding to trying circumstances but we are considering it in isolation at

the moment. Under the conditions during which the sympathetic system was evolved, increased activity in emergency states meant muscular work; to fight or to flee or to mate. This is still the case in the wild. In human society these situations also arise, sometimes disguised, but still calling forth the autonomic responses appropriate to the more primitive circumstances. It should be clear that sympathetic activity does not cause the increased muscular effort; nor does a lack of sympathetic activity prevent increased muscular effort. But greatly increased muscular activity in the absence of sympathetic arousal produces profound disturbances and damage to the body, sometimes resulting in death. Emergency conditions result in great muscular work willy-nilly. The sympathetic mechanisms ensure that this inevitable response does not harm the body. In this way and to this extent it may be said that the sympathetic system conserves the internal environment. It does this by:

(1) Reducing all activities that do not contribute to muscular work, e.g. vasoconstriction of the viscera, inhibition of gastrointestinal motility and inhibition of most glandular secretion.

(2) By facilitating all activities that aid muscular effort, e.g. increased heart rate, vasodilatation of skeletal muscle, activation of sweat glands, dilation of bronchioles, contraction of the spleen, secretion from the adrenal medulla.

The adrenal medulla warrants special consideration. Anatomically and embryologically, it must be considered to be a part of the sympathetic system, since the cells of which it is composed are simply postganglionic cells that have migrated and become extensively modified under the influence of the preganglionic sympathetic fibres supplying it.

The adrenal medulla secretes adrenaline and related compounds. In this way the circulating products of the adrenal medulla serve to prolong sympathetic effects after cessation of the neural stimulus, because in general adrenaline duplicates the responses that follow stimulation of postganglionic sympathetic fibres. Exceptions to this statement are (a) the generalized calorigenic effect, and (b) the glycogenolytic effect of circulating adrenaline. The adrenal medulla releases its secretions only under the special conditions of generalized sympathetic activation, not under resting conditions. Two special points about the sympathetic system are worth noting.

(1) There is a tonic discharge of sympathetic impulses to the blood vessel musculature in both skin and muscle. The impulses to the

muscle blood vessels have a vasodilator effect, whereas those to the skin blood vessels are vasoconstrictor. However, muscular exercise increases the sympathetic tone to the muscle blood vessels but decreases the sympathetic tone to the skin blood vessels, producing vasodilatation in both cases. This is the only known example of decreased sympathetic activity in muscular exercise.

(2) The sympathetic system discharges tonically to many other structures, e.g. the heart and the pupil, but there is no tonic discharge to the sweat glands, pilomotor muscles, gastrointestinal tract or adrenal medulla. The special circumstances designated "emergency" conditions by Cannon (1939) are required to produce sympathetic activation of these structures.

PARASYMPATHETIC SYSTEM

As with the sympathetic system, the anatomical arrangement of parasympathetic fibres (Fig. 45) suggests the function. Very short postganglionic fibres occur within the innervated organ, with the

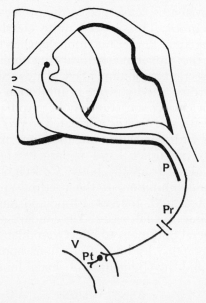

FIG. 45. Arrangement of fibres in the parasympathetic system. Preganglionic fibres (Pr) from cell bodies in the intermediate grey matter pass out through the ventral nerve roots into the pelvic nerves (P), and continue to the wall of a viscus (V) where they synapse with very short postganglionic neurones (Pt).

F

unimportant exceptions of the parotid and sublingual glands and the iris. The preganglionic fibres leave the cord in two discrete outflows. These two characteristics enable the parasympathetic system to produce highly local effects. This is correlated with a lack of unitary function, in distinction to the unitary, emergency response of the sympathetic system. If the parasympathetic system were activated in a generalized fashion there would occur at one and the same time constriction of the pupil, salivation, slowing of the heart, constriction of the bronchi, increasing peristalsis, contraction of the bladder, defaecation and engorgement of the erectile tissue. Such a collection of responses is so physiologically unrelated that the organism would be at a biological and social disadvantage in most situations. Accordingly, in addition to the local arrangements of the fibres there is complete absence of any parasympathetic counterpart to adrenaline. Acetylcholine, the parasympathetic neurotransmitter substance, is released at the postganglionic nerve ending inside the organ and is rapidly destroyed by the enzyme cholinesterase. Its action is not prolonged and generalized as is the case with adrenaline.

In very general terms it may be said that the cranial portion of the parasympathetic system is concerned in the protection and conservation of body resources. This is seen quite clearly with respect to gastrointestinal function. Proper nutrition depends to a very considerable extent upon the proper mechanical functioning of the gut and upon the proper secretions of alimentary glands. Similarly, the vagal influence upon cardiac activity is one of inhibition or conservation of a vital organ's powers. Constriction of the pupil and contraction of the ciliary muscle are also actions calculated to protect the body from the environment, with concentration upon internal processes. The sacral outflow on the other hand is largely concerned with the elimination of material from the body. Contraction of the bladder smooth muscle and inhibition of the urethral sphincter allow the voiding of unwanted fluid. Increased tone and motility of the colon favours the rejection of solid waste. A secondary and rather isolated function of the sacral outflow is to effect vasodilatation in the vessels of the external genitalia, leading to erections appropriate to reproductive activities and the elimination of sexual fluids.

Joint Actions

Most viscera are innervated by both divisions of the autonomic system, but the effects are not always antagonistic. Synergism of action is seen in stomach peristalsis, where each of the divisions may either stimulate or inhibit contractions. Similar joint action is associated with the salivary glands.

ANTAGONISTIC ACTIONS

Nevertheless, in most situations the two autonomic divisions do indeed exert opposite influences. Such antagonism is seen with regard to the heart rate, external genital vessel calibre, iris, ciliary muscle, bronchial calibre, intestinal peristalsis and urethral sphincter.

SINGLE INNERVATION

Some structures (sweat glands, pilomotor muscles, nipple, nictitating membrane muscle and blood vessels of skin and skeletal muscle) receive only sympathetic innervation. It is considered unlikely that any structure is innervated by the parasympathetic system only, although until recently it was not known that the ciliary muscle and the sphincter pupillae received sympathetic fibres.

DOUBLE EFFECT

The blood vessels of skeletal muscle receive only sympathetic fibres. Some of these have a dilator effect and others have a constrictor effect. Under normal resting conditions, the slight dilatation of muscle blood vessels (occasioned by unhurried limb movement, say) is brought about by a reduction of the tonic impulses in constrictor fibres. When rigorous muscular movement is required, the extensive dilatation is effected on a larger scale by an increase of the tonic impulses in the vasodilator fibres. (It should be borne in mind that the *maintenance* of vessel dilatation during exercise is largely due to the chemical effects of accumulated products of metabolism.)

Central Control of the Autonomic System

No precise account can be given of the anatomical pathways connecting supraspinal regions with autonomic outflows, for these have not been clearly demonstrated. Functional data make it clear that such pathways exist. There is no doubt that the Edinger–Westphal nucleus is a controlling site for the parasympathetic fibres of the third cranial nerve to the ciliary muscle. Similar certainty can be attached to the salivatory nuclei as the seat of vagal control of gut, bronchioles and salivary glands. Autonomic control of cardiovascular phenomena must be situated below the mesencephalic region, for transection at this level does not interfere with these functions. The most important cardiovascular controlling area seems to be in the *medulla* near the rostral end of the nucleus gracilis and the adjacent area postrema. Even so, it is well known that after the initial shock of spinal transection has worn off, vasomotor reflexes and the blood pressure both return to normal. Hence, there must be centres in the *spinal cord* capable of exerting tonic cardiovascular autonomic influences. Stimulation of various parts of the hypothalamus results in activation of the autonomic system. This is seen with clarity in regard to the sympathetic division, but is not so clear cut with respect to the parasympathetic division. It was for long claimed that stimulation of the anterior hypothalamus was effective in discharging only parasympathetic impulses, but more recent work suggests that the earlier results were due to spread of current to cells rostral to the hypothalamus. In any event, it is generally agreed that the hypothalamus does not play an important part in the tonic activity of the autonomic system. Rather, it superimposes higher control on the lower tonic mechanisms under special conditions and serves to balance the effects of the two autonomic divisions. The dorsomedial nucleus of the *thalamus* is reported to have some influence upon such autonomic functions as heart rate, respiration rate and temperature regulation. Anatomically this nucleus has well-known connexions with preoptic and hypothalamic areas. Many parts of the *cerebral cortex* evoke discharges in the autonomic system when stimulated (Fig. 46). Similarly, ablations of cortical regions result in autonomic effects. Most commonly the effects are upon heart rate and blood pressure, but cortical interventions have also affected salivation, piloerection, sweating, pupil diameter and bladder contractions. An excellent review of these localized effects can be found in Kennard (1949). Understanding of the role of the cortex in autonomic phenomena is at first sight made difficult by the facts that (a) the result of stimulation of any given point is not predictable, e.g. the blood pressure may be either raised or lowered, (b) very often the same effects are produced by stimulation or by ablation of a given area. In general terms, it seems that the cerebral cortex brings about the autonomic changes that are appropriate to the motor phenomena it is causing at that time. Indeed, it has been shown that stimulation of motor cortex can result in vasodilatory volume increase in the limb that moves as a result of the cortical stimulation. It is likely that the pathway for many such influences involves the hypothalamus, but not exclusively for stimulation of the pyramids also produces autonomic effects. Figure 46 shows the relation between various parts of the cerebral cortex and autonomic functions. It should be borne in mind that a great many of the functional changes are in ordinary circumstances closely connected with emotional states. Experimental neurosis in animals is accompanied by various cardiovascular disorders and it is common

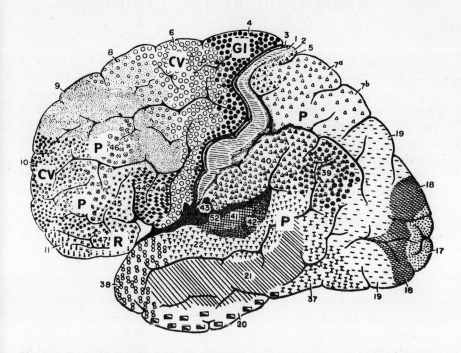

FIG. 46. Regions of cerebral cortex involved in autonomic phenomena. Stimulation or ablation gives cardiovascular (CV), gastrointestinal (GI), pupillary (P) and respiratory (R) changes. The human brain is given for convenience, but most of the experimental work has been done on the macaque.

knowledge that respiration and pulse rates, together with pupil and blood vessel diameters, alter considerably under conditions of psychic stimulation. Teleologically, one may consider that the cortex brings about visceral changes that are, in lower animals, appropriate to the motor activity that accompanies emotional states. Such states in the human are at various stages of remove from the more primitive forms and the motor activity is accordingly modified, but the ancient autonomic changes still occur, even though they are ineffectual (blushing) or inappropriate (loss of bladder control).

For an account of the role of the cingulate gyrus, see page 274.

CHAPTER 10

NEUROENDOCRINE RELATIONS

General

Over the last fifteen years one of the most rapidly expanding fields of neurophysiology has been the one involving the interrelations between the brain and the endocrine glands. Functional intimacy between the adrenal cortex and the sympathetic system (q.v.) is a long established piece of knowledge, but only recently has it become clear that in very many ways the central nervous system and the series of ductless glands form a functional unity. Classically the endocrines are looked upon as organs which produce hormones that circulate in the blood stream to have local (e.g. gonadal) or widespread (e.g. thyroidal) effects. In this view the organism is looked upon as without an environment; discussion is limited to internal events and is, in effect, concerned only with the mechanisms by which the *milieu intérieur* is kept constant. Such an orientation neglects the environment by assuming that it is constant. When such conditions occur, as for example in laboratory animal accommodation, there does indeed seem little need for the nervous system to be involved in endocrine phenomena. But in the real world of non-laboratory animals and in the semi-real world of civilized humans, the environment is by no means constant. The presence of food, oxygen and a mate cannot be counted upon continuously. Temperature and lighting vary regularly or irregularly and from time to time emotional vicissitudes disturb even the relatively calm constancy of university cloisters. Inconstancy characterizes the real world and for this the endocrine mechanisms must be brought in touch with changing conditions. This is done by the nervous system which detects and assesses external changes and orders the necessary hormonal (and other) adjustments. The biological hazards of the real world require a neuroendocrine system.

It will be seen below that the hypothalamus and the anterior pituitary gland are the most important structures in this system. When the anterior pituitary gland is separated from the hypothalamus, the endocrines function basally. That is, while still to some extent manufacturing and secreting hormones, they do these things at a very low level and maintain that level even when environmental exigencies are demanding a different level. By and large the basal activities of the endocrines are controlled by the negative feedback action of target gland hormones upon the anterior pituitary; as the tissues utilize the target hormones, so the blood level of these drops and this low concentration in the blood passing through the pituitary evokes the release of the appropriate trophic hormones. In general this does not apply to the gonads, for these rapidly pass into a quiescent state when the link between the brain and the pituitary is severed. It will be seen later that this is a reasonable consequence of the important role played in sexual behaviour by gonadal hormones acting upon the brain. Indeed it will be necessary to devote a part of this section to the ways in which various components of behaviour as well as the activity of the brain itself is affected by hormones. Several fairly recent reviews cover this field in detail (Harris, 1960; Campbell, 1963; Schreiber, 1963).

Neural Control of the Glands

HYPOTHALAMO-HYPOPHYSIAL CONNEXIONS

At the outset it must be clearly established that the median eminence of the tuber cinereum—long considered to be part of the hypothalamus—is really a component of the neurohypophysis. It certainly arises from neural tissue, growing down a little way to meet the adenohypophysis on its way up from the pharynx. But its reaction to vital dyes, its uptake of radioiodine, its cytology and its blood supply all indicate that the median eminence must be looked upon as the proximal part of the neurohypophysis. It will be seen that the median eminence plays a most important role in neuroendocrine integration.

The neurohypophysis is supplied by fibres that arise in the paraventricular and supraoptic nuclei of the hypothalamus (Fig. 47). Tracts from both nuclei join in the region of the median eminence and run back along the infundibular process to end in relation to the posterior lobe. A small tuberohypophysial tract is said to follow a similar course from the hypothalamic tuberal nuclei, but this is not seen clearly in many species. There is general agreement that the neural control of the posterior pituitary is mediated via these tracts of fibres.

Considerable controversy and not a little vituperation have been generated among those who have studied the nerve supply of the adenohypophysis. Harris (1948) has summarized the erroneous anatomical descriptions given from 1845 to 1945 of nerves reaching the anterior pituitary from a wide variety of sources. However, more recent and more cautious investigations including electron micro-

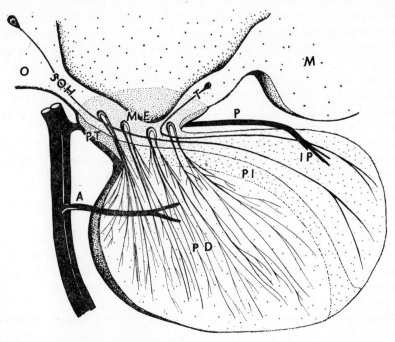

FIG. 47. Schematic drawing of the pituitary gland and its relations projected onto the sagittal plane. A, Anterior hypophysial artery arising from left internal carotid artery; IP, infundibular process; M, mammillary body; ME, median eminence; O, optic chiasma; P, posterior hypophysial artery, arising from right internal carotid artery; PD, pars distalis; PI, pars intermedia; PT, pars tuberalis; SOH, supraopticohypophysial tract; T, tuberohypophysial tract. (From Campbell, 1963.)

scopic studies have shown that earlier (and a few later) workers were misled by the presence of reticular fibres. The general opinion now is that any sparse nerve fibres that may be present in the anterior pituitary are vasomotor in function, not secretomotor, and as Harris (1948) has stated: *"the pars distalis of the pituitary may, in general terms be described as a gland under nervous control but lacking a nerve supply"*.

The other way in which the brain could be functionally connected to the anterior pituitary is by the portal vessels that traverse the pituitary stalk. These arise from a primary plexus of capillary loops in the median eminence and end as ramifications among the venous sinusoids of the anterior lobe. Since it could be shown that blood in the portal vessels passes downwards (not upwards as was thought at first) and since the system is present in all animal groups from cyclostomes to man (Green, 1951), the hypothesis was put forward that the hypothalamus forms one or more substances that pass down the portal vessels to the anterior lobe, evoking the release of trophic hormones (see Harris, 1955). Concentrated research in laboratories all over the world has amply confirmed this hypothesis, which is now accepted almost without question.

SEPARATION OF PITUITARY FROM BRAIN

In many normal animals there are cycles of sexual receptivity (oestrus) and fertility (ovulation). There is good evidence that such cycles—which include menstruation and ovulation in women—are profoundly influenced by environmental factors. Regularity of the cycle can be lengthened or shortened or the cycles abolished by changes in lighting, temperature or emotional situations. Again, a few mammalian forms do not ovulate cyclically but tend to have almost year-long oestrous periods and to ovulate in response to the psychic stimulation of coitus (rabbit, cat, ferret). Hence, environmental changes are able to influence the activity of the gonads (i.e. the release of gonadotrophic hormones). Environmental changes also have profound effects upon thyroid and adrenocortical activity especially with regard to emotionally stressing conditions. In these circumstances the thyroid gland (i.e. release of thyrotrophic hormone (TSH)) suffers inhibition which may be complete and the adrenal cortex (i.e. the release of adrenocorticotrophic hormone (ACTH)) is highly stimulated.

If the *anterior pituitary gland* is removed from the influence of the hypothalamus by transplantation to a distant site or by effective section of the pituitary stalk, none of the above reactions can be elicited. All endocrine glands atrophy (but not to hypophysectomized levels), sexual cycles cease and only a low level of thyroid and adrenocortical secretion occurs. Environmental changes of light, temperature, sexual stimulation or emotional stress are no longer followed by changes in glandular secretion. Atrophy occurs to some extent in the anterior lobe after stalk section but not to an extent that would explain the loss of function (Campbell, 1959); moreover, the return of pituitary transplants back to the sella turcica with consequent regeneration of portal vessel connexions is accompanied by return of function. It should also be noted that transplantation or stalk section does not abolish endocrine reactions to what has come to be called physical or systemic stresses. Depression of gonadal and thyroid function and stimulation of adrenocortical function follows any mechanical insult to the body, e.g. surgery, infection, ingestion of toxic materials, inanition. These agents appear to exert their effects by altering the composition of blood passing through the pituitary and do not require neural mechanisms.

Stalk section results in great atrophy of the *neural lobe* with reduction in its content of antidiuretic and oxytocic principles. Under these conditions the median eminence doubles its volume, shows an increase in neurosecretory substance and exhibits some degree of function (Campbell and Harris, 1957). These results are to be expected when it is realized that stalk section merely cuts the neurohypophysis into two portions, one of them still attached to its important neural origins. Only seldom, however, does the proximal portion retain enough activity to maintain its endocrine functions. "Neurosecretory substance" as used above refers to material with special staining properties that can be found under some conditions in the region of the supraopticohypophysial tract. It is thought to be a precursor of posterior pituitary principles formed in the supraoptic and paraventricular nuclei and passing down to the axons of those cells to the neural lobe. Some investigators believe it may be formed at any part of the axon (Christ, 1962). An excellent review of neurosecretion has been prepared by Ortman (1960).

Brain Lesions

In general terms the functional deficits in endocrine activity mentioned above may also be produced by suitably placed lesions in the brain. Caution is required in the interpretation of such studies for it is not easy to know whether an effective lesion has destroyed a regulatory site or has merely interrupted a pathway from a distant regulatory site. Hence the mapping of the nervous system with respect to endocrine function is still at a very early stage. The most obvious region to begin mapping was the hypothalamus and considerable attention has been paid to this area over the past few years. By and large, lesions of fair extent in the hypothalamus have an effect upon pituitary function similar to transplantation or stalk section, i.e. there is a panhypopituitarism. Smaller lesions have produced effects which are selective for particular hormones (Fig. 48).

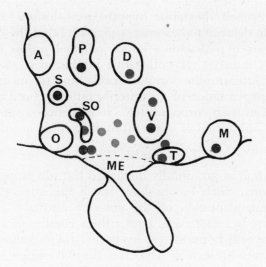

FIG. 48. Hypothalamic nuclei projected onto the sagittal plane with sites at which lesions affect the secretion of ACTH (blue), TSH (green) and gonadotrophins (red). A, Anterior commissure; D, dorsomedial nucleus; M, mammillary body; ME, median eminence; O, optic chiasma; P, paraventricular nucleus; S, suprachiasmatic nucleus; SO, supraoptic nucleus, T, tuberal nuclei, V, ventromedial nucleus.

Gonadotrophic Hormones

It seems that lesions in the region of the paraventricular nucleus produce a condition that is loosely described as constant oestrus, i.e. continuous vaginal cornification. Similar results follow more ventral lesions in the ventromedial nucleus and median eminence, but these may exert their effects by interrupting a descending pathway which is concerned with the release of luteinizing hormone (LH); it is likely that the lesions do not prevent the release of follicle-stimulating hormone (FSH). Lesions in the anterior hypothalamus just behind the optic chiasma have been associated with advancement of the time of vaginal opening in rats and of vulval swelling in ferrets, both of these results being interpreted as precocious puberty due to the destruction of a hypothalamic inhibitory region. In this view the normal hypothalamus retards the release of gonadotrophins from the anterior pituitary before puberty and during the anoestrous phase in animals with sexual cycles. When brain development is complete in the first case and when appropriate environmental conditions occur in the second case, the inhibitory effect is removed, hypothalamic stimulatory mechanisms come into force and pituitary gonadotrophin secretion is evoked. Posterior hypothalamic lesions, on the other hand, result in delayed pubescence, suggesting that the brake exerted by the anterior hypothalamus is not released unless the posterior hypothalamus is intact. Hypothalamic inhibition is also directed at the release of luteotrophic hormone (prolactin), for median eminence lesions or transplantation of the anterior pituitary both result in prolonged life of ovarian corpora lutea. No evidence is yet available for hypothalamic inhibition of other pituitary trophic hormones.

Thyrotrophic Hormone

TSH secretion is profoundly disturbed but not stopped by hypothalamic lesions. Such lesions have much the same effect as stalk section or transplantation of the anterior pituitary—reduction of thyroid activity to basal levels. Under these conditions a reduction in circulating thyroid hormone (as by partial thyroidectomy) does not result in enhanced release of TSH (i.e. thyroid compensatory hypertrophy). This fact, coupled with the finding that injections of thyroxine into the anterior pituitary reduce thyroid activity whereas similar injections into the hypothalamus do not, indicates that the pituitary is sensitive to increases in circulating target hormone and the hypothalamus sensitive to decreases. Most workers are agreed that to be effective the lesions must be placed in the anterior hypothalamus, just behind the optic chiasma.

Adrenocorticotrophic Hormone

ACTH secretion under resting conditions is not affected by hypothalamic lesions. Whereas such lesions are followed by atrophy of the thyroid gland, no adrenal atrophy has ever been found to accompany lesions in any part of the hypothalamus. Of course, lesions in the median eminence result in atrophy of the adrenal (and of all other endocrines) due to interruption of the portal system. Hypothalamic lesions, on the other hand, are very effective in reducing or abolishing ACTH responses to emotional stress stimuli. In the intact animal the brain–pituitary–adrenal axis is exquisitely sensitive to stressful situations. Even the mild procedure of picking up an animal results in increased release of ACTH. This stress response is absent when there are lesions either in the high anterior hypothalamus (above optic chiasma), in the anterior or posterior basal tuberal region or in the dorsomedial or ventromedial nuclei. Evidently more research is required to delineate precisely the role of various hypothalamic components in the several aspects of ACTH release.

There can be little doubt that, important though the hypothalamus undoubtedly is, other regions of the brain must convey information or instructions for the hypothalamic control of endocrine function. A beginning, but only a beginning, has been made in locating such other areas. Initially studies have been directed at structures which possess phylogenetic antiquity comparable to that of the hypothalamus—the limbic system (or rhinencephalon) and the reticular formation. These, of course, are also regions that have come into prominence in recent years from a purely neurophysiological point of view. Anatomically, they seem to be in an ideal position for participating in endocrine responses to environmental changes, for (a) they are interconnected, (b) each is connected to the neocortex, and (c) each is connected to the hypothalamus. Unfortunately the results obtained at the time of writing by lesions and stimulations of the limbic and reticular regions do not warrant any definitive conclusions. Similar remarks apply to other regions that have been sporadically studied such as the cerebral cortex and tegmentum. In general terms the higher regions of the nervous system seem to be able to exert either an excitatory or an inhibitory effect upon hypothalamic endocrine mechanisms, just as they have both of these effects upon hypothalamic control of autonomic responses (q.v.). Details of experimental results may be found in recent reviews (Campbell, 1963; Schreiber, 1963), where it will be seen that the many conflicting results highlight the urgent need for more research in this field.

STIMULATION OF THE BRAIN

As with lesions, so with stimulation procedures, the most obvious part of the brain to study in this field is the hypothalamus. Effects upon neurohypophysial function have been known since 1947 when Harris introduced the method of remote control stimulation of an induction coil chronically implanted on the skull. Stimulation of the supraopticohypophysial system by electrodes attached to the coil was routinely followed by release of both antidiuretic hormone and of oxytocin.

Gonadotrophic Hormones

These hormones are released in the rabbit in amounts sufficient to produce ovulation by a very brief stimulation (3 min) of the hypothalamus, whereas stimulation of the anterior pituitary gland for up to 7 h did not evoke ovulation. Similarly, rats treated with barbiturate on the day of pro-oestrus do not ovulate on the following day, but will do so if the anteromedial ventral part of the hypothalamus is electrically stimulated.

Thyrotrophic Hormone

TSH secretion can be increased within minutes by electrical stimulation of the anterior hypothalamus, as seen by enhanced release of radioactive thyroxine from the thyroid gland (Fig. 49). Stimulation of posterior regions do not have this effect. Since continued stimulation maintains a high level of TSH release in the presence of high blood levels of thyroid hormone, the hypothalamic mechanisms are evidently dominant over the negative feedback effects.

Adrenocorticotrophic Hormone

ACTH release is greatly enhanced by stimulation for a few minutes of several regions of the hypothalamus near the midline from anterior median eminence to mammillary bodies. As with TSH, hypothalamic control of ACTH secretion is dominant over the negative feedback mechanism.

With regard to extrahypothalamic regions much the same remarks apply here as in the above paragraph on this topic. There is urgent need for more research in this field.

BRAIN EXTRACTS

According to the neurohumoral theory of endocrine control, one or more substances is formed in the median eminence and passed down the portal vessels to the anterior pituitary gland. Therefore it is reasonable to suppose that, at least under some conditions, extracts of the median eminence could be made which would have a stimulating effect on the adenohypophysis. This has been shown to be the case. Median eminence extracts have been prepared, in various degrees of purity, that cause the release of ACTH (Schally *et al.*, 1960), TSH (Schreiber, 1961) and gonadotrophins (Campbell *et al.*, 1964). Thus, the actual existence of neurohumours has been demonstrated and each of these groups has shown that the active principles do not occur in other parts of the brain. The agent responsible for the release of ACTH has been the subject of intense biochemical investigation and is seen to be a peptide which will evoke easily detectable ACTH release in a dose of 0·05 μg.

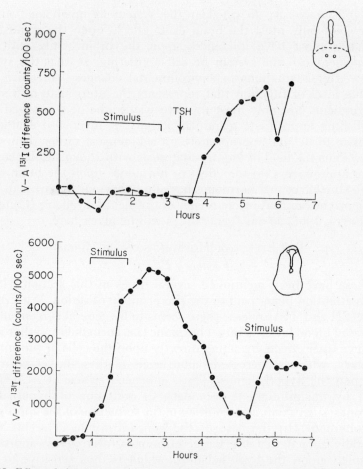

FIG. 49. Effect of electrical stimulation of the hypothalamus upon the release of thyrotrophic hormone (TSH) as indicated by the enhanced secretion of radioactive thyroid hormone. Upper curve, lack of thyroid response to electrical stimulation of posterior hypothalamus. Integrity of thyroid function shown by response to TSH injection. Inset shows horizontal section of hypothalamus with position of electrodes (circle) in mammillary bodies. Lower curve, thyroid response to two periods of electrical stimulation of the anterior hypothalamus. Inset shows site of electrodes (circles). (From Campbell *et al.*, 1960.)

Glandular Control of the Brain

It is beginning to make more and more sense to look upon the brain and the endocrine glands as a single system, quite apart from the natural bias among neuroendocrinologists. From such a point of view it is necessary to consider the system as involving two-way traffic. Not only must the brain exert effects upon the glands, but the latter must have influences upon the brain. Only with this arrangement can the system be self-regulating, so that the system tends—after adaptations to environmental changes—to return to a suitable level of function that represents the ideal state of a stable environment. Not only must this two-way traffic be concerned with establishing appropriate glandular activity, it must also enable the organism to behave appropriately, in a biological rather than social sense. Thus the field of inquiry that deals with the glandular control of the brain covers (a) the effect of hormones upon the brain itself, and (b) the effect that hormones have on behaviour by virtue of their action on the brain. A recent review of this field is available (Campbell and Eayrs, 1965) so only generalities will be given here.

THE EFFECT OF HORMONES ON THE BRAIN
Feedback Effects

These have been mentioned several times in this section without much attention being paid to the site or mode of action. With regard to ACTH and TSH release there seems to be general agreement that increased blood levels of target hormone (i.e. corticoids and thyroxine) produce their effects by acting directly upon the cells of the anterior pituitary, whereas decreased blood levels of these target hormones act upon the hypothalamus. Thus, enhanced release of ACTH and TSH by the pituitary is secondary to excitation of hypothalamic neurones, such excitation resulting in the formation of the appropriate neurohumour. In the case of the gonadotrophins it seems to be generally agreed that the target hormones (oestrogens, androgens) act solely upon the hypothalamus, which is thus sensitive to both increased and decreased blood levels. It seems reasonable to suppose that this is due, at least in cyclic species, to the important role of the target glands themselves. Whereas the thyroid and adrenal cortex change their basal activities mainly in response to external events and over short periods, gonadal (or at least ovarian) activity fluctuates in response to internal changes and over a fair amount of time. In other words, gonadal feedback is not so much a matter of quick responses and quick return to an equilibrium as a matter of slow routine, continuous rhythms.

A special case of gonadal feedback upon the brain involves the prepubertal animal and trespasses into the field of behaviour. It was shown many years ago that (a) male pituitary tissue implanted into the sella turcica of hypophysectomized females will support sexual cycles, and (b) pituitaries from newborn animals transplanted similarly would also maintain sexual cycles. Thus it was apparent that neither endocrine gender nor endocrine maturity is determined by the kind of pituitary tissue that an organism possesses; it seemed that the hypothalamus must control such matters. The assumption became fact when it was shown that a single injection of a small amount (5 μg) of testosterone into newborn rats permanently prevented the appearance of ovarian cycles or oestrous behavioural periods. If such treatment were delayed beyond about 5 days from birth, no effect was observed (Barraclough, 1961). The inference is that at birth in the rat the hypothalamus is sexually undifferentiated. In the untreated animal differentiation becomes complete at about 5 days from birth and the creature is henceforth endocrinologically female. If during these 5 days the hypothalamus is exposed to testosterone, differentiation of this kind does not proceed and the creature shows only anatomically female characters; it does not exhibit cyclic ovulation, has constant vaginal cornification and lacks all forms of sexual behaviour. From some points of view it does not seem appropriate to consider that such animals have been converted to males, for males do not have a virtual absence of LH and they do exhibit sexual behaviour. However, these ideas must be viewed in relation to results obtained on male animals. Harris (1964) has found that if male rats are castrated on the day of birth they show cyclic activity (in revolving drums) and cyclic cellular changes in abdominal vaginal transplants. Thus it seems as though the undifferentiated hypothalamus of these animals has been protected from the influence of testosterone and has proceeded to differentiate into the female pattern. There is a possibility that these phenomena may be limited to cyclic species, that the neonatal hormonal influences act not so much upon endocrinological gender but upon a neural timing mechanism. Neonatal hormone treatment of non-cyclic species (rabbit) does not have the effects described above (Campbell, 1964b), although it is also possible that the hypothalamus of the newborn rabbit has already become differentiated.

Excitability Effects

These have been demonstrated for all of the target gland hormones. This should not be in itself surprising, for since it is known that hormones affect the brain it is to be expected that the effects will be produced by variations in cellular excitation. What, perhaps, is surprising is that so many parts of the brain are so affected, including the cerebral cortex. There is general agreement that *thyroid hormones* affect brain activity with regard to both electroshock threshold and EEG. This is seen in the clinical states of hypothyroidism (myxoedema) and hyperthyroidism (thyrotoxicosis) and also in the experimental animal under conditions of thyroidectomy or thyroxine administration. No doubt exists that all of the effects, or most of them, do not originate from contingent changes in metabolic rate, for substances that raise this rate do not have the recorded neurological effects. These include a great depression of brain excitability in conditions of thyroid deficiency correlated with mental disturbance (myxoedema madness) and considerable increase in frequency and amplitude of brain activity in thyrotoxicosis, accompanied in severe cases by gross neurological dysfunction such as coma, bulbar palsies and athetosis. By and large it has been found that appropriate treatment returns both the electrical signs and the neurological responses to normal. An interesting and important aspect of thyroid–brain relationships is the effect of excess or deficiency of these hormones upon the newborn brain. It is well known that congenital hypothyroidism is accompanied by sluggish or absent intelligence and sluggish or absent α-rhythm (Fig. 50). Eayrs and his colleagues (see Eayrs, 1960) have examined the cortical histology of rats thyroidectomized or treated with thyroxine *in utero* and found marked abnormalities in both conditions. It was also found that if treatment were delayed until some days after birth, the abnormalities did not arise. Such observations provide a neurological basis for the necessity of early treatment of cretins, in whom the EEG is found to return to normal, in many cases with attainment of normal intelligence.

In the early days of rather promiscuous treatment with *adrenocortical hormones* and ACTH for manifold conditions, many conflicting reports were published. Some workers found these agents to have anticonvulsant properties, to raise the electroshock threshold and to depress the EEG. Other investigators reported lowering of electroshock threshold, excitation of the EEG and epileptiform convulsions sometimes terminating fatally. The present view seems to be that adrenal cortical hormones do not (as the thyroid apparently *does*) have a tonic effect upon brain excitability, but come into action when some other factor has induced a change in excitability. Under these conditions it is proposed that adrenocortical principles serve to return brain excitability to normal, to which end they either increase it or decrease it. There is some evidence that they exert their effects by acting upon sodium and calcium interchanges between cells and extracellular fluid. There is also evidence that they act not only upon the cerebral cortex but also upon the thalamus, limbic system and reticular formation. Clinically, disturbances of the EEG are seen also in hypercorticism and in adrenal insufficiency.

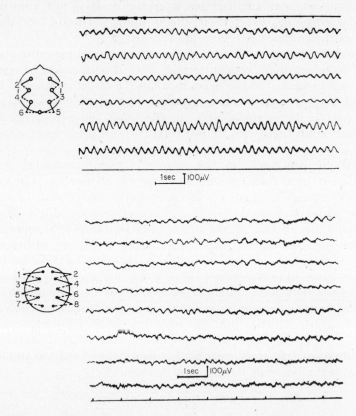

FIG. 50. Effect of deficiency of thyroid hormone on the human EEG. Upper-records taken at age 5 months. A regular, synchronous and symmetrical 4–4½ c/s θ-rhythm. Lower records taken after 4 months' treatment with thyroid hormone, 0·5 gr daily. More irregular 5–6 c/s rhythm with some fast activity. (From Nieman, 1961.)

No serious disagreement exists about the effect of gonadal hormones upon brain excitability. Many reports make it clear that oestrogens decrease electroshock threshold (EST) whereas androgens increase it. Even in untreated animals, the female is more susceptible to electroshock convulsions than is the male and the female's EST is even further reduced in the oestrous phase of the sexual cycle. No data are available about the site of action of oestrogens, but it has been shown that progesterone and testosterone depress the electrical activity of the hippocampus, limbic system and posterior hypothalamus. In large doses testosterone increases the sensitivity of the reticular formation whereas small doses decrease it. It is not known how gonadal hormones exert their effects upon the brain but there is some evidence that oestrogens are cholinergic.

Metabolic effects such as changes in oxygen consumption, alterations in electrolyte concentrations and disturbances of enzyme action are produced in the brain by all of the target hormones. In the case of *thyroid hormones* it is generally agreed that these play very little part in brain metabolism in the adult (largely carbohydrate reactions concerned with neural activity), but are important in the immature organism when the developing brain is actively engaged in anabolic processes; in the neonatal animal thyroid hormones stimulate oxygen consumption and enzymic dynamics. *Adrenal and gonadal hormones* have not yet fallen into any clearly defined category. Earlier workers claimed that ACTH and cortisone did not affect the metabolic rate of the human brain, but Gordan (1956) reports that adrenal and gonadal steroids reduce cerebral oxygen utilization in man and suggests that under normal circumstances these hormones exert a tonic inhibitor effect upon brain metabolism. This would explain the beneficial effects of such steroids in reducing the high cerebral oxygen consumption found in hypopituitarism, prepuberal eunuchoidism in the human and after prepuberal castration in animals. There appears to be no doubt that adrenal steroids are concerned with electrolyte exchanges, especially of sodium and it may be that sexual steroids have a similar action.

THE EFFECT OF HORMONES ON BEHAVIOUR

Over the years this topic has become one of the most vast aspects of neuroendocrinology and yet one of the most tantalizingly difficult to deal with definitively. Probably because behaviour has so many components it is hard to design experiments rigidly enough to satisfy the usual criteria of belief and interpretation. Nevertheless, light is slowly coming and a few facts and general principles may be tentatively considered. One major drawback to the inclusion of many experiments is that observations have been made on animals given an excess of various hormones. Under these conditions it is not easy to disentangle pharmacological from physiological effects. We have already seen that oversecretion or underactivity of various target glands in clinical conditions is frequently accompanied by changes in behaviour, but these instances do not tell us if the hormones play a part in normal behaviour—except non-specifically in their role of guardians of the *milieu intérieur*. Indeed with regard to both thyroid and adrenal hormones it is practically impossible to assign any specific normal behavioural role to them. Perhaps this is not surprising in view of the fact that their importance in the body is simply to maintain normal resting cellular activities and to assist the return to normal after any environmentally induced change. More convincing are the behavioural functions attributed to the gonadal hormones.

Thyroid Hormones

These have been administered to or removed (thyroidectomy) from experimental animals and observations made on discriminatory responses, acquisition and retention of conditioned reflexes, maze-learning and even spontaneous activity, with no clear results. There is an undoubted correlation between absence or reduction of thyroid hormone in the immature animal and the capacity to engage in various forms of behaviour (Eayrs, 1960). But this does not imply a specific behavioural role; it is simply a consequence of the fact that thyroid hormone is necessary for the proper histological development of the cerebral cortex.

Adrenal Hormones

As mentioned above, when given in large doses adrenal hormones cause considerable behavioural aberrations but there is no evidence that these actions are not purely pharmacological. It is highly probable that, as with thyroid hormones, under normal conditions the adrenocortical hormones have no more (and no less) action on behaviour than, say, glucose or amino acids.

Gonadal Hormones

These fall into quite a different category. There is no disagreement that the feedback of gonadal hormones upon the brain plays a dominant part in sexual behaviour. We have already seen (p. 169) how androgens act upon the undifferentiated hypothalamus to determine, among other things, the type of sexual behaviour exhibited by the adult. It is also clear that in the adult cyclic female the onset of sexual receptivity is correlated with the action of oestrogen upon the brain. Ovariectomized cats fly into a rage if a male is brought within their purview, but such cats show the reverse behaviour and mate if a tiny amount of oestrogen is implanted within the posterior ventral hypothalamus. Their whole reproductive tract is atrophic and the vaginal smear is completely bereft of cornified cells, so evidently all that is required for behavioural (as opposed to endocrinological) oestrus is a proper level of gonadal hormones. In male animals the results of applying testosterone to the hypothalamus are not so clear because the male rat does not usually show anoestrous behaviour. However, injections of testosterone into various hypothalamic nuclei is reported to be followed by exaggerated and abnormally rapid components of maternal and sexual behaviour. Such findings provide a key to the neurological basis of the well-known fact that ovariectomy or castration results in deficits in sexual behaviour in many species, correctable by appropriate hormone therapy. Thus with regard to gonadal hormones there is no question that the behavioural effects are due to pharmacological mechanisms or arise simply because the animal is in a healthy endocrine state. The hormones actually modulate the specific central mechanisms of sexual behaviour. An excellent and exhaustive review of the role of hormones in mating behaviour is available (Young, 1961). A reversal of parental behaviour occurs when rabbits are treated with steroids during pregnancy (Campbell, 1964a). Data of an electrophysiological kind have been presented by Sawyer and Kawakami (1961). These authors detected a change in the EEG of the female rabbit after coitus, coincident with behavioural depression and the same changes could be induced by administration of LH. FSH did not have this neural effect. Since it is known that coitus in the rabbit stimulates the release of LH but not of FSH, it seems highly likely that the rabbit's postcoital behavioural reaction is actually caused by the LH released during coitus. Hence the neuroendocrine sequence associated with coitus in the rabbit would appear to be (a) coitus activates neural elements which release neurohumour into the portal vessels; (b) the neurohumour stimulates the secretion of LH from the anterior pituitary; (c) this hormone causes ovulation and at the same time depresses the brain's activity, bringing the formation of neurohumour to a stop and inducing quiescent behaviour. The after-reaction can be induced by electrical stimulation of the hypothalamus and rhinencephalon. When this is done after treatment with one of the 19-nor steroids (oral contraceptives) it is found that the threshold has risen enormously (Fig. 51). After such treatment the animals will copulate but not ovulate, suggesting that the neural thresholds concerned with oestrous behaviour are unaffected by the progestogen, whereas the thresholds for endocrine activity were raised beyond effective limits. The same elevated after-reaction threshold, sexual areceptivity and pituitary inhibition is produced by progesterone. This seems to offer

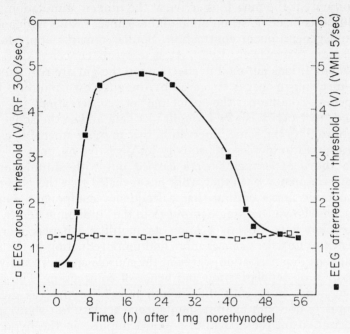

FIG. 51. Differential effect of norethynodrel (17α-ethinyl-5(10)-estraenolone) on the EEG after-reaction and EEG arousal thresholds in the rabbit. (From Sawyer and Kawakami, 1961.)

an explanation for the anoestrous behaviour and gonadotrophic depression that occurs during pregnancy, while the corpus luteum maintains high blood levels of progesterone.

Supplement on Visceral Functions

Autonomic Mechanisms

Phenomena at Nerve Endings

In the preceding section practically all that was said about what happens at autonomic nerve endings was that sympathetic fibres release adrenaline and parasympathetic fibres release acetylcholine. The matter is not as simple as this. The effect produced on smooth muscle by excitation of an autonomic nerve is not invariably the same but frequently depends upon the state of the muscles. Stimulation of sympathetic fibres in the splanchnic nerve causes hyperpolarization of intestinal muscle with consequent inhibition of contraction only if the muscle is active at the time of stimulation. When the muscle is inactive, stimulation of these fibres results in depolarization and generation of contraction. Similar remarks apply to vagal stimulation (van Harn, 1963). It is easy to conceive that under normal conditions autonomic effects upon the gut are regulated by a servo-mechanism that is triggered by the gut's own motility. Under emergency conditions the principle of conservation of energy demands that peristalsis be brought to a halt, and so the active gut is immobilized by the same innervation that in more amenable circumstances serves to increase its activity for digestive purposes.

The above experiments were carried out with stimulation at a constant frequency but other work has revealed that the phenomena at autonomic nerve endings has a frequency component. Gillespie (1961), has shown that single impulses in the autonomic nerves to the rabbit colon have no effect upon its motility, whereas increasing frequency of impulses causes more and more reduction in the rate of spontaneous depolarization waves in the muscle and eventually leads to cessation of depolarization and hence of contraction. The reverse phenomenon occurs with the smooth muscle of the vas deferens. This muscle does not exhibit spontaneous activity but shows partial depolarization on the arrival of a single impulse in the hypogastric nerve; successive impulses produce a summation of depolarization and at 40 mV the muscle contracts. Burnstock and Holman (1963) have reviewed the data concerning the mechanism of transmission at autonomic junctions with smooth muscle and conclude that it is essentially similar to the mechanism at the junction of somatic nerve and voluntary muscle (see p. 14). One of Cannon's many contributions to autonomic physiology was his finding that for a variety of organs maximal sympathetic effect was obtained with frequencies of stimulation from 15 to 25/sec and maximal parasympathetic effects at frequencies of 25–35/sec. An extensive review of autonomic neuro-effector transmission has been provided by von Euler (1959).

Phenomena in the Ganglia

One remarkable property of autonomic ganglia is that they show fatigue under conditions of repetitive stimulation. When preganglionic nerves are continually stimulated the response of the effector organ gradually declines and this can be shown to result from a progressive decrease in action potentials in the postganglionic nerve as more and more ganglion cells become fatigued beyond the point of acting as impulse generators (Larrabee and Bronk, 1952).

In the previous section it was stated that by definition the autonomic nervous system is entirely efferent. The rationale for this definition is the belief that afferent fibres subserving autonomic reflexes are the same ones as those subserving somatic reflexes. This view seems to be true for higher regions but may have to be modified for some of the outlying ganglia. Despite several claims to the contrary, most authorities are now agreed that no sensory fibres enter the paravertebral ganglia. The position is not so clear with regard to such ganglia as the mesenteric and coeliac. Several pieces of evidence, both anatomical and functional, indicate that some intestinal reflexes are mediated entirely within the autonomic system. Destruction of preganglionic fibres leaves some synapses intact in these ganglia and gastrointestinal reflexes remain operative. Moreover when the postganglionic nerves from these ganglia are cut, some fibres remain undegenerated, indicating that the cell bodies are in the gut wall (Kuntz, 1953). The presence of receptors in the gut wall has been demonstrated by Iggo (1955), who reports that their axons travel in the vagus nerve. Further, when the central stump of a cut hypogastric nerve is stimulated, orthodromic impulses are initiated in intact autonomic nerves on the same and opposite sides; study of degeneration in the distal part of the nerve indicated that the cell bodies of the afferent fibres must be in the inferior mesenteric ganglion (Job and Lundberg, 1952). Hence the overall picture is that receptors in the gut send axons directly to autonomic ganglia, there synapsing with cells that supply the region near the receptor and also with cells whose axons pass to unknown higher regions. Incidentally, doubt has been raised that the intrinsic nerve plexuses of the gut are essential for intestinal motility. Pieces of isolated jejunum from which the plexuses had been removed, still exhibited rhythmic contractions in response to distention (Evans and Schild, 1953), suggesting that the smooth muscle of the gut, like cardiac muscle, may have an inherent capacity for periodic contraction.

Neurosurgeons have for some time been unhappy about the results of various operations for partial sympathectomy inasmuch as the results have seldom come up to expectation. Following the textbook descriptions of autonomic anatomy, competent neurosurgeons have carried out their operations in the hopes of complete sympathetic denervation of a part of the body, only to find postoperatively that the sympathectomy has been effectively incomplete. A clue, and possibly a full explanation of this anomaly, comes from the careful anatomical work of Boyd, which he has reviewed (1957). This work pertains to what have come to be called (in Boyd's view, "unfortunately") inter-mediate sympathetic ganglia (Fig. 52). These appear to occur in a

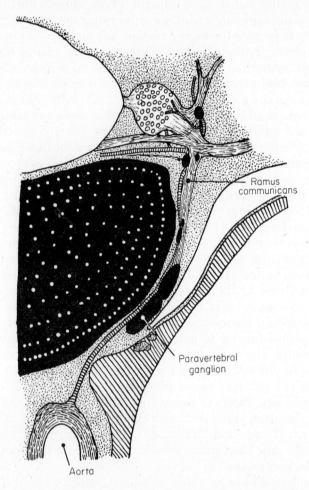

Ramus communicans

Paravertebral ganglion

Aorta

FIG. 52. Camera lucida drawing of a section through the second lumbar vertebra in a 100 mm crown-rump length human foetus. Six "intermediate ganglia" are shown in relation to the lumbar nerve and to a ramus communicans. The largest of the interme-diate ganglia is almost confluent with the paravertebral sympathetic ganglion. (From Boyd, 1957.)

scattered and random fashion in the region of the paravertebral ganglia and ramus communicans. Boyd points out that intimations of the existence of intermediate sympathetic ganglia have appeared in the literature since 1845, but no one hitherto took them very seriously. In general terms these "extra" ganglia occur in the cervical and upper thoracic segments and in the lumbar and lower thoracic segments. The midthoracic and sacral regions have few or no intermediate ganglia. The pre- and postganglionic connexions of these ganglia are still obscure, but nonetheless they should be borne in mind by anyone who is in any way associated with human autonomic surgery.

PHENOMENA IN THE SPINAL CORD

The impression may have been given in the earlier part of this section (although safeguards were stated, too) that the sympathetic system acts in a widespread and diffuse manner. It is better to think this than to believe it behaves as discretely as the parasympathetic system. Nevertheless, a truer idea of sympathetic function involves the understanding that under some conditions the sympathetic system can have localized actions. After all, it seems sensible that a mechanism which is in its entirety of great use during emergency conditions should have some of its components available for non-emergency use. Such localized actions are well seen in some of the experimentally elicitable spinal autonomic reflexes. By stimulating particular regions of the spinal cord, quite limited sympathetic effects can be produced. For example, stimulation of the fourth thoracic segment results (autonomically) only in a rise in arterial blood pressure. When the stimulation is taken a little higher, to T1 to T3, the blood pressure effect does not occur, but pupillary dilatation is produced. Many of these localized spinal effects can still be elicited after section of the spinal cord and thus seem to be complete in themselves but can be modulated by higher regions and integrated thereby into the total response.

It would be a mistake to look upon the autonomic system as something isolated from the somatic nervous system. Not only do higher regions control both of these systems at the same time, but they also interact at lower levels. Stimulation of the splanchnic nerve gives rise to impulses in all somatic nerves to the body wall, from T3 to L3 (Downman, 1955) on both sides of the body. No doubt these viscerosomatic interactions account for such responses as contraction of abdominal wall muscles when abdominal viscera are stimulated.

Autonomic Cortex

Cortical influences upon visceral phenomena have been reviewed in the earlier part of this section and there it was pointed out that many of these influences are thought to be mediated via cortico-hypothalamic connexions. There is little doubt that at least some visceral changes evoked by manipulation of the cortex do not involve the hypothalamus. Stimulation of the medullary pyramids has been shown to cause cardiovascular changes, sweating, pupillary changes and contraction of gut and bladder (Landau, 1953). Since the fibres in the pyramids have originated in the cerebral cortex it seems clear that the latter structure is able to activate autonomic effectors independently of the hypothalamus.

Cerebellum

There is considerable evidence that the cerebellum exerts its effects via the hypothalamus. In a primary sense, stimulation of the cerebellum resulted in changes of cardiovascular and respiratory activity. Involvement of the hypothalamus is suggested by the results obtained when the cerebellum was stimulated during attacks of hypothalamus-induced sham rage (see p. 268). There was immediate inhibition of both behavioural and visceral phenomena, which returned when cerebellar stimulation was stopped. It is likely that the cerebellum is not restricted to any one division of the autonomic system, for both sympathetic and parasympathetic effects on the pupil have been produced.

NEUROENDOCRINE MECHANISMS

Neural Control of the Glands

The role of the hypothalamus in endocrine phenomena has been described in some detail in the earlier part of this section. Some attention could now be given to non-hypothalamic structures. Important though the hypothalamus undoubtedly is, it must not be looked upon as a primary region for control of the endocrines. The available evidence shows that the anterior pituitary gland is able to function reasonably well under resting conditions, except for gonadal function in cyclic animals. But it would be short-sighted to believe that the hypothalamus is solely in charge of the cyclic mechanism or of the other endocrine responses to environmental change. The reasonable view is that external changes impinge upon the hypo-thalamo-hypophysial equipment via the mediation of higher brain regions. Studies in this field are very sparse and no firm conclusions can as yet be drawn. Speculation, however, can be valuable if guided by rational principles rather than by sheer intuition and various workers have postulated extrahypothalamic regions as being involved in glandular physiology and have carried out experiments to support their ideas. The limbic system has been a favourite collection of structures because of its connexions with both higher and lower structures. Septal regions, amygdaloid nuclei, hippocampus and fornix have been implicated, by stimulation or by lesions, in the release of ACTH (Endroczi *et al.*, 1959). With regard to TSH release, the fornix and habenula nuclei are said to be involved (Szentagothai and Mess, 1958). Olfactory bulb, amygdaloid nuclei and septum appear to be in some way related to secretion of gonadotrophic hormones, possibly by way of the mammillary bodies (Sawyer, 1960). It would seem likely that various parts of the limbic system exert specific effects upon separate endocrine mechanisms. Yet it is well known that some pituitary responses are non-specific, especially those related to emotional stress. A likely candidate for the mediation of such responses is the reticular formation which, though it may show some degree of specificity, is undoubtedly largely a non-specific region. Since the reticular formation is acted upon by all of the senses, since it receives information from the cortex and since it relays to the hypothalamus, it would be strange indeed if this large collection of midline neurones had no part to play in endocrine phenomena. Considerable attention is being paid to the reticular formation currently and it is said to have a role in ACTH secretion (Moll, 1959; Slusher and Hyde, 1961; Giuliani *et al.*, 1961) and gonadotrophin secretion (Critchlow, 1958). So far it has not been shown to be related to the release of TSH, which may be because this trophic hormone is secreted at a lower, not higher, rate during stress. It is rather disappointing that the available evidence to date suggests that the neocortex has very little if any role to play in neuroendocrine responses that accompany emotional stresses.

Glandular Control of the Brain

Possibly the most exciting future studies in this field will be concerned with work designed to determine the fundamental nervous changes that occur when hormones act upon the brain to produce behavioural alterations. There is ample evidence that most of the hormones have the capacity to alter brain excitability but this is a rather indirect and non-specific characteristic. More valuable is the knowledge that is accumulating with regard to the production of actual changes in nerve cells, especially during the brain's developmental period. The capacity of adaptive behaviour in adult life is severely impaired by thyroidectomy at birth (Eayrs and Lishman, 1955) and this seems to be related to the marked effects upon neuronal organization of this experimental intervention. The size of cerebral cortical cell bodies, of their dendritic processes and of the associated neuropil are clearly and measurably altered by an absence or an excess of thyroid hormone during gestation in the rat (Eayrs, 1965). The physico-chemical mechanism is thought to be related to the nerve cell's power to synthesize protein at a critical stage of development. In the absence of such protein anabolism the cells are permanently deficient in their capacity to engage in synaptic connexions. This, of course, raises cogitations about the minimum amount of thyroid hormone necessary during immaturity for normal adaptive behaviour in the adult. The extreme of cretinism is familiar enough both in incidence and in aetiology; but one may wonder how many cases of maladaptability may be due to a lesser and unrecognized deficiency of thyroid hormone during development.

Part V

Higher Functions

CHAPTER 11

CORTICAL ORGANIZATION

The cerebral cortex is the latest development in the central nervous system. It becomes progressively more extensive throughout the mammalian order until in man, it is said, the area of cerebral cortex is approximately 2 yd². Forty per cent. of this is frontal lobe, 21% temporal lobe and 17% occipital lobe. Although a consideration of the cerebral cortex is necessary in conjunction with the study of several different higher nervous functions, it is convenient in this section to focus attention in a general way upon this structure alone.

Histology

Unlike the cerebellar cortex, the cerebral cortex has a variable histological appearance. An expert neurologist, given a section of a small part of the cerebral cortex can make a reliable estimate of its region of origin. Not only the cell disposition, but also the thickness varies. In the region of the anterior central gyrus it is about 4 mm thick, whereas at the occipital poles the thickness is reduced to about 1·25 mm. The average thickness is 2·5 mm. However, detailed examination would be out of place at this juncture. Instead a more generalised account will be given with emphasis on functional pattern rather than anatomical appearance. An excellent detailed account is given by Cajal (1955).

Classically, there are six alternating layers of cell bodies and cell fibres. Actually, cell bodies *and* fibres occur in all layers, but the various types of cells tend to become arranged in a fairly definite stratified pattern. Afferent fibres are of three kinds.

1. Fibres from the lower regions enter the cortex and ascend to layer IV (Fig. 53, W). These fibres are activated by weak or brief stimuli. In layer IV they branch and synapse with several *granular* cells (hence this layer is called the internal granular layer). Axons from the granule cells descend to layer V where they synapse with the bodies of large *pyramidal* cells (hence, large pyramidal cell layer or ganglion layer). Axons from the pyramidal cells descend to sub-cortical regions and also to other parts of the cortex.

G
185

2. With stronger or more persistent stimuli, fibres are activated which ascend to layers II and III (Fig. 53, S). In layer II, synapses occur with small *granular* cells (hence, external granular layer). In layer III, the afferent fibres connect with small pyramidal cells (hence, small pyramidal cell layer). Axons from the granular cells of layer II and from the pyramidal cells of layer III descend to layer V and synapse with large pyramidal cells there. Again, these pyramidal cells send axons to subcortical regions and to other parts of the cortex.

3. Recurrent collaterals from the granular cells in layer IV ascend to layers II and III and synapse with the granular and pyramidal cells in those layers (Fig. 53, C). Thus, weak or brief stimuli, while effecting the discharge of layer IV granular cells (which in turn cause the discharge of layer V pyramidals) also sensitize the cells in layers II and III. This increased central excitatory state represents the concept that the higher cells are already "aware" of what is happening elsewhere when and if stimuli arrive through their own afferents.

That a single afferent fibre synapses with several efferent cells makes plain the fact that it is possible and probable that numerically the output from the cortex is greater than the input. Certainly, the information arriving in any single fibre is spread over an area of cortex, even if not all the cells in that area discharge.

Dendrites from the cell bodies in layers II, III, IV and V ascend in layer I (Fig. 53, D). Afferent fibres from other parts of the cerebral cortex ("association" and commissural fibres) also ascend to layer I and synapse with the dendrites of the lower-lying cells. The inter-meshing of axons and dendrites gives an overall net-like appearance, hence the name plexiform layer. It is likely that wherever an axon and a dendrite cross in proximity there is a potential synapse.

Layer I therefore serves to sensitize the efferent components of a particular region according to information received from distant parts of the cortex. The output from the pyramidal cells of layer V is not simply a result of specific information arriving in the afferents to layers II, III and IV, but is the result of these impulses arriving in a neuronal network *already in a certain pattern of excitation* as a consequence of events in remote parts of the cortex. Thus it is in layer I that the highest level of cerebral integration occurs.

A few other histological elements remain to be dealt with. Fusiform cells occur in layer VI (spindle cell layer or multiform layer) with

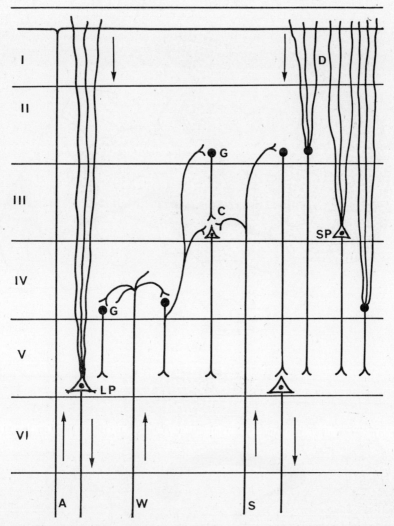

Fig. 53. Diagrammatic representation of the histology of the cerebral cortex. Weak stimuli enter by fibres (W) that ascend to layer IV and synapse with granular cells in that layer. Stronger stimuli enter by fibres (S) that reach layers II and III, synapsing with small pyramidal cells (SP) and granular cells (G) in the respective layers. The granular cells of layer IV synapse with the large pyramidal cells found in layer V (LP). They also send collaterals to the cells in layers II and III, so that weak stimuli are able to raise the central excitatory state of the small pyramidal cells. Dendrites from the pyramidal cells and from the granular cells of layer II ascend to layer I (D). In this outermost layer the excitatory state of the local cells is raised by impulses arriving from distant parts of the cortex over association fibres (A). Transmission of information occurs between the horizontal axons of the association fibres and the vertical dendrites of the local cells. The net effect of threshold stimulation is the discharge of effector impulses along the axons of the pyramidal cells.

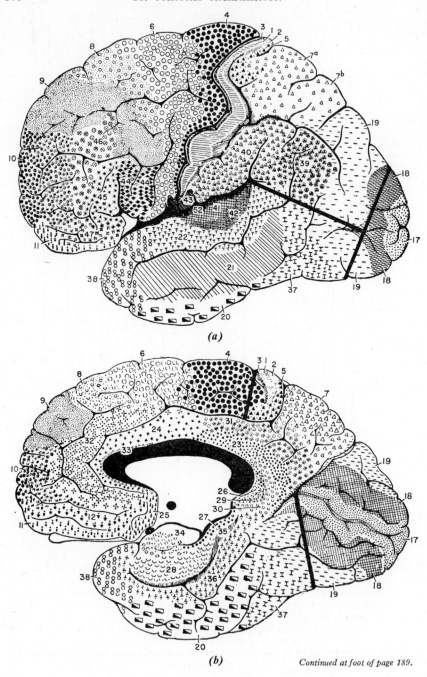

(a)

(b)

Continued at foot of page 189.

axons that run towards the periphery; their function is unknown.
Two cell types are found which are not limited to any one layer.
There are the "short axon cells", whose axons remain in the same
layer as the cell body; they serve to raise the central excitatory state
of neighbouring cells and hence effect *horizontal* spread of information. Secondly, there are the "cells of Martinotti". These are
distinguished by having axons which travel centrally to synapse with
cell bodies in higher layers. Their dendrites are activated by recurrent collaterals from pyramidal cells. They provide a mechanism for
reverberating circuits, i.e. they serve to continue the sensitization
after the stimulus has ceased. Differences of cytoarchitectonics have
caused the cortex to be divided into many numbered areas (Fig. 54).

METHODS OF MAPPING THE CEREBRAL CORTEX

Although the idea of specific areas of cortex is very old—Aristotle
had, of course, made statements about it—yet until 1870 scientists, as
opposed to philosophers and suchlike, believed that the cortex
functioned as a whole, as a homogeneous structure. It was in 1870
that Fritsch and Hitzig showed that electrical stimulation of the
precentral gyrus caused movements of the opposite limbs. In some
ways this was unfortunate because, although it raised the concept of
localized action, it also generated the idea, which became more and
more entrenched, that each little bit of cortex did its own job, all
alone. Modern evidence shows less and less dependence upon small
areas for specific functions. A new concept of cortical function is
arising in which *levels* of activity are more important than areas. It
would not be too great an exaggeration to say that all or at least many
parts of the cortex are involved in all functions, but some parts come
into particular circuits at different stages and with different levels of
dominance. There is not yet enough evidence available to make such
a generalization certain. Nevertheless, fewer confusions will result

Continued from previous page.

FIG. 54. The lobes of the cerebral hemispheres. A, Lateral view. The central fissure,
lying between areas 3 and 4, separates the frontal from the parietal lobe. Other lines of
demarcation are drawn rather arbitrarily except for the points of origin at the occipital
notch and where the lateral fissure meets the supramarginal gyrus. B, Medial surface.
The occipital lobe is separated from the parietal lobe by the parieto-occipital fissure, and
from the temporal lobe by the arbitrary line drawn from the occipital notch to the rostral
end of the calcarine fissure. Parietal and frontal lobes are separated by the arbitrary line
drawn from the central fissure to the cingulate sulcus. Cingulate gyrus is considered to
be part of the "limbic lobe". The dividing lines are superimposed upon the cytoarchitectonic maps of Brodman.

if this idea is held tentatively in view when considering any cortical function in a scientific manner. Historically, however, it is important to know of the methods that have been used for mapping the cortex (Table III).

TABLE III

Methods of Mapping the Cerebral Cortex

1. Histological

(a) Cytoarchitectonic
(b) Post-traumatic degeneration

2. Destruction

(a) Surgical
(b) Electrical
(c) Chemical

3. Stimulation

(a) Electrical (suitable in conscious human)
(b) Chemical

4. Recording

(suitable in conscious human)

(a) "Spontaneous"
(b) Central stimulation effects
(c) Peripheral stimulation effects

1. *Histological*. Fritsch and Hitzig's discovery led a number of histologists to apply aniline dyes to the cerebral cortex, after they had been rejected as useless for other parts of the nervous system, and the result was the beautifully selective cell staining that is so familiar to us today. It was found that some areas of cortex, while of uniform structure, were different in cellular architecture from other regions. The efforts of these workers have led to the cytoarchitectonic maps (Fig. 54) which do not carry in themselves the answers to problems of brain function. But they were not useless, for degeneration studies (e.g. using the Marchi method) based upon them gave the earliest clues to cortical connexions with other structures and so paved the way for functional experiments.

2. *Destruction* of cortical regions began with plain *surgical* techniques. Various parts of the cerebral cortex were removed and observations made on functional deficits. Though gross destruction

was the rule, much useful information accrued from such work. Some information on the human cortex came from accidental injury to various regions. Much more discrete mapping of the cortex has become possible with the introduction of *electrolytic* means of destruction. It is now possible to destroy a very few cells or fibres and so assess much more finely the contributions to function of small regions. Destruction, often temporary (and therefore repeatable in the same animal), by *chemical* agents in the form of local or general anaesthetics, has also helped to map the functional areas of the cortex.

3. *Stimulation* has been employed from the days of Fritsch and Hitzig, at first rather crudely with considerable spread of stimulus, and then with finer electrodes until now it is possible to stimulate a single nerve cell body or nerve fibre. The detailed studies of Woolsey's group on localization in the motor areas illustrate the possibilities of the method. *Electrical* stimulation in the conscious patient undergoing brain surgery has provided most of the experimental information obtained about the human cerebral cortex. *Chemical* stimulation, usually with strychnine and its derivatives, has been employed to good effect, especially in the studies on inhibitory areas. Although only applicable to the surface of the cortex, this method is easy to carry out, fairly localized in action and temporary in effect.

4. *Recording* the electrical activity in various parts of the cortex is the most recently introduced method. The early gross recordings obtained by EEG instruments were found to be unsuitable for scientific studies because the apparatus was shown to be affected by activity in subcortical structures. Once again, techniques and materials have been refined to the point where records may be taken from a single nerve cell body or nerve fibre. Three main lines of investigation are followed with the recording technique. *"Spontaneous"* electrical activity involves recording the activity of various regions without experimental intervention, i.e. under normal, but controlled living conditions. *Central stimulation* is applied to the cortex or to subcortical regions, and any consequent activity recorded from other regions of cortex. Connexions to regions of known function have thus been established. *Peripheral stimuli* are given and records made of consequent cortical activity. In this way, cortical regions involved in the various sensory modalities have been mapped.

Association Areas and Fibres

Association involves the phenomenon of information or instructions being carried from one part of the cortex to another or to others, without the intervention of subcortical regions. The term arose before it was known how very widespread is the cortical radiation to lower regions and how widespread is the radiation from lower regions to the cortex. Many observations that were thought to exhibit this type of association have subsequently been found to include a subcortical relay. Thus the term "association area" does not have a very precise meaning. Another and perhaps more useful orientation is to look upon association areas as places where more than one type of information (say auditory together with visual) meet and are integrated to produce an appropriate response (say, head and eye movements towards or away from something heard and seen).

ASSOCIATION FIBRES

On the other hand, association fibres are well known and easily demonstrable, often to the naked eye, by gross dissection. They may be defined as fibres that begin and end in the cortex. But this does not mean that the regions of cortex in which they begin or end are necessarily association areas in the sense that they communicate only with other parts of the cortex. An arcuate association fibre (running to layer I) may have its cell body in the somatic sensory gyrus and its termination in the primary motor gyrus. Neither of these gyri are traditionally considered as exclusively association areas. Fibres that fall into this category may be classified as follows.

1. *Short fibres*. (a) Intracortical. The horizontal part of these fibres lies deep in the cortex; they unite fairly widely spaced gyri. (b) Subcortical. The horizontal part lies superficially; they unite adjacent gyri, e.g. the arcuate fibres just mentioned, running between sensory and motor gyri.

2. *Long fibres* (Fig. 55). These form fairly thick bundles and run deep in the cortical white matter. (a) Uncinate. Linking the orbital gyri of the frontal lobe with the rostral part of the temporal lobe. (b) Inferior occipitofrontal. Between the lobes named and occurring close by the lentiform nucleus. (c) Superior occipitofrontal. Similar to previous bundle but lying close to the caudate nucleus. (c) Cingulum. Short fibres making up a long bundle which unites various parts of the cingulate gyrus with the hippocampal gyrus. It lies between the

cingulate gyrus and the corpus callosum. (e) Superior longitudinal fasciculus. This bundle, although running from front to back, tends to connect the more lateral parts of the cortex. (f) Commissural fibres: (i) Corpus callosum connecting the neopallium of one side

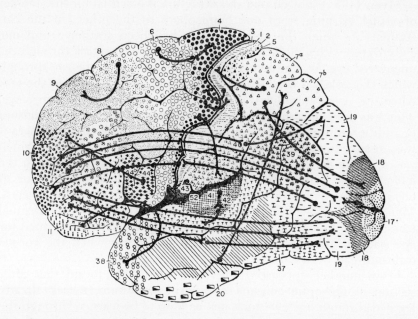

Fig. 55. Connexions of some long association pathways, projected onto the lateral surface of the cerebral hemisphere. They lie deep in the white matter of the cortex and may well be at least partly composed of short chain fibres that unite intermediate regions.

with the neopallium of the other, *not* in equal degrees throughout its length. (ii) Anterior commissure. This has two limbs, the anterior of which connects the olfactory bulbs together; the posterior limb unites the middle temporal gyri. (iii) Hippocampal commissure, connects various parts of the rhinencephalon.

Function of Association Fibres

Because of their deep-seated locations, most collections of association fibres do not lend themselves to direct experimentation. The corpus callosum, however, is more accessible and some information is available about its function. In man the corpus callosum has been completely sectioned without any obvious deficit, subjective or objective; patients have been able to type, tap-dance and play the piano under these conditions. In lower forms, more subtle tests have demonstrated an interhemispheric transfer function for the corpus callosum.

Myers (1955) showed that this structure is essential for the transfer of visual learning from one hemisphere to the other, in the cat. Animals in which the optic chiasma had been sectioned and one eye covered with a blinker were able to learn a visual task through the uncovered eye. When the blinker was transferred to the eye through which the task had been learned, the animal still performed the task when the visual stimulus was presented to the hitherto covered eye. This was not the case after complete section of the corpus callosum in addition to section of the optic chiasma. In these circumstances it was possible to condition through say, the right eye, a response which was opposite and incompatible with a response learned through the left eye. The animal would then respond to the same stimulus in one of two opposing ways, depending upon which eye was uncovered. Myers and Henson (1960) made similar studies in monkeys on manual tasks, and in much the same way it was found that a task learned for one hand could not be transferred to the other when the corpus callosum had been cut.

From another approach, Sperry et al. (1956) found that after section of the optic chiasma and corpus callosum, a task already learned through one eye, took just as long to be learned through the other eye as if the animal had never before been presented with the experimental situation. It was further found that effective transfer from hemisphere to hemisphere would occur if even a few millimetres of any part of the posterior half of the corpus callosum were left intact.

Whether it is reasonable to believe that somewhat similar functions are carried out by the other association bundles, is still a matter of opinion. However, it does seem that experiments involving lesions of these deeply lying bundles must be designed to detect rather subtle changes, since the corpus callosum-sectioned animal appears perfectly normal to casual observation and to routine neurological tests. It is highly likely that interhemispheric connexions are much more numerous than is indicated by the visible bundles, and also that many such connexions are not isotopic, i.e. not running between analogous points in each hemisphere. Lesions in the occipital lobe result in degeneration pathways to several parts of the opposite hemisphere, not just of the opposite occipital cortex (Fig. 56).

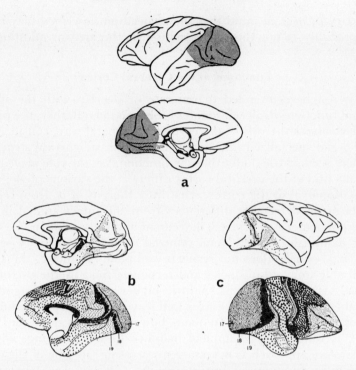

Fig. 56. Commissural connexions between the occipital lobes. (a) Lateral and medial views of the monkey's brain to show the extent of cortical ablation. (b) Medial view of the sites at which degeneration was found on the side opposite the ablation (top) and the corresponding cytoarchitectonic areas according to Brodmann (bottom) (c) Lateral view showing degeneration found on the side opposite ablation, together with the corresponding cytoarchitectonic areas. (From Myers, 1962.)

Association Areas

It is likely that association areas do not exist, in the sense of projection solely to another part of the cortex. If the definition is made non-exclusive, so that association areas become those which connect directly with other parts of the cortex *and*, possibly, with other structures, then it is likely that all parts of the cortex are association areas. Most probably all or many parts of the cortex project to several other parts, not necessarily with discharging impulses, but with information which changes the central excitatory state of distant regions thus "keeping them informed" of overall events. Nevertheless, in a rather vague but quite useful way, it is possible to relate some cortical regions fairly specifically with others. It is simply necessary to bear in mind that the association described may not be and probably is not the only function of the area in question (see p. 204).

Functions of the Cerebral Cortex

It is not here intended to reiterate or overlap with the specific cortical functions dealt with under other sections. Rather, the present aim is to assess the role of the cortex in a general way, considering it as an organ specialized in different form from subcortical structures.

There seems little doubt that the function (i.e. the role played in an animal's life) of the cerebral cortex differs at the various phylogenetic levels. Removal of the cortex, what little there is of it, from reptiles, results in no detectable differences from the intact animal in such crude phenomena as primary movement and sensation. In one of the lower mammals, say rat, total removal of a whole primary sensory area—e.g. visual—does not result in complete blindness; the animal is still able to avoid obstacles and recognize food by the use of sub-cortical visual mechanisms. A little higher up the scale, in say the dog, ablation of the visual cortex still leaves the ability to distinguish between light and dark. In man, however, removal of the visual cortex is followed by complete inability to see anything. Thus, a comparative approach is necessary in assessing the role of the cortex in any given function, and great care must be exercised when tentatively comparing results obtained in animals with results that might occur in man.

Further, it seems likely that at any given phylogenetic stage the cortex (as a whole and as separate regions) exhibits different levels of function, different degrees of contribution to functions. A particular area may contribute a great deal to one function, not so much to another and even less to a third function. Much of this present attitude to the cerebral cortex stems from the work of Lashley (1929), who studied the relationship between the cortex and the rate of learning and retention of learning in rats. Six main points arise from these experiments.

1. Whatever part of the cortex was removed, there was a slowing of the learning rate.

2. Removal of equal amounts of cortex produced equal degrees of slowing, irrespective of the region from which the ablation was made.

3. The contribution to the learning process made by any given area of cortex was non-specific. Removal of the *visual* cortex produced

a slowing of the rate of learning, but not by a visual mechanism. Blinded rats (eyes removed) did not exhibit retardation of learning, but a slowing occurred when their visual cortex was ablated. These findings indicate that the primary sensory areas of cortex in the rat at least, exert effects on learning that are independent of the area's specific modal function.

4. The degree of slowing of learning was proportional to the amount of cortex removed, irrespective of the region removed. Greater degrees of retardation followed the removal of greater amounts of cortex, even when the larger ablations were made up of removals from widely spaced regions. These findings led Lashley to propose his "mass action" theory of cortical function. This says, in effect, that *for some activities* the cortex functions as a whole, non-specifically and as a single organ.

5. It was found that the mass action principle applied also to specific areas as well as to the whole cortex. Rats were trained to a habit of brightness discrimination; then the visual cortex was surgically insulted. The time required to relearn the habit was proportional to the amount of visual cortex removed, independently of the place from which it was ablated. Similar results were obtained with the other modalities. Hence, each primary sensory area exerts a mass action with regard to *retention* (i.e. memory) of learned habits in that modality. It should be noted that, for example, in brightness discrimination, only the visual cortex exerted this function. Total mass action effects were not observed inasmuch as removal of other parts of the cortex did not affect retention of brightness discrimination. Here, then, is a higher level of specificity of function than with regard to maze learning.

6. With visual pattern discrimination the response was made to depend upon detailed characteristics of the stimulus. Under these conditions ablation of a small, particular part of the primary visual cortex was as effective in abolishing the response as if the whole visual cortex, or indeed the whole cerebral cortex, had been removed. Once again, we see greater localization of function than in brightness discrimination.

These latter ideas lead to a principle that is even more important than the mass action theory. It seems that *the more specialized* the activity, the more localized the function. Put in another way, the highest levels of cortical localization involve the lowest levels of function. This is seen quite clearly in the detailed maps of the highly localized sensorimotor areas—mere "perceiving" and "moving". Whereas it is not possible to point to a given area of cortex as being *the* area for "learning" or *the* area for "memory".

These observations were made in the rat and it has already been pointed out that extrapolation to other species in this matter is a dangerous procedure. Later workers have confirmed that Lashley's findings apply also to the dog and cat, but in all three species the brain has one highly pertinent difference from man, the relative lack of areas that are not concerned with primary function. The phylogenetic series shown in Fig. 57 indicates the enormous difference in

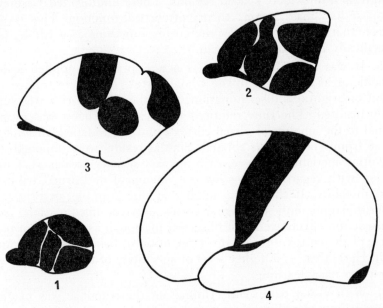

FIG. 57. Schematic representation of the relative proportion of primary cortex (black) to association cortex (AC) in various species. 1. Rat, 11% AC. 2. Rabbit, 22% AC. 3. Monkey, 64% AC. 4. Man, 86% AC.

this respect between the brain of man and that of sub-human creatures. Monkey cerebral cortex begins to approximate the human condition at least inasmuch as there are large areas that do not seem too closely tied to primary function. This makes the work of Pribram (1955) of great relevance to the present discussion.

Pribram ablated various non-primary (i.e. "association") areas of the monkey cerebral cortex and observed the changes produced on learning responses. It was found that removal of a great many regions had no effect on a variety of test situations. However, the following regions were found to be concerned.

1. Removal of the postero-infero-temporal region resulted in loss of learned visual discrimination.

2. Removal of the occipito-parietal region interfered with the learning of habits based upon somaesthetic stimuli.

3. Removal of the antero-temporal region abolished or reduced the animal's ability to learn tasks with olfactory or gustatory stimuli.

4. Removal of part of the frontal region resulted in abolition or impairment of learning delayed-response reactions, *irrespective of modality*. This seems to indicate that the role of the frontal areas is of a different order or level from the other regions inasmuch as its associations are non-specific for sense modality, and inasmuch as it is concerned with the "higher" function of time discrimination. So, as in the lower forms, it appears that in the monkey the level of localization of function decreases as the function becomes of a higher order.

At this point it is convenient to review in general terms the various subdivisions of the cerebral cortex. More detailed analysis of the role of the cerebral cortex in higher functions, especially in man, will be given in the sections immediately following. It will be seen that the most rational view of the function of the cerebral cortex is that it is not so much concerned with mere sensation and mere movement but serves to elaborate, associate and refine a variety of concurrent sensory information, so that its significance can be truly assessed with respect to past experience and used to generate precise, effective, skilled, motor responses, and to arouse ego-satisfying subjective affections.

Subdivisions of the Cerebral Cortex

The several ways of subdividing the cortex are shown in Table IV. Much of the terminology seems to be unnecessary except for those concerned with the minutiae of anatomical structure, but there is no harm in being at least aware of the applications of the terms because this sometimes avoids misunderstanding about functional divisions. For example, there is a widespread feeling that the archipallium appears at first and alone in the reptiles, that at a higher level the archipallium is joined by the palaeopallium and that at the highest

TABLE IV

Subdivisions of the Cerebral Cortex

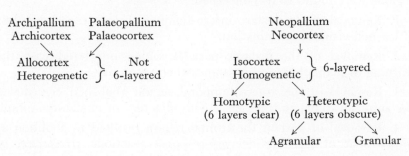

evolutionary levels a neopallium is added. This is not the case. At the earliest phylogenetic appearance of cerebral cortex in the reptile, all three types are present at once. The terminological distinction is concerned with the phylogenetic level at which the fullest development of each type occurs. Archipallium is fully evolved in forms where palaeopallium and neopallium are still rudimentary. Similarly there are animals in which both archipallium and palaeopallium have reached full development while the neocortex is primitive. The archipallium and palaeopallium ontogenetically do not pass through a stage where six cell-layers are formed (see Histology, pp. 185–189). For this reason either of the terms allocortex or heterogenetic cortex is applied to cover both of them. By and large the archipallium includes the structures that are, or were, predominantly concerned with olfactory phenomena—olfactory bulb and tract, paraolfactory area, anterior perforated substance, hippocampus and entorhinal cortex. Palaeopallium seems to be involved in the sexual sphere and is largely made up of that part of the hippocampal gyrus called the pyriform cortex. Neopallium covers the remaining major parts of the cortex; it passes through or remains in a stage where six cell-layers are formed, hence it is called isocortex. Where the six layers are still clearly defined in the adult (somatic, auditory sensory areas) the regions are said to be homotypic cortex; where adult development obscures the layering (visual, motor areas), the term heterotypic is applied. Most of this terminology is of great importance in cortical histological studies, but where function is involved the rather crude nomenclature of lobes and areas is more in keeping with the known facts, which do not allow very precise marginal lines to be drawn (Fig. 54).

FRONTAL LOBE

This comprises the neocortex that lies in front of the central sulcus. It contains the following main functional areas.

(a) Area 4, the precentral gyrus, is the main origin of the voluntary motor pathways (corticospinal tract) travelling mostly to the opposite body musculature (see p. 110).

(b) Area 4s, a strip lying anterior to area 4, is claimed to exert suppressor functions indirectly upon the motor activity generated by area 4 (see p. 118).

(c) Area 6, is quite large and occurs rostral to area 4s. It connects with areas 4 and 8 on the same side and with areas 4 and 6 on the opposite side. There are also several subcortical connexions. Its functions are not precisely understood, are definitely involved in motor phenomena and seem to be very much concerned with the functional interconnexion of parts of area 4 (e.g. forearm with upper arm) to bring widely spaced body musculature into synergism in the process of learning activities such as piano playing.

(d) Areas 44 and 45, occur in the frontal operculum. They are involved in speech mechanisms.

(e) Area 46, lying antero-dorsally to area 45 is important in the control of eye movements.

(f) Area 47 is a small region near the orbital surface. It appears to have autonomic functions inasmuch as stimulation or ablation results in defects of temperature regulation, peristalsis, respiration and blood pressure.

(g) Areas 9, 10, 11 and 12 (prefrontal cortex) have many connexions with other parts of the brain. Several association bundles occur wholly within the prefrontal cortex and others connect this region with the thalamus and the parietal, temporal and occipital lobes. It is said that the thalamo-frontal radiations (from the dorsomedial nucleus) are concerned with the affective tone that accompanies sensation. Connexions to the hypothalamus explain the experimental findings of autonomic changes following stimulation of the frontal regions. Thus the association in the prefrontal cortex of information from various parts of the cerebrum, the affective tone and the visceral phenomena, together suggest that these frontal parts of the cortex are important in the mediation of emotional behaviour (see p. 279).

PARIETAL LOBE

This term covers the regions of cortex enclosed by the central sulcus, parieto-occipital fissure and a line drawn from the centre of the latter forward to the posterior end of the lateral fissure. Its main functional areas are these:

(a) Areas 1, 2 and 3 occupy the postcentral gyrus and form the primary end station for somatosensory information. Collectively they are sometimes called somatic sensory area I. This area should not be looked upon as essential for all forms of somatic sensation; its destruction results in very great, but not complete sensory loss. The sense of vibration, for example, remains fairly well developed under these conditions. By and large, areas 1, 2 and 3 receive information from the opposite side with a little ipsilateral supply (see p. 56).

(b) Areas 5 and 7 occur in a position posterodorsal to the post-central gyrus. They are connected with the pulvinar and lateral thalamic nucleus and with several cortical areas. It seems that these regions may be looked upon as having a somatosensory recognition function, inasmuch as lesions of areas 5 and 7 result in asteriognosis, where the patient is unable to recognize objects by handling them although there is no primary sensory deficit. The posterior part of area 7 is involved in eye movements (see below).

(c) Area 19 occurs posterior to the somatosensory association area and extends downwards to the base of the brain and around onto the medial surface. It is connected with area 18 on both sides, with area 7 and with the superior colliculi. Most well known are its functions in eye movements, which are related to the visual following of moving objects.

(d) Areas 39 and 40 form the angular and supramarginal gyri. They have a great many connexions to other parts of the cerebral cortex, explaining their function as association areas. Lesions in these regions are accompanied by one or more associational deficits— agraphia, alexia and severe speech disturbances. These areas are also intimately concerned with awareness of the body and its parts. Small lesions may be accompanied by a subjective loss of one limb; larger lesions may result in hemidepersonalization (where the patient believes he has only half a body) or even complete depersonalization (in which the patient is convinced that he has no body at all).

TEMPORAL LOBE

This forms the ventrolateral part of the brain from the temporal pole back to the occipital notch and up to the line that separates it from the parietal lobe. It has the following main functional areas.

(a) Areas 41 and 42 occur on the superior temporal gyrus. They form the primary end station for auditory information. A two-way connexion occurs with the medial geniculate body and association bundles connect with other cortical regions (see p. 193). The superior temporal gyrus is not exclusively concerned with primary audition. Stimulation of its rostral end in man is accompanied by sensations referrable to the vestibular sense, such as vertigo. In addition, stimulation of the superior and lateral surfaces has produced complex hallucinations that are involved in the phenomena of consciousness (see p. 253).

(b) Area 22 lies adjacent to the primary auditory area and represents a most important association area. Lesions in area 22 produce severe defects when bilateral, but also result in disturbances when unilateral. The patients have no primary auditory defect but are partially or completely unable to understand what they hear, even when speaking themselves. Hence, area 22 is an auditory recognition region (see p. 188). Area 22, especially its superior part, also has ill-defined motor functions.

(c) Area 37 lies at the posterior end of the temporal lobe adjoining area 19. Little is known about its functions with clarity but it seems to be an area in which a predominantly visual input is associated with auditory and somatic information to form complex patterns of multi-modal interpretation.

(d) Area 38, at the rostral pole of the lobe, is inextricably bound by association fibres to nearby regions of temporal lobe, especially areas 21 and 22, and to the hippocampal gyrus, uncus and amygdaloid area. It cannot sensibly be considered in isolation from these other parts. From experimental (see Kluver–Bucy Syndrome, p. 275) and clinical (see p. 260) observations, it is clear that the temporal pole region is intimately involved in the mechanism of recent memory. That motor functions are here integrated with experiential records is indicated by the highly prevalent epileptogenic foci in the region of the temporal pole. As might be expected from its connexions with the limbic system, the amygdaloid area of the rostral pole has olfactory functions. From the observations made on patients with lesions of this region it seems to be concerned with the affective tone produced by odours.

OCCIPITAL LOBE

This is the posterior pole of the brain, lying behind a line drawn from the parieto-occipital fissure to the occipital notch on the lateral surface of the hemisphere; on the medial side, it comprises the region bounded by the parieto-occipital fissure and a line drawn from the anterior end of the calcarine fissure down to the occipital notch. An account of its major areas follows.

(a) Area 17 occurs towards the occipital pole, and in man is only just visible on the lateral surface of the brain, although it is easily discernible on this surface in lower forms such as the monkey. In man, area 17 has its greatest extension on the medial surface, where it runs above and below the calcarine fissure. It is the primary end station for visual information (see p. 75).

(b) Area 18 is situated just rostral to area 17 on the lateral surface and has a medial prolongation superior and inferior to the medial disposition of area 17. It is sometimes called the parastriate area because it is beside the area that contains the stripe of Gennari (striate area, area 17). It has intimate connexions with areas 17 and 19 on the same and opposite sides, and has long associative connexions with various parts of the frontal, parietal and temporal lobes. Subcortical connexions occur between area 18 and the tectal and mesencephalic regions. The latter connexions explain the production of eye movements on stimulation of area 18. However, it would seem that the most important function of area 18 is visual recognition. Patients with extensive lesions in this part of the brain are not able to name or state the significance of things that they quite obviously can see (visual agnosia). Stimulation or irritative lesions in the human result in rather formless visual hallucinations, although rather more definitive visions are seen (of the spatial or temporal perseveration type) when the lesion extends to the adjacent parts of the occipital and temporal lobes. From what has been described above, it is evident that area 18 has another function besides visual recognition, viz. to relay information to some association areas of the other lobes.

SUMMARY

From the foregoing account, it can be seen that the cerebral cortex of man is made up of two main functional types: (a) the primary sensory and motor areas, and (b) the association areas. It should also be apparent that association areas should be considered from two points of view.

1. They do not simply associate thinking or sensation but serve to bring together into a physiological continuum both sensory and motor phenomena, so that the associative assessment of immediate

sensory inputs and past experience does not occur as a neurologically academic issue, but is correlated with appropriately integrated motor responses to ensure that the organism behaves in a suitable manner. Clinical evidence is abundant that dysfunction of the association areas is not only accompanied by disorders of sensory orientation, but is also manifested in, to be mild, unusual behaviour (see p. 275).

2. They do not all exhibit the same level of association. Indeed, some could be called *primary association areas* (e.g. area 18); these are concerned with the association of information in one sensory mode with information in the same sense modality that has arrived in the past (recognition, memory). Others could be called *secondary association areas* (e.g. area 37), in which the current information in several modalities is associated, together with the recognition information from the primary association areas, thus contributing towards a behavioural response that is experientially appropriate to the multi-modal sensory input, i.e. to the total external situation. Other areas could profitably be looked upon as *tertiary association areas* (e.g. areas 9–12). These are not concerned with the association of primary or secondary sensory inputs; nor are they involved very much in the behavioural responses to such inputs. It is in the tertiary association areas that subjective phenomena appear. Here, an affective tone is generated to accompany the activities of the other areas. In other words, the tertiary association areas are the ones involved in emotional responses; they are at least a part of the seat of subjective justification for the apparent motivation of overt behaviour. They help to provide the *rationale* for irrational responses.

It is perhaps ironic that nothing in the above description of the latest neurological apparatus has any exclusive application to man. Though it has generally been agreed that man differs from lower forms in his ability to think in abstract terms, i.e. to remove his ego from the situation and to assess it impersonally according to purely logical rules, yet no anatomical basis has been demonstrated for this ability. There is no neurophysiological basis, as yet, for the *rationale* of rational behaviour. It is by no means unreasonable to ask to what extent might rational behaviour be merely group-justified emotional behaviour.

Spontaneous Electrical Activity of the Cortex

In various earlier sections it has been pointed out that nerve cells are seldom, if ever, inactive. What we look upon as activation of a set of neurones is usually an increase in the activity that was present to begin with. Very often it is not merely the passage of impulses along a nerve fibre that determines whether an effector organ will be put into action. It is the frequency of impulses that is the operant factor, and it has been shown over and over again that nerve fibres to and from inactive muscles and glands are carrying low-frequency impulses even while the organs are inactive. Activity of the organ is accompanied by raised frequency of impulses in the nerve fibres that supply it. In much the same way, recording electrodes in various parts of the central nervous system demonstrate that considerable electrical activity is going on in some subcortical nucleus or in the cortex even though nothing effective seems to be coming of it. No known sensory input is reaching the active region and no known results are flowing from it. This type of activity is said to be "spontaneous", although all are aware that it does not arise out of nothing. No explanation of the generation of spontaneous activity can be given. Its slow, rhythmic character has, however, led to a set of theories. Some workers favour the idea that waxing and waning biochemical changes, metabolic reactions, are the source of fluctuating levels of excitation in the nerve cells in which such reactions are taking place. Other workers consider that reverberating circuits, with impulses having to cross synaptic resistances, give rise to periodic high and low phases of cellular excitation. Yet others believe that the biochemical changes would be too slow to account for the rhythms found, and that neuronal circuits are not involved because waves of excitation have been shown to pass over a cut made in the brain substance. Some workers propose that spontaneous rhythms arise solely from electrical sources, ion exchange and spread of eddy currents. For the electronically minded reader it may be mentioned that the rhythmic activity in single units has been compared to the function of a sawtooth relaxation oscillator. Interaction of the overlapping electrical fields of several such units gives rise to a rhythm of excitation that is slower than that of the single units and which could be comparable with actually observed rhythms.

α-RHYTHM

When the brain is at rest, inasmuch as the organism is not paying attention to anything, electrodes upon the scalp or cortex pick up a rhythmic activity that has a frequency of about 10 c/s. This is the α-rhythm and is most noticeable over the posterior parietal and occipital cortex, though it may spread to more frontal regions. It is a feature of recordings made from this region in a wide variety of animals, the frequency differing slightly with species.

α-Rhythm frequency also varies among individuals of the same species. The variation in frequency in the human population is very wide even among normal people (8–17 c/s, average 10 c/s) and indeed in rare individuals it is lacking.

As soon as the organism begins to pay attention to something— either an external stimulus or internal thinking—the α-rhythm ceases and the record shows faster, asynchronous activity (Fig. 58). However, there are some people in whom the α-rhythm persists even with the eyes open and the subject paying visual attention to the environment. Normally the α-rhythm is blocked when the eyes are open and

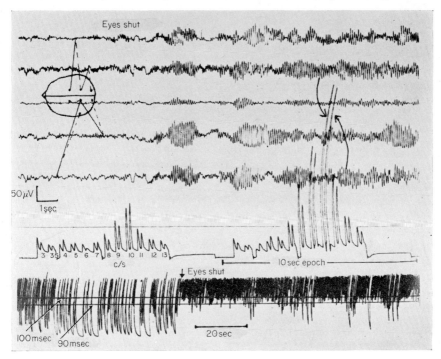

FIG. 58. An example of the classical effect of eye closure on α-rhythm in a normal subject. The upper five traces were recorded from electrode sites shown in the diagram in the upper left corner. These five "primary traces" show the typical burst of α-activity as the eyes are closed, followed by marked amplitude modulation, the α-rhythms being most prominent in the posterior occipital derivations. The sixth trace representing the frequency analysis, indicates the presence of two components at 9 and 10 c/s. The seventh trace, that showing the period analysis, indicates the presence of wave intervals varying from 90 to 110 msec. (From Grey Walter, 1959.)

patterned visual stimuli are being received. If frosted glass is placed before the eyes so that light but not pattern enters, then the α-rhythm is not blocked or is only slightly reduced in amplitude. Several components have been identified in the original α-rhythm described by Berger (1929). These components can be separated by use of orthogonal electrode chains. This arrangement of electrodes frequently shows one component to be dominant in one area of cortex and another component dominant elsewhere. Again in people with persistent α-rhythm, one component is most apparent when the eyes are shut, while another component continues when the eyes are open. Similarly, where the subject has an α-rhythm of 10 c/s with the eyes closed and then is given a mental problem, still with the eyes closed, the frequency may rise to 11 or 12 c/s. It seems as though the synchronous activity of occipital cells is disturbed when they come into use for visual functions. A given subject's normal α-rhythm is extremely stable, fluctuating in value by about 0·5 c/s. Even though it is well known that ethyl alcohol has a profoundly disturbing effect on cerebration, yet even in a state of considerable inebriation the α-rhythm changes by only about 1 c/s. Similarly, drugs which markedly stimulate the brain also have just such a small effect upon the α-rhythm. If the subject is exposed to a flickering light of the same frequency as his own α-rhythm, then the spontaneous rhythm becomes more sharply synchronized. With flicker stimuli at frequencies different from the subject's own α-rhythm, evoked potentials are superimposed upon the spontaneous rhythm. Electrodes placed upon different areas of the cortex show that when the eyes are shut the α-rhythm does not appear in all parts at the same time. It usually begins in anterior regions and then arises in more posterior regions until it reaches the posterior limit of the brain. Such features have given rise to the conception that the α-rhythm represents a scanning sweep by which the association areas examine the primary areas for evoked activity. The fact that the rhythms are so nearly constant also suggests that it might act as a timing mechanism. It must not be thought that the α-rhythm necessarily originates in the cerebral cortex, for recordings made with electrodes implanted below the cortex register a similar kind of spontaneous activity.

θ-RHYTHM

In children and in emotionally disturbed adults the parietal and temporal areas exhibit an apparently spontaneous rhythm of 4–7 c/s. This θ-rhythm appears at the onset of emotional frustration, lasts for about 20 sec and then disappears. It persists however, over long periods in psychopathic individuals. Some workers believe that the θ-rhythms represent a scanning sweep in search of emotional pleasure. The θ-rhythm practically disappears during a pleasurable experience and rises abruptly at the conclusion of such an experience.

β-RHYTHM

Generalized activation of the normal adult brain, especially under conditions of emotional tension, is associated with an electrical rhythm that has a frequency of rather more than 14 c/s. This β-rhythm is also considered to represent a scanning sweep of the brain. It is believed to be concerned with the analysis of sensorily evoked patterns of activity. This analysis leads to a concentration of the electrical changes involved in the efferent activity that forms the response to the stimulus.

δ-RHYTHMS

Brain rhythms with a frequency of between 1 and 3·5 c/s are assigned to the delta group of brain waves. In normal adults the δ-rhythm can only be detected during deep sleep. In children how-ever, up to the age of about 12 years the δ-rhythm is a normal com-ponent of the EEG. Persistence of the δ-rhythm beyond the age of about 12 is usually associated with a kind of immaturity which is characterized by a tendency to be easily led. It is by no means un-usual for this rhythm to be particularly marked in the waking EEG of young criminal delinquents. Under these latter conditions the δ-rhythm seems to arise in the right temporo-occipital region and is hardly at all disturbed by sensory stimulation. In the normal child, on the other hand, the δ-rhythm of the waking EEG is localized bilaterally in the occipital lobes. Moreover, it is highly distorted by sensory stimulation. In adults the presence of typical δ-rhythms is to be taken as an indication of deep-seated midline organic disease of the brain. The involvement of subcortical midline structures in the genesis of the δ-rhythm is also indicated by the ease with which it can be suppressed by the administration of compounds which activate the midbrain reticular formation. It should be clear that either stimulation or inhibition (e.g. by disease) of the midbrain reticular formation will interfere with the transmission of non-specific sensory information to the cortex. Since it is a disturbance of non-specific (rather than specific, as with the other rhythms) sensory input that affects the δ-rhythm, there has arisen the interpretation that the δ-rhythm is not, like the other rhythms described above, a scanning sweep device, but has some overall protective function. Grey Walter (1953) has termed this the phylactic hypothesis. In his view "it is reasonable to conjecture that some mechanism may exist to constrain or restrict the influence of conditions likely to initiate excessive and persistent activity".

SPONTANEOUS BURST ACTIVITY

This term has been applied to a component of the brain's spontaneous activity which persists during *deep* anaesthesia, when all other rhythmic activity is suppressed. It takes the form of rhythmic bursts occurring at intervals of 8–12/sec. Recordings of greatest amplitude are obtained from the association areas of the cortex, the trace being far less marked over the primary areas. It has been shown (Dempsey and Morison, 1943) that spontaneous burst activity is not dependent upon transcortical connexions (since circumsection does not affect the rhythm) but is generated by spontaneous activity in the dorsal medial nucleus of the thalamus. Disruption of subthalamic sensory pathways does not abolish spontaneous burst activity, therefore this phenomenon originates in the spontaneous activity of the thalamic nucleus itself. While spontaneous burst activity is being recorded, stimulation of a peripheral nerve evokes an action potential that is superimposed upon the 8–12 c/s rhythm. Hence, the thalamocortical pathways that evoke spontaneous burst activity are different from those that transmit the information from the sensory channels. This might be expected from the fact that sensory evoked potentials are obtained by stimulation of the ventral lateral nucleus of the thalamus, whereas spontaneous burst activity is produced only when the dorsal medial thalamic nucleus is stimulated. It was once thought that the spontaneous activity of the dorsal medial nucleus was due to a cortico-thalamic pathway. However, it has since been shown that the activity in the dorsal medial nucleus persists after removal of the cortex. Although, no explanation can be given for the genesis of the spontaneous activity of the dorsal medial nucleus of the thalamus, it would seem that this nucleus may serve to maintain the association areas of the cortex at a low, stand-by level of excitation in readiness for handling information from the primary cortical areas.

PROJECTION ACTIVITY

It has been stated above that spontaneous burst activity is the sole remaining component of the EEG when the organism is *deeply* anaesthetized. At a lighter level of anaesthesia the spontaneous burst activity is present with another component that takes the form of a random and irregular activity. This component of the EEG is recorded most distinctly from the primary projection areas of the cortex; hence it has been called projection activity. As with the spontaneous burst activity, so with projection activity circumsection in the cortex is without effect, whereas disconnexion from the thalamus results in abolition of the activity. In this case, however, it has been shown (Morison and Dempsey, 1943) that the ventral lateral nucleus is the thalamic region involved. Simultaneous recordings from this nucleus and primary cortex show almost identical traces under conditions of light anaesthesia. As would be expected from the fact that the ventral lateral nucleus is concerned, disruption of subthalamic sensory pathways results in the disappearance of projection activity. It seems reasonable to believe that the origin of projection activity lies in the spontaneous discharge of receptors that was described in the section on Sensation (pp. 35–95). Such spontaneous receptor activity, occurring in the absence of stimuli, would serve by means of the projection activity to maintain the primary areas of cortex at a stand-by level of excitation, ready for the handling of a peripheral sensory input.

FAST RHYTHMS

Various workers have identified components of the EEG which are characterized by low amplitude and high frequency. These components are seen most clearly in the lightly etherized animal, occur in all parts of the cortex and have frequencies of 30–80 c/s. Since this fast activity persists after the disruption of thalamocortical connexions it is considered that, unlike all the other spontaneous cortical activities so far mentioned, it is not dependent upon subcortical structures but is generated and maintained solely within the cortex. Bremer and many more recent electroencephalographers are of the opinion that all nervous elements possess the power of spontaneous rhythmic activity. It is believed that the fast rhythms represent this intrinsic power of cortical cells. The spontaneous or induced activity of subcortical structures then modulates fast activity to give the complex multi-component trace seen in the normal EEG.

CHAPTER 12

CONDITIONING

There are two basic kinds of reflex. One is inborn, instinctive or unconditioned, a familiar example being a salivatory response to the presence of food in the mouth. Stimulation of the taste buds excites a straightforward nervous loop from periphery to central mechanisms and back to the periphery, this time along secretomotor fibres innervating the salivary glands. The second fundamental kind of reflex is not present at birth but is acquired or conditioned. Within the same field as the above example, an illustration would be salivation at the sight of food. A particular pattern of activation in the visual system becomes somehow linked with the inborn gustatory mechanisms and produces activation of the salivatory secretomotor fibres without the presence of taste bud stimulation. This process of developing responses to remote stimuli is what is meant here by conditioning. At the outset it is important to be aware that conditioning occurs very frequently in the absence of experimental intervention.

Natural conditioned reflexes are those which are formed under ordinary living circumstances, such as a salivating response to the sight of food already mentioned. A moment's reflection will reveal an enormous number of somatic approach and avoidance responses that have been acquired in the normal process of additive living experience. In order to study the properties of conditioned reflexes it is useful deliberately to establish them in the subject, animal or man. Such experimental kinds are *artificial* conditioned reflexes. A classic example is Pavlov's elicitation of salivation in dogs by auditory stimuli. We should note that there appears to be no really basic difference in the mechanisms of the two kinds of conditioned reflex, although artificial cues take rather longer to establish than natural ones. Hence, data obtained in the study of artificially induced conditioned reflexes are readily applicable to natural conditions.

Establishment of a Conditioned Reflex

This requires first and foremost that there exist an unconditioned mechanism that leads to the response envisaged. The essence of conditioning is that an "extraneous" stimulus pathway is made to impinge upon an already present, innate stimulus pathway. The extraneous or conditioned stimulus is applied at the same time as (or shortly after) the innate or unconditioned stimulus (US). In the establishment of a natural conditioned reflex (CR) this is inevitable for normal animals. When animals eat, they see the food in front of them. A single instance of simultaneous stimuli is sometimes enough to establish a natural CR, especially of the nociceptive type. Artificial CRs usually require several such presentations, the number increasing with the modal remoteness of the conditioned stimulus (CS) and the complexity of the CR. No CR is established if the CS *follows* the US. As Grey Walter puts it (1953, p. 111), "if the dinner bell is to be of any use it must be rung before and not after dinner". For much the same reasons the CS must not occur *too long before* the US. If the time interval between the two stimuli is great, the subject does not associate them, just as primitive peoples attribute childbirth to celestial bodies; 9 months is too long for them to associate cause with effect.

Another very important factor in the establishment of a CR is that the various other sensory stimuli impinging upon the subject must be normal. Pavlov, trying to be scientifically methodical, carried out his early experiments in circumstances that eliminated as far as possible all stimuli except his US and CS. He discovered that when he placed his animals in the "insulated" box, the lack of normal stimuli was itself a conditioned stimulus. Ideally, CRs are established by training under the animals' normal living conditions; no extra stimuli and no removal of stimuli. Such ideal circumstances are not always possible.

Maintenance of Conditioned Reflexes

Once a subject has acquired a response to the application of the CS alone, it will continue to respond maximally on a few occasions and then the degree of response will gradually fall, with subsequent presentations of CS, until no response is forthcoming. It is as though the nervous system decides that there is no permanent association between the two stimuli after all. If the dinner bell is regularly sounded but no dinner served, the bell becomes just another sound, with no particular significance. On the other hand, if the US is presented at intervals, the CS retains its significance and the reflex can be maintained over indefinite periods. Even though the dinner bell does not always precede a meal, it will continue to raise expectations if a meal is provided every now and then. It is as though the nervous system is not going to risk the loss of a dinner if the odds are not too badly placed.

Types of Conditioned Reflex

Apart from the division into natural and artificial categories, it is useful to distinguish CRs on the basis of remoteness of the CS. So far the reflexes we have discussed are of the *primary* type. In these, a CS has replaced a US–sound of a bell has assumed the secreto-motor role of taste-bud stimulation. Provided this CR is properly maintained, it is possible to treat it as an existing pathway and to make another CS impinge upon it. Such a *secondary* CR might, for example, utilize a flash of light to elicit salivation, even though the visual stimulus had never been presented with the unconditioned stimulus food. Secondary CRs are established by presenting the secondary conditioned stimulus (CS′) at the same time or just before the primary CS. In a similar manner it is possible to establish *tertiary* CRs, in which a third conditioned stimulus (CS″) is presented with the CS′. These are easily established for defensive responses to nociceptive stimuli, but seem to be inapplicable to alimentary reflexes. Perhaps there is an inbuilt extension of possibilities for defensive reactions to match the wide range of natural nociceptive indicators. It should also be remembered that although for experimental purposes some simple response is observed, yet all CRs involve a complex of responses. Even the simple alimentary forms involve not only salivation but also jaw, head and limb movements, vocalization, etc. Under natural conditions the complexity of nociceptive responses parallels the complexity of remote stimuli signifying danger. But there appears to be a limit to conditioned flexibility, inasmuch as attempts to establish fourth order or quaternary CRs have not been successful.

Another type of CR is the *trace reflex*. When the CS is regularly applied at a certain distance in time from the US, then when the CS is given alone the CR occurs at that same time interval afterwards. For example, if the presentation of a green triangle is routinely followed by an electric shock 30 sec later, then eventually the animal takes evasive action 30 sec after the triangle is presented, doing nothing very much in the meantime. In other words, although there is no apparent change immediately after the application of the CS, yet there must be some *trace* in the nervous system which only becomes evident when a certain amount of time has passed. Somewhat similar are the *time reflexes* in which a period of time is itself made a CS. A simple example is established by feeding an animal at intervals of, say, 1 h. When the food is no longer given, the animal salivates every hour. Evidently, something is happening in the nervous system during this hour even though no external evidence can be seen. Such time intervals may be quite extensive. That great ethologist Konrad Lorenz (1954) records how one of his many dogs came to spend its weekends at a local public house, because the titbits were plentiful at such times. Of course, non-temporal cues may have informed the dog when Saturday came around. A more complex example, perhaps, is the waking response of old soldiers who continue for years after discharge to rouse themselves at an early hour to the non-existent call of a bugle.

Properties of Conditioned Reflexes

By and large, conditioned reflexes exhibit certain properties, no matter what the mode of conditioning or what the type of response. The existence of such a set of common characteristics, of course, supports the view that all (or most) CRs have a common central mechanism. In other words, conditioning is an unspecific property of the central nervous system. Although it is necessary to deal with each property separately, it should at all times be remembered that this tabulatory description is about different aspects of *one* great neural mechanism, the conditioned response. We will first consider the properties as viewed externally (i.e. in behaviour) and then survey the information available on the fundamental neural mechanisms.

EXTERNAL INHIBITION

This is a property that was discovered very early in the history of CRs. Any fairly strong and unfamiliar extraneous stimulus—a loud noise, a flash of light, sudden movements—abolishes the response to the CS. If such a stimulus occurs at several trials, it loses its inhibiting property and the CS once again is followed by the CR. It seems that the unfamiliar stimulus (which, as mentioned above, may also be a *lack* of something familiar) acts as a US and activates an unconditioned "exploratory reflex" which being one of the strongest innate responses competes with the response under test. The entire CR neural mechanism is inhibited by an external (i.e. different) neural mechanism. The sight of food rarely excites hunger in the person with external anxiety; exploratory cogitation of a worrying kind effectively dampens the appetite.

INTERNAL INHIBITION

Under this heading come several forms of inhibition of CRs which have the common feature that the inhibition occurs *within* the CR neural mechanisms.

EXTINCTION

This term is applied to the phenomenon mentioned above, where repeated application of the CS alone is accompanied by a gradual decline in the degree of response until finally no response is evoked. Sometimes an extinguished CR will return after a short rest from the CS; it can also be elicited by a sudden extraneous stimulus (disinhibition). But the ideal way to keep a CR in existence is to give the US from time to time in conjunction with the CS. This is the procedure of *reinforcement*, the process of maintaining the subject's expectations. Just such a mechanism of extinction led to the downfall of the boy who cried "wolf" too often.

CONDITIONED INHIBITION

When a CR has been established to one CS and then another conditioned stimulus (CS') is applied *with the first* on several occasions but without any reinforcement with the US, then CS will continue to evoke the response when given alone, but not when given together with CS'. The secondary stimulus has become a *conditioned inhibitor* and the whole phenomenon is a *negative conditioned reflex*. In human affairs it is possible that this mechanism is involved in selective impotence. The CS (say, erotic visual stimuli) is much the same whether originating in wife or mistress, but the CS' (say, auditory stimuli) usually has a different significance in each. The CS alone may rouse libido (as it docs, to fruition, in the case of the mistress) but when CS and CS' occur together the CS' acts as a conditioned inhibitor due to previous experience of non-reinforcement.

DELAYED INHIBITION

Consider first the simultaneous CR. In this the response is established by giving the CS and the US more or less immediately—a quick ring of the bell and the food at once available. When the CS is given alone then the response (in this case salivation) has only a very short latency; salivation starts as soon as the bell starts. If, however, the response is established by giving a long CS (say, bell for 30 sec) before presenting the US, then when the CS is given alone, the response does not appear until the end of the CS. The subject does not salivate or move at the first sound of the bell. Some process of internal inhibition, due to the previous delay in reinforcement, holds up the response for 30 sec. The integrated human being does not try to wrench open the drawer of a slot machine immediately after depositing the coin.

DIFFERENTIAL INHIBITION

This has proved a most useful property of CRs in the study of perceptual discrimination in many species and all sensory modalities. If a subject has been conditioned to a precise stimulus, say a pure tone of a certain frequency, or light of a particular wavelength, then a response will be obtained with stimuli of roughly the same numerical value. If the conditioning tone was 100 c/s, then 80 and 110 c/s will evoke the CR. But if such a range of tones is presented to the subject and only one of them regularly reinforced, then the subject eventually responds only to that frequency. The other frequencies have been differentially inhibited. By gradually decreasing the interval between two such stimuli a point is reached where differential inhibition does not occur. Both stimuli, say 100 and 103 c/s, regularly evoke the response. The assumption is that the subject cannot perceive any difference between the two stimuli; his powers of auditory discrimination are limited to a difference of 3 c/s in that frequency range. Studies of this nature are not limited to determining the degree of discrimination in each of the sense modalities. They have been extended to sub-modalities, so that data are available, for example, to compare the levels of discrimination of pitch, loudness, rhythm and timbre. Similar techniques have been used to study the retentive powers of the subject. The highest level of sound intensity discrimination in man can be demonstrated only when the stimuli are given within a few seconds of each other. Discrimination is still evident in the dog when the second sound is presented a day after the first.

IRRADIATION OF INHIBITION

Consider the situation where a CR has been established to two CSs, say a pure tone and a flash of light. Each of these applied alone will elicit the response. Now let one of these stimuli, say the tone, be converted to a conditioned inhibitor by a process of non-reinforcement; the tone is not now followed by the response. To produce irradiation of inhibition, the tone is now applied just before the flash. Under such conditions the flash of light no longer evokes the CR. If the tone is applied a fair time before the flash, then the flash still triggers the reflex. There has been a temporal irradiation of inhibition from the auditory pathways to the visual pathways. Similar irradiation of inhibition can be demonstrated within one modality, e.g. a buzz can be made to inhibit the stimulus qualities of a pure tone or a coloured light may be used to inhibit the effect of a flashing white light. In the field of tactile receptors, activation of one area can be made to inhibit the effect of activation of a neighbouring area. It should be noted that the inhibitory effect really does radiate from the centre of inhibition and takes time to do so. Decay of this inhibition is also radial and a function of time. It seems as though stimulation of the inhibitory receptors causes a process of inhibition to spread gradually from the centre and then to shrink back again. Note carefully that the inhibitory process starts to spread out only when the inhibitory stimulus *ceases*. The inhibitory stimulus must be given before, not during the excitatory stimulus (see Positive Induction, below).

INDUCTION

Under this heading come two properties which have the common feature of involving mutual interactions of excitatory and inhibitory conditioned stimuli.

Negative Induction

This name is given to the procedure by which an inhibitory stimulus is made even more inhibitory—as measured by the number of trials required for the stimulus to become excitatory again by repeated reinforcement with the US. This increased inhibitory power is induced simply by applying the inhibitory CS just after the excitatory CS, followed by immediate reinforcement.

Positive Induction

This is the term applied to the procedure by which an excitatory stimulus is made even more excitatory—as measured by the intensity of a quantitative response. To do this, a CR is established such that one CS (say, a buzzer) is made excitatory in the usual way and another CS (say, a flashing light) is made first excitatory and then inhibitory by non-reinforcement. If, now, the two stimuli are applied simultaneously, a bigger response is obtained than when the excitatory stimulus is applied alone. It seems as though inhibitory processes in one neural mechanism, in this case visual, contemporaneously raise the excitability of other neural mechanisms, in this case auditory. When the inhibitory stimulus is stopped, then irradiation of inhibition (see above) occurs and the augmentation of the excitatory stimulus is abolished. It is likely that the alternation of "waves" of positive induction and irradiation of inhibition, spreading and shrinking throughout the nervous system, forms a constant and important feature of the neurology of conditioning. It may also be the case that such phenomena constitute a basic property of the sensory apparatus under all conscious conditions.

SYNTHESIS OF STIMULI

The properties now to be described have a special importance because they are the experimental counterpart of situations that approach rather more closely to natural conditions. Seldom, possibly never, is an animal presented in real life with a single stimulus. Even if an environmental change involves only one modality (which is rare), there is always a complexity about the stimulus which is not reproduced in pure tones, pure colours, etc. Although pet dogs soon become conditioned to the sound of their names, the response is poor or absent when the name is spoken by a stranger; something in the quality of the voice is an essential part of the stimulus. In addition, the CNS is constantly receiving information over the proprioceptive pathways. It is appropriate now to consider the experimental data on the synthesis of several stimuli in the same modality applied simultaneously.

A conditioned response is easily established in the usual way to the sound of a musical chord. If the tonic chord of C major be used, then the response follows when the three notes C, E and G are played together. Further, if any one of these notes is sounded, the CR will be evoked. There will be no response if, say, the note B or F or even F# is sounded. Similar results are found with combinations of different rhythms and with such "chorded" stimuli in other modalities. Evidently the nervous system is able to discriminate between the different notes of the chord and to synthesize them into a compound stimulus. Each of the separate stimuli is recognized as forming a part of the compound stimulus.

Consider now the use of simultaneous stimuli in different modalities. Much the same kind of thing occurs as before. A subject can be made to respond, say, to a coloured light, a buzzer and a tactile stimulus applied simultaneously. But now a difference is noted from the effects of stimuli in the same modality. One of the components of a multimodal compound stimulus is always dominant. If a compound stimulus consists of a visual and auditory component, then the auditory stimulus applied alone will evoke the response; but the visual stimulus applied alone will not. Similarly, with somatic

H

modalities, if a compound stimulus is composed of tactile and thermal elements, then the tactile one alone evokes the response, but the thermal one does not. It would be tempting, on this evidence, to believe that the non-dominant mode is playing no part in the CR when the compound stimulus is applied. This is not the case.

Suppose that a CR has been established to the simultaneous presentation of a visual and an auditory stimulus. As we have said, if the visual component is applied alone, no response follows. Now suppose that the effective auditory stimulus is presented several times without reinforcement. Then it, too, becomes ineffective and will no longer evoke the CR. The surprising fact is that if these two ineffective stimuli are now applied together, then the response occurs. Thus, although it seems at first sight that the visual stimulus is playing no part in the effect of the compound stimulus, and although it seems on second sight that no effects are produced by each of the ineffective stimuli separately, nevertheless both stimuli on both occasions must be having some non-observed effect. When these two non-observed changes in the nervous system occur together, then the new neuronal activity gives rise to the observed response.

Now we should consider the situation where compound stimuli are spread over time, i.e. where the components are given in (reasonably rapid) succession. It is abundantly evident that many species are able to synthesize separate stimuli into a specific order. Taking a single modality, a CR can be established to the notes of a chord played one after the other, e.g. C, E, G. The response will not follow the application of any one of these notes alone. When the notes are played in the reverse order (G, E, C) the response *is* evoked, and this may suggest that the subject is discriminating the mere intervallic nature of the stimulus rather than a specific order. However, either of the two sequences can be made ineffective by non-reinforcement, leaving the other sequence still effective. Similar findings occur when the components fall into different modalities; for example, a light, a tone and a touch will evoke a response when applied sequentially but no single stimulus will do so. Hence the nervous system is able to synthesize ineffective separate stimuli into an effective sequential compound stimulus, discriminated from other sequential combinations of the same stimuli.

Internal Events

The above information has been obtained by observation of animal behaviour. This is highly important work and throws a good deal of light on the neural mechanisms of conditioning. Nevertheless it is of prime importance to follow these behavioural studies with investigations of the changes that occur in the nervous system itself. Modern techniques make such studies possible and this field is showing rapid advances. Here follows an outline which will serve to indicate the methods used and to emphasize the general view that many parts of the brain are involved in conditioning, not, as once thought, only the cerebral cortex. (See also Learning, pp. 226–245.)

By and large, information on the internal events associated with conditioning have been obtained by the classical methods of lesions and stimulations in various parts of the nervous system. More recently, the additional powerful tool of recording the activity in single cells and fibres with microelectrodes has contributed many fertile pieces of information. These methods have been applied under various conditions: (a) during the establishment of a CR; (b) during the performance of an established CR; (c) during special performances such as discrimination. The following summary of the available data is drawn largely from the excellent review of the subject by John (1961).

RETICULAR FORMATION

This old widespread system appears to be involved in just about everything that happens in the nervous system and conditioning is no exception. Recording electrodes in the midbrain reticular activating system (RAS) show the occurrence of increased electrical activity during the establishment of a CR. It would be expected that the application of any stimulus would have this effect since all sensory pathways send collaterals to the RAS. This knowledge, coupled with the fact that lesions in the RAS do not abolish the acquisition or retention of CRs nor affect discriminatory ability, might suggest that the RAS is not significantly involved in conditioning. The same impression might arise from the knowledge that when a CR has become well established, the CS no longer causes increased electrical activity in the RAS. Even so, there are one or two pieces of data which prevent the RAS from being dismissed so summarily. Stimulation of the RAS may, depending upon the overall conditions, evoke an established CR in the absence of the CS or may inhibit an established CR in the presence of the CS. Such stimulation certainly enhances the possibilities in differential conditioning and it will abolish neurotic inhibition. By and large, it would seem that the RAS contributes to the acquisition of a CR by adding its non-specific spread of information to the specific recepto-thalamo-cortical information system. On the first few occasions when the CS is presented, it presumably evokes the alerting reaction (see Consciousness, pp. 246–255). Then, as the pattern of the CR is laid down, the non-specific alerting reaction gives way to the more specific response required by the US. At this stage there is no great point in having the RAS activated by the CS; the RAS becomes habituated and the CS no longer raises its electrical activity. Naturally, the more alert the subject is during tests of differentiation, the finer will be its discriminatory powers. Hence, where such capacities are called for, activation of the RAS would be an advantage. Apart from the improvement in differentiation caused by stimulation of the RAS, further evidence is provided by the fact that recordings during differentiation responses show that slow, irregular waves of excitability pass through the RAS. It is difficult not to look upon this as part of a scanning mechanism. One should not be too concerned at the apparent ineffectiveness of lesions in the RAS. Lesions destroying the whole of it would also destroy life; lesions destroying most of it would abolish consciousness. Lesions that are compatible with life and consciousness are apparently too small to produce observable effects upon the acquisition and retention of CRs. Non-specific systems can frequently be severely reduced in size without notable functional deficits.

RHINENCEPHALON

Modern research frequently indicates that the rhinencephalon is not a collection of structures that together form a unitary system. Interaction among the parts there may be, but some parts do not seem to be too closely linked with the others. For present purposes, however, no attempt will be made to "map" the rhinencephalon. In general terms, the available evidence suggests that the role of the hippocampal system in conditioning is largely inhibitory. Lesions do not affect the process of acquisition of CRs, whereas electrical stimulations of various regions have completely abolished the subject's ability to be conditioned. Previously learned CRs are not evoked during stimulation of the rhinencephalon. Nevertheless, during acquisition and during performance there is a detectable increase in the electrical activity of rhinencephalic structures.

HYPOTHALAMUS

Once again, here is a single anatomical term used to describe what is clearly becoming recognized as a physiological complex. In several fields it is apparent that different parts of the hypothalamus have different functions, and this is evident in the field of conditioning. Lesions in the posterior hypothalamus have little effect on acquisition of CRs. Interference with the mammillary bodies, mammillo-thalamic tract and other parts results in serious defects in both retention and acquisition. Stimulation of hypothalamic regions may evoke a previously learned CR, which may be of the approach or avoidance variety. Recording electrodes show that the CS produces electrical potentials in the hypothalamus both during acquisition and during subsequent performance. That is, there is no evidence of hypothalamic *habituation* to the CS as there is with the reticular formation. If it be remembered that the hypothalamus plays a major role in autonomic regulation, it is not too difficult to assess the part it plays in conditioning. The CR, whether in the process of being established or already entrenched, must be accompanied by appropriate changes in visceral functions. Thus the CS, even when the alerting systems have become used to it, must continue to activate hypothalamic mechanisms. On the same thesis, hypothalamic lesions will interrupt these mechanisms and so make the acquisition or performance of CRs difficult.

THALAMUS

Surprise would be the immediate reaction to any suggestion that the body's major sensory relay apparatus played no part in conditioning. Direct evidence shows that it is of considerable importance in several aspects of conditioning. Without going into the details of thalamic anatomy, it can be said that lesions in this structure impair or abolish both acquisition and retention of CRs. Stimulation in the midline prevents the acquisition of CRs but does not affect retention, whereas lateral thalamic stimulation results in a loss of retention. Recording electrodes have demonstrated the occurrence of increased, rather generalized electrical activity on the first few presentations of the CS. This becomes considerably localized when the CR is established. The overall view seems to be that the thalamus has an importance (a) in relaying sensory information in specific modalities to the appropriate higher structures, and (b) in a less specific manner where established CRs are concerned.

CEREBRAL CORTEX

Once upon a time it was thought that the cerebral cortex was the only structure of any real importance in conditioning, apart from the pathways that bring information to it and take instructions from it. More modern findings, such as those concerning the reticular system, require a modification of this view. Even so, it is worth remembering that the cerebral cortex is the latest development of the vertebrate nervous system, and although it does not render lower structures vestigial, yet it has unique properties that are essential for the "higher" functions. Perhaps it is not too important for any one facet of any one higher function. But it is required for the totality of sensible, organized and non-automatic directive living.

There seems little doubt that some very simple visceral responses can be conditioned in the absence of the cerebral cortex. This is not the case if the discussion is restricted to the much larger and more important responses that involve behaviour of one sort or another. No acquisition of new behavioural CRs and no performance of established CRs occurs in the wholly decorticate subject. Partial ablations involving the primary sensory areas abolish the ability for conditioning within the modality involved. With passage of time after, say, an ablation of auditory cortex, there is partial recovery in ability to acquire auditory CRs, but not if much is called for in the way of discrimination. Ablation of parts of the frontal cortex, at least in monkeys, seems to have a non-specific (i.e. not related to modality of CS) effect in abolishing conditioned avoidance responses. When the region of cerebral cortex that corresponds to the US is stimulated, application of the CS produces the response. But the CS is ineffective if the region of cortex corresponding to it (e.g. visual cortex in the case of a light CS) is stimulated while it is being presented. Evidently the extraneous stimulation of the CS cortical region in some way prevents the proper organization of the sensory information being brought to it from the receptor. Recording electrodes show a widespread increase in cortical electrical activity during the setting-up of a CR. This must be largely due to radiation of post-synaptic information from the reticular activating system. As with this latter structure, there is marked cortical habituation to the CS once the CR is well established; yet the CS continues to raise the activity in certain regions of cortex. Once again, this is to be expected, since the CS is no longer serving as a non-specific alerting stimulus but has become specifically associated with a particular response.

All this evidence leaves no doubt that the cerebral cortex is doing something in the field of conditioning. Quite what it is doing remains to be discovered. Its functioning involves subcortical rather than transcortical connexions, for circumsection of the CS region has no effect upon the CR whereas undercutting the CS region abolishes the CR. This may simply reflect the cutting off of afferent information channels, but there are reasons for believing that efferent disconnexions are also partly responsible for the effect.

CHAPTER 13

LEARNING

The last place where one ought to find philosophical deliberations is in a textbook of neurophysiology. However, since many original papers and several reviews contain matter that can only come under the heading of philosophy, it is not entirely out of place to present here a consideration of what is meant by learning—before passing on to examine the neural basis of it. Perhaps the broadest definition is that learning is involved whenever an organism can do something now that it could not do in the past. This definition would therefore include under learning the acquisition of the various types of motor co-ordination: walking, grasping, conveying objects to the mouth, even such a simple affair as standing up without falling over. From these elementary forms of motor learning, the above definition would pass on to muscular activities that are, perhaps, more acceptable as examples of accomplishment such as talking, dancing, playing of musical instruments or the various manual crafts like wood-carving and sculpture. Another view would separate all of the above activities as the development of skills and would look upon learning as the specialized, directed and appropriate use of such skills. Those with the latter outlook would include among learned activities such acquisitions as direction-finding in mazes, pedal-pressing in test-boxes, sensory discriminations of many kinds and avoidance responses in devices like the shuttle-box. Others consider that even this type of complex behaviour should be looked upon as quite distinct in form and mechanism from novel abilities that involve only a minimum of sensorimotor skill, such as the learning of a foreign language, mathematics or the collected data and principles of a scientific discipline. Quite obviously, the scale of learning covered by all of the above definitions is reflected in the phylogenetic scale of animals, with the highest part of both scales applying to man. If learning is to be looked upon as including all of the above activities, it is clear that no branch of the animal kingdom can be said to lack the ability to learn. Transition from behaviour involving many errors to behaviour in which every move, literally, under natural conditions is in the right direction, is characteristic of the development of all animals from Protozoa upwards. The only real distinction is that the kind of learned behaviour becomes more complex with ascending phylogeny and, presumably, a more complex neural basis has been evolved in parallel fashion. Hence much of the search for the neural mechanisms of learning has been a search *not* for the processes underlying learning itself, but for those underlying the particular kind of learning under test. Once it is recognized that learning—in the broadest definition given above—is an intrinsic property of any animal cell, then learning in the senses given subsequently above is seen to consist in the combination of the learning capacities of groups (perhaps thousands) of cells into patterns that are especially appropriate to various forms of behaviour.

Components of Learning

Very clearly, in the course of evolution some cells have become specialized to play a pre-eminent role in learning. In general terms one can say that these are the nerve cells. While every nerve cell seems to have the ability to learn—in the broadest sense of acquisition of new capabilities—it is still a matter of conjecture whether some nerve cells, those in a particular region, have a kind of super-specialization that enables them to play a necessary and sufficient role in learning as defined more specifically above. In other words, although there can be little doubt that neurones in, say, the pyramidal system can learn (by changes in chemistry and morphology) in such a manner that new motor acts become possible, it is pretty certain that these neurones are not essential for the "higher" types of learning such as acquiring skill at chess. Nevertheless, even if there are places in the CNS where groups of cells are specially adapted to higher learning capacities, we may be sure that they are dependent upon a great deal of the rest of the nervous system. Learning, whatever it may be and wherever it is located, involves a set of ancillary functions.

It is difficult, for example, to conceive of learning taking place under conditions of complete sensory deprivation. Few would disagree that the overall ability to learn is likely to be reduced in proportion to a reduction in sensory powers. Hence, for an organism to learn properly—not just one particular task, but all the tasks that naturally come its way—it needs must have complete integrity of the sensorium. (This does not apply under some artificial conditions, see p. 197.) Again, apart from personal introspection, the only way in which we can examine learning in organisms is to see how they behave in certain conditions, so we study their motor response to significant stimuli. Hence, to us as observers, for an animal to learn properly it must have an intact and adequately experienced motor system. Further, these two functions—sensory input and motor output—must be brought together in a highly non-incidental manner.

Somehow the significance of patterns of excitation of the sensory system must be appreciated and their meaning communicated precisely to the appropriate motor mechanisms. Without such an intermediate integrating and transposing "transducer" there would be no learning, no novel accomplishments, but only automatic, stimulus-response behaviour. True, it is apparent that *after* learning has been accomplished there is a measure of automaticity about many pieces of behaviour. It may well be that the "transducer" device is only necessary *during* the process of learning and can be dispensed with at a later date. Indeed, some neurologists believe, on the basis of the effects of brain injury, that some parts of the brain may be essential in children, while much learning of many kinds is going on, but that these parts gradually become less essential and less functional with advancing age. Despite the obvious decline with age of the efficiency of the sensory and motor systems, these deficits are not marked until senility, so that it is much more likely that it is the "transducer" mechanism that exhibits fairly early failure. This would provide a neurological basis for the principle in psychology that ability to learn decreases with age. Another component of this phenomenon may be gradual failure of memory.

Memory must play a most important part in any type of learning, however the latter is defined. Presumably learning cannot occur unless some kind of memory "traces" are left in the CNS on successive confrontations with particular stimuli. Memory is more fully dealt with in a later section (p. 256); here we may pass lightly over its mechanisms and simply note that, however it happens, a record is made that can be re-examined at a later date and compared with a re-presentation of the sensory pattern. More than that, several records are made at the same time. Not only is the stimulus pattern remembered but there is also recall of the motor response which was made last time and the effects of that motor response with, possibly, remembrance of the emotional attitude that accompanied this piece of past behaviour. Short acquaintance with patients suffering from some forms of temporal lobe damage, in which recent memory lasts only a few seconds, is enough to convince anyone that the neural mechanisms of memory are absolutely essential to even the simplest kind of learning. Such patients have not lost their memory and they have not lost whatever they have learned in the past; they have lost the capacity to memorize and the capacity to learn. Whether the two capacities are neurologically inextricable cannot yet be told, but several aspects of memory seem to separate it from learning, at least to the introspective view. We are all aware that we are able to remember things that do not seem to have been involved in any learning task. Indeed, some workers consider that the entire sensory input is recorded and can be recalled under suitable conditions such as hypnosis.

Another component of learning and one which is rarely mentioned, probably because its neurological basis is so vague, is that of incentive. Workers in the field of behaviour provide a quite strong reason why their test animals should behave in the required manner. The animals are starved, for example, before being put into food-reward situations, or they are given unpleasant sensory stimuli unless they operate the investigator's test device. If the animals are fed at the usual regular intervals, they "learn" (i.e. they start to behave as the investigator wishes) with considerable difficulty or not at all. In general terms, as far as experimental behavioural studies are concerned, learning does not seem to occur, or occurs with difficulty, however intact the brain may be, or however high in the scale of animals it is, *unless some sort of satisfaction is the subjective end point.* In other words, what the animal really *learns* is not the appropriate motor response to a significant stimulus, but the association between a sensorimotor phenomenon and a reward. It does not learn to do something; it learns that if it does something of which it is already capable it will obtain satisfaction. As intimated above, the neurological basis of satisfaction is something upon which only the most unwary neurologist would venture to pontificate (but see Emotional Behaviour, pp. 267–280) but little contact with animals is necessary, to say nothing of personal insight, to realize that satisfaction of one kind or another seems to be at the root of every piece of learned behaviour— whether in animals or man, whether in the sane or the insane. The behaviour may not be appropriate; it may not bring the desired reward; but it is undoubtedly generated by the desire for reward. Clearly, the satisfaction does not have to be in material form. The psychological term "endogain" and the pleasure-pain principle both represent a sort of sublimated satisfaction that accounts for most human behaviour that is not directed at the more material rewards of food and sex. Thus an important ancillary to the learning process is whatever neural mechanism is responsible for subjective desires. It can at once be seen that when this mechanism exists only in an elementary form (e.g. in reptiles), then only the most elementary types of learning will occur—even if the neural equipment for more advanced learning is present in the organism. Leaving all that is meant by "sublimation" on one side, it is generally agreed that the most important brain regions in the generation of incentive and the acceptance of reward are the old regions—hypothalamus and rhinencephalon—so we must beware of carelessly assuming that only the newer higher regions of the brain are concerned with learning. However, "high" the nervous system of man, and however "intellectual" he may consider his learning to be, it is likely that the basic mechanism of incentive is the same in him as in the lizard.

Thus it becomes clear that many parts of the CNS are associated with, if not an integral part of, the learning process. Nevertheless, each of these parts is made up of groups of cells with similar (but probably not identical) functions. Understanding of the learning process itself, therefore, becomes a matter of understanding what happens in single cells when they become capable of new activities. Understanding of complex behavioural responses becomes a matter of understanding how the changes in all of the single cells involved become linked together, which includes knowing *where* they come together, or in other terms which parts of the brain are involved. The treatment of these topics below will deal first with the kinds of behavioural responses that are routinely studied, then with the brain regions that may be involved and lastly with the possible mechanisms by which single cells and groups of cells may come to exhibit the property of having learned something.

Types of Learning

CONDITIONING

It is difficult when surveying the literature to avoid the impression that to many, and perhaps to most workers learning and conditioning are equated, inasmuch as although other terms (see below) are sometimes applied, the technique used is of classical conditioning type. Investigators in the field have applied the term "Type I" learning to conditioning procedures that are strictly Pavlovian. In this form, a conditioned stimulus that would not normally evoke a response is made to do so by being applied several times simultaneously with an unconditioned stimulus that *would* be expected to produce the given response. The famous example is the pairing of presentation of food with the sounding of a bell to produce the response of salivation, evoked eventually by the bell alone. Type I learning, therefore, raises the pertinent query as to whether this form of neural association should properly be included under learning. Can an organism sensibly be said to learn to salivate, i.e. to perform an involuntary response? Of course, Type I learning need not have visceromotor phenomena as the end-point; the animal might "learn" to walk towards a box when the bell rings. But it is as well to bear in mind that the term Type I learning is sometimes applied, without qualification, to both voluntary and involuntary acts and it is for the individual to decide for himself exactly what he will accept as learning.

When the unconditioned stimulus is of an unpleasant character, an electric shock for example, the procedure is called Type II learning. At first glance there may seem to be no essential difference between Type I and Type II learning. A clue to the distinction is given by the alternative term—"instrumental learning". The animal's response in Type I learning is not instrumental in its acquisition of a reward—there is no guarantee that salivation will be followed by feeding. However, in Type II learning the response, which is usually some kind of motor evasive activity such as jumping, is indeed instrumental in the obtaining of a reward; the jump ensures absence of electric shock. In the beginning these terms were applied to the above-described forms in which "avoidance" responses were the end-point. Since then, Type II learning has come to include procedures that are not based upon evasion but which still demand a motor response that leads to the reward. Hence, Type II learning is now applied to such activities as lever-pressing or maze-wandering leading to acquisition of food. However, it is not at once apparent that these two forms of Type II learning are really similar. Few would doubt that the first type—the avoidance kind—represents something very close to the traditional requirements for conditioning. There are the usual four components: *unconditioned stimulus* (electric shock, say) which normally gives an *unconditioned response* (jump when shocked), a *conditioned stimulus* (a bell, say) and a *conditioned response* (jump at sound of bell). In the situation where the animal is required to press a lever in order to obtain food this pattern is not present. What could be called the unconditioned stimulus (the food) would not normally evoke the response of lever-pressing, which therefore cannot be considered as an unconditioned response. Further, there would seem to be no conditioned stimulus at all, inasmuch as nothing like the bell is involved. This leads to the inevitable conclusion that there is no conditioned response. It is difficult to see how a situation of this kind can be said to have anything at all to do with conditioning in the usual sense. However, many workers apply the terms "operant conditioning" or "trial-and-error conditioning" under these circumstances. Perhaps this is because it is felt that conditioning may justifiably be extended to include all situations in which some kind of association occurs between a particular sensory input and the reward obtained by a particular voluntary act. There can be little doubt that the lever-pressing rat comes to associate this activity—which he begins of his own accord and for no special reason except his hungry restlessness—with the sudden appearance of a food pellet. Similarly, the maze-wandering rat begins to wander for no very special reason and comes to associate a certain sequence of right and left turns with the sudden availability of food. It is for the reader to decide for himself whether he will apply the term "conditioning" to all situations that involve sensory-motor-visceral associations. If this connotation is accepted it would seem that the term's denotation would include just about every form of learning that is conceivable, since association is one of the several essential components of any learning procedure.

IMPRINTING

Fairly recently discovered is a form of learning that cannot be induced experimentally, but can be modified in various ways. Only a few species have been studied in this respect, but the principle probably applies to very many, including the human. It seems that the developing nervous system passes through a phase where it is particularly sensitive to a specialized sensory input. The impact of the sensory stimuli is to "imprint" upon the growing brain a pattern of behavioural response that lasts for a very long time, possibly for life. The most famous example is that given by the ethologist, Lorenz, who showed that at a certain stage of development ducklings respond to the moving mother's call by following her. The mother duck can be replaced by any other moving object and provided it makes a sound and is presented to the ducklings at the proper time, they will follow it for a good part of their lives, even in preference to their mother. If the presentation of the natural or artificial stimulus is made too early or is delayed beyond a certain, quite short, period, then the effect is not produced and the ducklings do not habitually follow anything. Evidently then, nerve cells that were not able to (or at any rate did not) generate a precise form of behaviour, suddenly and permanently exhibit that capacity not as an inevitable corollary of development, but as a result of a collision of genetic determinants with temporally accurate and appropriate excitation.

Delayed Responses

One of the biggest problems that confront behavioural neurophysiologists is to devise tests that can be applied to animals and yet will deliver information on the kind of "higher" learning that goes on in at least some humans. Such higher learning involves the use of ideas, concepts, the imagination—thinking on a level vastly more complex than mere association. One way in which investigators have tackled this problem is to examine the ability of animals to make delayed responses. In these studies the animal is first of all taught which of two stimuli is the one that brings satisfaction and is then made to wait some time before being allowed to choose between the two stimuli. Some workers have failed to discern the conceptual nature of such tests and look upon the procedure as a simple modification of discrimination conditioning with the delay period giving an additional assessment of recent memory. However, it must be admitted that in delayed response investigations, the higher animals have superior performance and also that such responses seem to be selectively disturbed by lesions of the frontal lobes, which many consider to be the dominant regions in ideation.

Serial Learning

In the continued attempt to increase the complexity of learning tasks, workers have devised methods by which an animal can achieve satisfaction only after carrying out a series of responses. Not only do these experimental situations require the animal to perform several actions, but they must also be performed in the right order. It could be said that tasks of this kind must involve ideation even if only with regard to temporal or spatial pattern and hence may approach more closely to "higher" forms of learning.

Another factor which should constantly be kept in mind when cogitating upon published behavioural work is that most of it is based upon the number of trials required to establish the desired response. Quite clearly, if an experimental intervention such as a brain lesion or stimulation doubles or halves the number of times an animal needs to be presented with a situation before it is able to perform the task efficiently, something of considerable importance has been discovered. However, it would be a grave mistake to look upon such results as giving any information whatever about the essential features of learning. Experiments based upon numbers of trials yield data concerning the *rate* of learning, not the degree of nervous integrity required for learning to occur. It should not be assumed that one and the same neural mechanism is responsible both for the ability to learn and for the ability to learn at a certain rate. Unless an inordinately large number of trials is still not enough for an animal to learn a task after intervention, it cannot be properly stated that the intervention has destroyed the neural basis of learning.

Brain Regions Involved

One of the most important lines of neurophysiological research has been concerned with discovering which parts of the brain are essential for various types of learning. It was natural that a good deal of attention was paid to the cerebral cortex since learning was looked upon very much as a "higher function". The results of this attention have been disappointing. Lashley's work on maze-learning in partially decorticate rats has already been described (see p. 196). From this it seemed that even such simple tasks as those involved in Lashley's mazes required an intact cerebral cortex for optimal learning. The idea became widespread that learning involved the setting up of "circuits" within the cortex and in some quarters there was considerable disappointment when it was shown that quite complex tasks can be accomplished by such creatures as the octopus which possess nothing remotely similar to the complex mammalian cortex. It now has to be admitted that learning as such is not a prerogative of corticate animals. Nevertheless, no one would doubt that learning in the absence of adequate cortex is limited to the simplest tasks. Undoubtedly the higher structures are more important in the higher animals, but this may only become apparent when complex learning tasks are investigated. With lower forms, such as the rat, a most remarkable level of activity (see Behaviour, pp. 267–280) remains after removal of the whole forebrain, leaving just the midbrain and hypothalamus—and these separated from each other (Woods, 1964)—but such animals show no evidence of learning. It will be convenient to consider the CNS at various levels and to examine what evidence is available as to its role in behaviour.

Spinal Cord

Despite a few claims to the contrary, the concensus of opinion appears to be that not even the simplest components of learning can be demonstrated in the spinal cord. Evidently this view is based upon a definition of learning that includes nothing simpler than complex skilled acts as seen in instrumental conditioning. From the point of view of the more fundamental definition—that includes the acquisition of control of the motor system—learning must occur at spinal levels, so that preferred routes of impulses occur between the pyramidal neurones and the ventral horn cells. Learning at the spinal level then, is restricted to the development of basic motor skills that are available for application in higher learning processes.

SENSORY NUCLEI

Lesions in the thalamus have almost always had a deleterious effect upon learning capacity, but by and large no thalamic nuclei are specifically involved. Naturally, destruction of the nucleus subserving a particular sensory mode, e.g. the lateral geniculate body, has a most serious effect upon learning which requires the integrity of that form of sensation, e.g. visual tasks. With regard to stimulation, the situation is different. A stimulus which is destined (by experimental design) to become the trigger for a learned task produces, after a series of presentations, a rhythmic discharge in the ventral anterior and central median nuclei at a frequency of 5 c/s. The significance of this is unknown. In the modality of audition it has already been pointed out in the section on Sensation (pp. 35–95) that complex neural events occur at several levels in this system and auditory learning is no exception. If a particular sound is repeatedly presented to an animal, it initially induces evoked potentials in the cochlear nuclei and in the medial geniculate bodies; these electrical responses then cease to be evoked (habituation). However, if the same sound is then used as a conditioned stimulus by pairing with an unconditioned stimulus, such as electroshock to the skin, the evoked potentials in the cochlear nuclei and medial geniculate bodies return. Evidently, these lower levels of the sensory system are able to evaluate the significance of any particular stimulus and can avoid habituation. This capacity, perhaps, explains the fact that electrical stimulation of lower levels (such as parts of the thalamus and midbrain) can be made into a conditioned stimulus by pairing with a suitable peripheral unconditioned stimulus. Whether such subcortical stimuli reach consciousness is a moot point, but it seems likely that they represent a sensory input that differs from other conditioned stimuli simply in being generated at a higher point in the system than the receptors.

LIMBIC SYSTEM

One of the most important recent reorientations in neurophysiology is the realization that the ancient components of the limbic system are not to be relegated to primitive functions only, but must be considered whenever a higher function is being examined. As yet, no clear picture can be drawn of the role that limbic structures play in learning—any more than with other parts of the brain—but the available data show them to be definitely implicated. Lesions of the septum do not seem to affect the ability to learn, but they have frequently impaired the capacity for recall; rather surprisingly, animals with septal lesions exhibit an enhanced rate of learning conditioned avoidance responses. Lesions in the amygdaloid nuclei reduce the rate of conditioned avoidance response learning but have no effect upon recall. In both the amygdaloid nuclei and in the hippocampus (Fig. 59), an auditory conditioned stimulus produces evoked potentials of large amplitude with a frequency of 40–45 c/s. With various types of trigger stimulus, waves of new electrical activity sweep through the hippocampus during the interval that separates the conditioned from the unconditioned stimulus. No explanation of these limbic responses readily presents itself, although one may suppose that they are intimately related to concurrent events in the neocortex and reticular formation.

RETICULAR FORMATION

It has been pointed out in the section on sensory phenomena that all modalities send collaterals to the midbrain reticular formation. Hence it can occasion no surprise that stimuli which are destined to become trigger events in learning produce, as all stimuli do, excitation of the reticular formation, This excitation plays an important role in the maintenance of consciousness and in the alerting reaction. But mere repetition of any given stimulus is rapidly accompanied by habituation in the reticular formation, so that excitation no longer occurs, or occurs to a much lower degree. When the repetitive stimulus is paired with an unconditioned stimulus, however, and hence takes on the properties of a conditioned stimulus or trigger, then excitation of the reticular formation continues. Under these conditions it takes the form of rhythmic waves of activity sweeping through the reticular formation at a rate of about 5 c/s. Rather interestingly, this response seems to be in some way related to other incoming stimuli, for whereas the effect may outlast the conditioned stimulus by as long as a minute

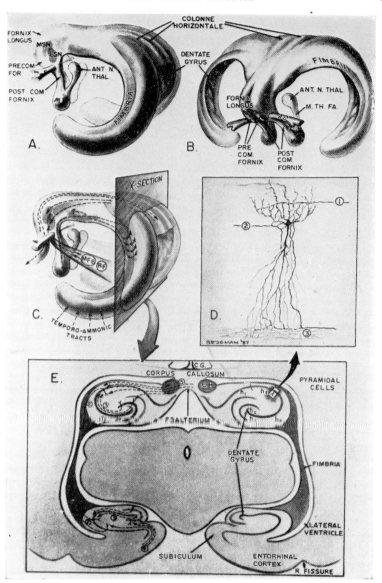

FIG. 59. Diagrams of the hippocampus of the cat. A, From the left side. B, From the front. C, From the left side with conduction paths superimposed. D, Terminations of afferents about a hippocampal pyramid; 1, from the alveus, 2, from dentate granule cells, and 3, from the temporo-ammonic tract. E, Schematic cross section at level shown in C; 1, afferents from the fimbria to the dentate gyrus; 2, axons of pyramidal cells; 3, dentato-pyramidal fibres; 5, fibres from the colonne horizontale and psalterium; h_1 to h_5 show the approximate locations of pyramidal neurone fields. (From Green, 1960.)

when the test animal is in the "test box", the response disappears
almost immediately when the conditioned stimulus is given in some
other locality. It rather looks as though the "test box" situation
generates stimuli which have also become conditioned without the
experimenter's volition.

CEREBRAL CORTEX

It is understandable, but unfortunate, that much more work has
been aimed at examining the role of the cerebral cortex in behaviour
than has been applied to subcortical structures. Probably, as mentioned above, this is due to a preoccupation with the idea that the
cerebral cortex must have a vast importance because of its size in man,
notwithstanding the abundant evidence that most of man's activities
and probably all of lower animals' activities are generated by subcortical structures and only modulated or modified by cortical mechanisms.
Studies upon the cerebral cortex are of very great value, provided the
role of the cortex is properly understood. The mere fact that no kind
of stimulation in any part of the cortex has ever evoked a learned
response should be sufficient evidence, *for the moment*, that the
cortex does not play an essential role in learning beyond the
acquisition of simple motor co-ordination. Few would doubt that the
cortex is of prime importance in mediating the precise form in which
learned phenomena are expressed. It evidently also contains mechanisms able to effect the highest degree of differentiation of stimuli and
selectivity of response. In these ways the cortex has a dominant role
to play in the subtleties and nuances of learned behaviour. But, as
pointed out above, in the absence of cortex learning remains; only
the superficial, i.e. useful but not essential, aspects are absent. Even
with the large amount of effort put into the problem, no good description of cortical functioning during learning can be given. It is to be
hoped that future research, perhaps more operationally orientated,
will produce meaning for the following meagre and ill-understood
data. (For an account of more basic studies of cortical neuronal organization and learning, the reader should consult the section on Neuroendocrinology, pp. 158–175.)

In many experiments, total ablation of the cortex has had practically
no deleterious effect upon the simpler forms of learning, i.e. Type I
conditioning. Severe defect and often total abolition occur when decorticate animals are subjected to Type II learning procedures, especially
those that demand evasive action. Non-specific removal of up to 50%
of the cortex has little effect upon simple learning, even up to the

point of a motor response such as bar-pressing. More complex tasks are correspondingly more sensitive to cortical ablations, and animals with about 30% loss of cortex may completely lose the power to learn tasks that involve traversive movements such as shifting keys along vertical and horizontal grooves in Perspex sheeting.

As mentioned in the section on cortical organization (p. 185), loss of specific sensory areas of cortex have different effects at different levels of the phylogenetic scale. In the higher animals this intervention completely abolishes the capacity to learn tasks in which the trigger stimulus is in the modality of the ablated region unless these tasks are of the simplest kind, such as intensity discrimination. Even with this type of learning, there are usually abundant signs of poor retention. In man, the situation is worse in that even very simple tasks are learned with difficulty or not at all. This has been known for a long time with regard to the special senses and has recently been shown to be true for somatic modalities. A penetrating wound that destroyed the hand region of somatosensory cortex prevented the individual from learning tasks with that hand (Ghent *et al.*, 1955). There is little doubt, however, that all or most of these effects, at least in higher animals are due to interference with sensation rather than with learning mechanisms as such.

The only studies on what are traditionally considered to be association areas have been carried out in the region around the primary visual cortex, area 18. The remarkable findings are that destruction of this area does not affect the animal's ability to learn and retain efficient performance in visual colour or form discriminatory tasks. Evidently, in the absence of area 18 the animal is still capable of relating fairly complex visual stimuli to the reward provided. This may be a consequence of the rather primitive type of reward (food). As pointed out above, auditory signals activate the limbic system and it is reasonable to assume that visual stimuli do this also and that where crude, visceral rewards are at stake, the ancient limbic structures are more concerned than the neocortex. The prestriate cortex (area 18) may apply its associating powers to the *interpretation* of complex visual stimuli that are discriminated on a crude basis elsewhere. Even the regions in the posterior part of the parietal lobe that are believed to have important associating functions can be ablated without much effect upon learning capacity.

The frontal lobes have been rather more rewarding. Ablations in this region are routinely followed by deficiencies in learning, without modal specificity. Once again, such lesions have little effect upon the learning of simple tasks but are more important when the task requires some rather special activity such as traversive movements. Delayed responses—which are considered to be an estimate of rather higher learning—are very adversely affected, though some observers believe that this is due to a defect in attentiveness. It is claimed that if great care is taken to avoid distracting conditions monkeys with frontal lobe lesions are able to perform delayed response tasks as efficiently as intact animals. This region of cerebral cortex also seems to have a special role to play in inhibition—a fact that will occasion little surprise, perhaps, to those who have witnessed the personality changes following frontal leucotomy in man. In monkeys trained to refrain from certain actions (negative response) following the presentation of a stimulus, frontal lobe lesions are accompanied by a positive response to the stimulus; their ability to restrain themselves is greatly diminished. Serial learning—again looked upon as representing a higher form of accomplishment—is adversely affected by very large ablations anywhere in the cerebral cortex, but quite small lesions in the frontal lobes cause animals trained in this way to make faulty reactions, such as carrying out a response before it should be done (anticipation) or repeating a response instead of going on to the next one (perseveration).

Stimulation of almost any part of the cerebral cortex (but *not* the motor areas) can be made into a trigger stimulus by pairing with an unconditioned stimulus. Hence, animals are able to learn to make correct responses when a part of the cerebral cortex experiences enhanced excitation, irrespective of what role such excitation plays under normal conditions provided it does not directly control the motor apparatus. The effect does not depend upon transcortical connexions for circumsection of the "conditioned area" does not affect the efficiency of the response; undercutting, however, destroys the effect. A full discussion of this topic is to be found in the review by Wells (1963).

During the process of learning the spontaneous electrical activity of the cerebral cortex undergoes several changes. It is well known that the occipital cortex (and to a less extent other parts of the cortex) exhibits, in the quiet, eyes-closed state, rhythmic waves of excitation whose frequency varies from about 10 c/s in man to 5–20 c/s in animals. This is the α-rhythm. Also well known is the fact that mere opening of the eyes, allowing light to enter, causes the α-rhythm to disappear, with a latency that is proportional to the intensity of the light. It must be clearly realized that it is the α-*rhythm* that disappears, not electrical activity; the basic resting rhythm of the species under investigation is replaced by another rhythm (see below). This so-called α-blocking response also occurs with stimuli in other modes and with a concentration of attention. Any kind of new and unfamiliar stimulus will also result in cessation of the α-rhythm, hence a stimulus that is destined (by experimental design) to become a trigger for action initially has this effect. New stimuli that do not become conditioned are followed, on repetition, by habituation and eventually no longer cause α-blocking. By and large it seems that trigger stimuli cause α-blocking to appear first in parietal association areas and later in the region related to the corresponding sensory mode. Most workers feel that α-blocking is a secondary event to the primary one, which is activation of the mid-brain reticular formation. In the section on Consciousness (pp. 246–255) it will be seen that any sudden sensory input causes the midbrain reticular formation to discharge excitatory impulses to many parts of the cerebral cortex. Such a widespread discharge serves to bring a sleeping animal back to consciousness or to bring a drowsy animal to the alert state. Clearly this mechanism must be of great importance in learning for the latter would hardly be expected to occur efficiently unless the subject were alert. Thus it can be seen that the initial effects of a stimulus are to produce diffuse and non-specific excitation of the cortex, which automatically displaces the α-rhythm.

Continued repetition of the stimulus results either in habituation (if the stimulus remains unassociated with meaningful events) or in enhanced excitation of a more specific nature. When the new stimulus is repetitive on a short-term basis, e.g. a flashing light or very low-frequency sound, then the appropriate part of the cortex shows evoked potentials that are synchronous with the frequency of the stimulus. When synchronous activity is produced in this manner the cortical cells are said to be "driven"; hence, with a flashing light there is said to be "photic-driving" of the cells in the visual cortex. If such a short-term repetitive stimulus is made to become a trigger for a learned response, it frequently induces a quite new rhythm of cortical activity independent of the stimulus-frequency. Conditioned stimuli of this kind in the human have shown frequencies that range from 5 to 30 c/s and most workers seem to be agreed that these new rhythms occur in parallel fashion with the development of any particular piece of learning. Indeed, the degree to which such new rhythms are established is frequently taken to correspond to the degree of completion of a conditioning process.

SUMMARY

From the above data, there can be no doubt that various parts of the cerebral cortex have some sort of part to play in learning, especially when something rather complicated—either sensory or motor—is involved. Exactly what part it plays and for how long are still matters for cogitation. Sperry (1945) has suggested that when the cortex does play a role in learning, it may do this only while learning is actually taking place, and that when the response has become automatized the controlling regions are subcortical. According to Pribram (1963) an essential feature of learning (and other higher functions) is the capacity of the CNS to compare incoming signals with experimental stores to see if there is match or mis-match. Only in the latter situation is there any novelty about the organism's response, including whatever internal responses are at the root of learning. It is reasonable to assume that much or all of the stored data is "in" the cortex and that at least one of the functions of the cortex is to carry out the comparison procedure in search of mis-match. When matching occurs, it may well be that the responsibility for the known (i.e. learned) appropriate response is placed in the control of subcortical structures. If this be true then the experimental procedure of determining the number of trials required for perfect response is really a measure of how long it takes for the cortex to achieve perfect (or near-perfect) matching and to relegate the actual performance to lower levels, retaining only slight interest as an inspectorate. This lends even more support to the argument that the role of the cortex may have been grossly overestimated and subcortical structures most unjustly dismissed from attention.

Neural Basis

At the very outset of a section under this heading it must be admitted that no precise factual account can be given of the neural basis of learning. The best that can be done is to consider some of the speculations of workers in the field and to give some idea of the lines along which current research is proceeding. Only recently, with the advent of refined electron micrographic and electrophysiological methods, has a deeply rooted pessimism been removed. Earlier workers were either of the kind who speculated wildly on a minimum of experimental data or of the type who worked hard and long to collect the facts and despaired that understanding would ever come. A more temperate attitude has for some time been discernible, characterized by a patient reappraisal of old data, painstaking search for new facts, guarded speculation and a sustaining degree of optimism that the neuronal changes underlying learning will eventually be understood. In general terms, speculation and research have centred around two main lines of thought, which will be dealt with now.

SYNAPTIC MODIFICATION

A highly attractive idea to many neurologists is the concept that learning (and other higher functions) is fundamentally due to changes in the phenomena at the synapse, leading to alterations of synaptic resistance. In simple terms the idea is that at any particular neuro-neural junction a certain set of conditions pertains in the "unused" state. Such conditions include the number of dendrites, the number of synaptic end-knobs, the area of the postsynaptic cell body, the thickness of the presynaptic axon and all other features that are pertinent to the transmission of information from one nerve cell to another. The "unused state" really means the condition of the junction when the two neurones have hardly been used at all. The general thesis is that repetitive use of a neuro-neural junction (as in the process of learning) causes another set of conditions to obtain at that synapse. These other conditions—which have actually been demonstrated to occur when a junction is stimulated a great deal—include increase in the number of dendrites, swelling of the dendritic terminals, increase in diameter of the axons and increase in number and length of axon side-processes. Conversely, when a junction that has been actively stimulated is allowed to remain unused for a time, these conditions are reversed and the general effect is a decrement in all features that aid neuro-neural transmission.

In addition to the changes in neurones outlined above, there are features of neuroglial organization that have led some investigators to implicate these in learning (and other) processes. Careful studies of these "supporting" elements have shown that they are capable of developing processes in an amoeboid fashion. The close application of neuroglia to neurones and their enormous numbers suggests that these processes could come to lie between two neurones, i.e. to bridge synaptic junctions. From one point of view, the projection of neuroglial processes into synaptic spaces would reduce the ease of neuro-neural transmission by acting as mechanical or chemical barriers. (It has been claimed that a cholinesterase is present in at least some neuroglia.) From another viewpoint, regarding at least the oligodendroglia as having a predominantly metabolic role, the interposition of glial processes between and around nerve cells might have an advantageous effect upon learning. This matter is dealt with in fuller detail in the section on Memory (pp. 256–266), but here we may note that the neurochemists have clearly demonstrated an increase in ribonucleic acid (RNA) content of activated nerve cells, whereas in the closely associated oligodendroglia the amount of RNA is decreased. Further, it has been shown that after a learning procedure, appropriate changes occur in the concentration ratios of specific nucleotides (Hyden and Egyhazi, 1962). Such findings have led to the fertile speculation that learning is fundamentally a matter of the biochemical effects that nerve impulses have upon neurones. No longer can the nerve impulse be looked upon as a piece of excitation that simply traverses certain paths in the CNS and eventually ends up in an effector organ. It may exert very important effects within the CNS. Briefly, the theory (Smith, 1962) is that nerve impulses cause enzyme induction in the neurones through which they pass, thereby causing the latter to change their protein production in such a way that specific geometrical patterns of protein molecules are formed. It is this pattern that represents the memory trace that is so essential to the learning process. If this theory be true, then it seems clear that the oligodendroglia may well have an essential part in these biochemical interactions.

NEURONAL CIRCUITRY

Explanations of learning based upon alterations in neuronal circuits have been popular since Pavlovian times, and some workers believe that learning will eventually be shown to consist in biochemical changes and circuit alterations working together. Pavlov considered that in the process of conditioning, irradiation of excitation (see p. 218) in the cerebral cortex sets up preferential conduction paths between the region concerned with the unconditioned stimulus and the region involved with the conditioned stimulus. The fact that vertical cuts in the cortex between two such regions have no effect upon a learned response seems to be adequate evidence for dismissing this theory as stated, but leaves intact the possibility that the preferred path is reflected from one cortical area to the other by some subcortical structure. Similarly, the idea that fields of excitation come to surround cortical areas is difficult to accept, partly because the imagination boggles at the complexity of the overlapping (but presumably not interacting) fields that would have to exist in a well-educated organism, and partly because neither implanted conductors nor insulators have had any effect upon learned responses.

The widespread occurrence of circuit arrangements that allow for reverberation of impulses from an axon back to the cell body has given rise to the speculation that this phenomenon explains learning. While only few workers would look upon this as the complete mechanism, it could evidently form a most important feature of learning since the latter must be based upon the passage of nerve impulses, and reverberating circuits reinforce whatever effect was produced by the initial impulse. Also, it must not be thought that reverberation is confined to single neurones. There is no doubt that it occurs also in neurone chains, so that repetitive excitation can pass back from a remote cell to the beginning of the chain.

Several other tentative explanations have been put forward, but these do not seem to have sufficient evidential basis to warrant discussion except at the most advanced levels. Recently, the mathematically-minded neurophysiologist has entered the field and there is already an unwieldy number of symbolic "models" of various brain functions including learning. The reader interested in these is referred to the excellent volume edited by Wiener and Schade (1963).

CHAPTER 14

CONSCIOUSNESS

From the neurophysiological point of view it is necessary from the beginning to beware of subjective definitions of consciousness, with which texts of philosophy and psychology abound. It is easy to feel that there is something significant in such statements as "consciousness is awareness", "consciousness is the appreciation of environmental stimuli", or in the words of William James, "consciousness is the function of knowing". Useful as these statements may be in explaining mental phenomena in a non-material manner, they are neurophysiologically tautologous. To say that "consciousness is awareness of the self and the environment", is saying nothing that is not already self-evident. Concepts such as the above arise from the abstract approach to consciousness. There are three reasons why earlier investigators used an introspective, abstract approach: (1) experimental techniques were inadequate for anything but abstract studies; (2) consciousness was by and large looked upon as an attribute restricted to the human species, and (3) most germane, it was truly realized that consciousness is indeed an abstraction. Consciousness, like beauty, like blueness, like happiness, is in the mind of the beholder and nowhere else. What exists outside the mind of the beholder is a collection of material substances and events which give rise to the subjective impression of consciousness. Advances in the neurophysiology of consciousness began to occur only when workers studied directly this collection of material substances and events.

Sleep

It was recognized very early in man's intellectual history that the state of consciousness is sometimes absent. Such a condition is called unconsciousness and it occurs in several forms from natural sleep through anaesthesia and coma to death. It would be appropriate at this point to consider very briefly the characteristics of natural sleep so that it may be readily distinguished from the other forms of unconsciousness. In *natural sleep* there occurs a slowing of the heart rate and regular respiration; the metabolic rate is reduced and the carbon dioxide tension of the blood rises, so that the kidney excretes a more concentrated, more acidic urine; the eyes are usually closed and the pupils exhibit a slight constriction; Babinski's sign is positive; quite frequently the posture is more or less characteristic (e.g. man, horse, bird, cat, dog). Animals that normally sleep standing up could not maintain the erect posture in coma or anaesthesia for the supporting reflexes would be abolished. Perhaps the most useful and most easily demonstrable character of natural sleep is that the organism can be awakened by physiological stimuli, hence the extensive trade in alarm clocks. Several theories have been put forward to account for sleep, but most of them do not bear close analysis and none of them has good experimental support except the purely neurological ones. An early idea that is still part of the general explanation was put forward by Pavlov. He postulated that negative conditioning (q.v.) produced a widespread process of internal inhibition. Nearer the present day mark were the findings of von Economo in the disease that bears his name. Von Economo noticed that in encephalitis lethargica, a syndrome accompanied by a condition that closely approximates natural sleep, there were lesions in the posterior hypothalamus. Experimental support for these findings came in the work of Hess. It would be appropriate to consider this in more detail here, before passing on to the mechanisms of consciousness.

THE TROPHOTROPIC REGION

Hess (1929) and his colleagues have described a "trophotropic region" in the cat. Medially it is bounded by the massa intermedia, caudally by the habenulo-interpeduncular tract, and rostrally by the mammillo-thalamic bundle. Its lateral limits were difficult to define because of the nearness of the thalamus. This region was electrically stimulated in normal cats fitted with EEG leads and the result was a progressive decrease of activity or gradual loss of consciousness. With 1 min stimulation the animal would sit or lie down; with 2 min stimulation the cat would curl up into a restful posture; with 3 min stimulation the animal would go to sleep. Such behaviour is very close to what is observed when the animals go to sleep spontaneously. There is no sudden collapse, but instead the slow adoption of a normal posture and a quiet lapse into unconsciousness. Further, the EEG tracings were significant. The desynchronized waking trace changed to the synchronized form when stimulation was applied. Ordinary physiological stimuli could be used to awaken the animal behaviourally and to return the EEG trace back to the desynchronized form.

So it rather looks as though *stimulation* of neurones in this region of the brain is able to induce a state indistinguishable from natural sleep. Once started the state continues as with natural sleep until a stimulus brings it to an end. It was asked whether the electrodes might have caused some kind of damage leading to inhibition. But the same techniques applied to other parts of the brain always caused excitation and anyway the effects of an electrolytic lesion would be expected to be permanent. In this regard it has also been pointed out that lesions in the trophotropic region do not interfere with the induction of normal sleep. This may be due to the diffuse nature of this part of the brain; lesions large enough to destroy most of it would be incompatible with life. Again, it could be that natural sleep does not involve Hess's hypnogenic area. We shall return to this point after dealing with the available data regarding consciousness.

SPINOTHALAMIC PATHWAYS

This term is used here to denote the classical sensory pathways, both somatic and special. From the receptor a neurone passes to the CNS; a postsynaptic fibre runs to the thalamus and from there a tertiary fibre carries the information to the sensory cortex. Interest in the spinothalamic systems with regard to consciousness stems from a discovery by Bremer (1935). He found that a midbrain section resulted in a state of sleep in front of the section, both behaviourally and with respect to the EEG trace. At first glance, it was reasonable to assume that the condition of the *"cerveau isolé"* was due to the interruption of spinothalmic pathways. But careful study showed that this was not the whole story. For example, destruction of thalmic regions or sensory cortical areas did not result in any lack of consciousness. Similarly, it was well known clinically that complete section of the spinal cord at high levels in man was not accompanied by any detectable decrease in awareness. Therefore, it was apparent that something other than or in addition to the classical sensory pathways is involved in the maintenance of a waking state.

MIDBRAIN RETICULAR FORMATION

A chance discovery by a worker of wisdom and experience led to the modern concept of consciousness. Magoun (1950) and his colleagues, about 1949, noticed that drowsy or sleepy animals would become alert or awake if the midbrain reticular formation were stimulated. The term reticular activating system (RAS) covers an anatomically rather diffuse meshwork of fibres and cell bodies, the limits of which

are difficult to define and which seem to expand in proportion to the
number of investigators working on reticular matters. Reference
should be made to modern anatomical works for topographical
details. It should be emphasized at the beginning that the RAS is not
exclusively concerned with matters of consciousness. A recent review
(Jasper, 1958) indicates the extent to which reticular regions are
implicated in neurophysiology.

Magoun's observations showed that excitation of the RAS resulted
in an immediate behavioural change from the drowsy to the alert,
accompanied by appropriate changes in the EEG trace. This phenomenon has been called the alerting response, activation reaction,
desynchronization response and blocking reaction. The EEG changes
closely resembled the traces seen when a sleeping animal is aroused
by normal external stimuli. Hence, it was thought important to examine
in a physiological manner the relation between the RAS and the
classical spinothalamic sensory pathways. With recording electrodes
in the RAS, animals were subjected to various peripheral stimuli,
e.g. clicks for auditory modality, electroshock to sciatic nerve for
somatic modality. It was found that the application of such stimuli
induced electrical activity in the RAS. The response was more wave-
like than spike-like and had a rather long latency, suggesting that the
recorded activity originated in some multi-neuronal organization.
When two different kinds of stimuli, such as the click and the shock,
were given in succession, in any order, each stimulus produced a
response in the RAS, but the second of the pair gave an attenuated
response. This is evidently an example of occlusion and implies that
both modalities were sending information to the same neurones. All
modalities of sensation have now been tested in this way and all give
similar results. These findings show clearly that there is some kind
of connexion between all sensory pathways and the RAS.

Investigating this relationship further, various workers have
studied the effects of lesions in various species, including man (Fig.
60). Their findings are quite harmonious. Lesions in the anterior part
of the RAS result in permanent coma with a hypersynchronized EEG
that is unaffected by peripheral stimuli, however strong. Such lesions
did not interrupt the classical spinothalamic pathways. Hence the
integrity and activity of these pathways is not sufficient to maintain
consciousness. Lesions placed ventrally and dorsally to the RAS,
clearly interrupting the spinothalamic pathways, did not affect the
EEG trace, not did they produce any behavioural signs of impaired
consciousness. These findings show clearly that the integrity of the

classical sensory systems is not essential for the maintenance of an awake condition.

Single-unit recording from the RAS has shown that there is tonic electrical activity in all of the neuronal elements so far studied. Magoun and his colleagues have suggested that the waking state,

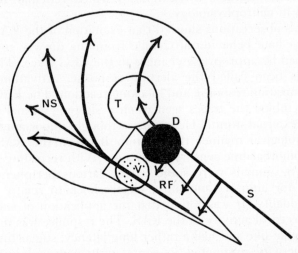

FIG. 60. Diagram to illustrate the major mechanism of consciousness and the alerting reaction. The sensory input (S), both somatic and special, reaches the thalamus (T) and is projected in a specific fashion to the primary areas of the cerebral cortex. Dorsal lesions in the brain stem (D) which interrupt this specific pathway do not affect consciousness. Nerve fibres from all sense modalities send collaterals to the reticular formation (RF), from which information is relayed in a non-specific manner to many parts of the cortex (NS). Ventral lesions in the brain stem (V) that do not interrupt the specific sensory pathway produce a state of sleep or drowsiness.

i.e. the conscious state, is maintained by impulses passing by *collateral* branches from the classical sensory pathways to the reticular forma-tion (Fig. 60). The RAS is thereby caused to transmit tonic impulses by anatomically unknown routes to the cerebral cortex. Electrical recording from the cortex shows that the output of the RAS is very widespread but principally to the so-called association areas. Bremer's condition of *encephale isolée* becomes understandable now. Midbrain section prevents a large part of the RAS from relaying information to the cortex, and in the absence of such information the cortex goes to sleep as seen by EEG traces.

In some ways it would seem that anaesthetics act as a kind of temporary midbrain section. This has been shown by inserting recording electrodes into the cerebral cortex and into the RAS. Arduini and Arduini (1954) found that when the *waking* cat was presented with an auditory (click) stimulus, activity was generated in both the primary auditory cortex and in the RAS; but when the animal was *anaesthetized*, the click no longer produced an action potential in the RAS whereas the cortical spike was undiminished. It seems likely therefore that a range of conditions resulting in unconsciousness may be due to depression of RAS activity. There is evidence that such drugs as chlorpromazine exert their tranquillizing effects by means of a partial depression of the activity of the RAS. It is, of course, possible that additional mechanisms are also in operation when anaesthetics and tranquillizers are producing their effects.

One point to be noticed is that in the above experiments on anaesthetized animals, the creatures would ordinarily be described as unconscious, i.e. *unaware* of the click stimulus. But the primary auditory cortex reacted in an apparently normal fashion to the external sound. This point will be taken up again later.

THE CEREBRAL CORTEX

From what has been said so far, the implication is that arousal from sleep or a drowsy state is produced by, firstly in time, sensory impulses passing to the RAS by collaterals from classical pathways and, secondly in time, by impulses passing from the RAS to the cortex. This explanation of consciousness brings the cortex into the situation at the end. Some of Bremer's more recent work indicates that this is an oversimplification. He showed (1953) that electrical stimulation of any point on the cortex results in increased electrical activity of the RAS. Further, if a sensory stimulus and a cortical stimulus are applied in succession in any order, then the second stimulus is followed by an attenuated action potential in the RAS demonstrating occlusion. As with different sense modalities so with somatic and cerebral inputs —they both impinge upon a common neuronal network. Further evidence that the cerebral cortex is involved in consciousness comes from experiments in which a primary sensory area (say auditory) is ablated. Modal stimuli (in this case, sounds) do not waken such a preparation from normal sleep, whereas stimuli in other modalities continue to do so. Hence, while the cerebral cortex may not be sufficient to maintain consciousness, it is evidently necessary.

Bremer proposed that the explanation outlined at the beginning of the previous paragraph is incomplete. What must be added is the concept that the cortex plays a part in its own arousal and maintenance of wakefulness by means of cortico-reticular impulses. On this basis, consciousness involves a centralization, modification and diffusion by the RAS of information brought to it either directly by collaterals from the classical sensory pathways, or indirectly after the infromation has passed through the thalamus and circulated through the cerebral cortex. There seems to be no reason to suppose that cortico-reticular impulses must have an immediate sensory antecedent. Purely cortical activity—thinking—may give rise to information being sent to the RAS. Such a mechanism may underlie the condition of psychogenic insomnia. Cortical activity due to some such reason as anxiety may maintain a ceaseless bombardment of the RAS and so maintain the arousal for long periods. Such cortico-reticular mechanisms also afford an explanation for the long-known and everyday experience that *significant* stimuli of low intensity (e.g. baby crying) can arouse a person under conditions where non-significant sounds of much higher intensity (e.g. traffic noises) do not. During sleep it is likely that external stimuli excite the RAS in the usual way and that the RAS relays the information to the cortex. Only if cortical examination of the stimuli attributes importance to them does a cortico-reticular flow occur and arousal result. These discriminative mechanisms may be restricted to nervous systems of the more sophisticated, i.e. primate, kind.

THE CENTRENCEPHALIC SYSTEM

Postulation that the cerebral cortex exerts a role before the end of the sequence of events that maintains consciousness recalls the findings of Penfield (1951) in the human. This neurosurgeon has for many years obtained the co-operation of patients undergoing brain operations. His results have led him to put forward ideas that are highly relevant to the problem of consciousness, inasmuch as the patients were able to describe what they were conscious of. Further, these findings bring to the study of consciousness something rather more definite and tangible than mere wakefulness. They involve both perception and affect.

Electrical stimulation of the primary sensory regions of the cerebral cortex in the unanaesthetized patient produced awareness of primary sensations. The patients reported seeing flashes of light or colours when the visual cortex was stimulated; buzzes, clicks and sighs with stimulation of auditory cortex; tinglings, numbness and phantom movement with stimulations of the somatic sensory area. Vertical cuts through the cortex around the stimulated regions did not affect the production of "hallucinations". Hence it seemed unlikely that transcortical connexions were involved. Penfield suggested that the awareness of primary sensation is not a purely cortical phenomenon. If the cortex is concerned at all, it does not receive information from its primary areas directly, but via some subcortical structure. This structure Penfield called the "centrencephalic system". Little wisdom is required to appreciate the similarities between the hypothesized centrencephalic system and the later experimentally demonstrated reticular activating system.

Perhaps the most intriguing of Penfield's findings were obtained when the superior and lateral surface of the temporal lobe were stimulated. Under these conditions the patients were conscious, not of primary sensations, but of coherent, well-organized sense data. They did not see flashes but saw trees, houses, people; they did not hear clicks, but heard a voice singing or a piano playing. Usually several sense modalities were involved so that the patient experienced an integrated continuum made up of all the sensory components that a real scene would have. No element of the bizarre or fantastic attaches to the "temporal lobe hallucinations". Reality of this kind would be expected when it is realized that the hallucination produced by temporal lobe stimulation is something that the patient has actually experienced in the recent or distant past. The patient remembers having had that experience before on some specific occasion. He does not report a song being sung in a general, vague sort of way. He reports that he can hear a song being sung in all particulars as he heard it once before. It is being sung by the same person, at the same tempo, with the same accompaniment and often with the same visual surroundings. Each hallucination is sharply defined as an isolated incident, with no overlapping or montage effects, and each hallucination carries with it the particular effect—joy, sadness, surprise—that was present on the original occasion. When the same spot on the temporal lobe was stimulated a second time shortly after the first, sometimes the same hallucination appeared. But if a longer period elapsed between the two stimulations, then an entirely different scene from the patient's past was enacted. Hence, it is not the cortical neurones themselves that contain the "sensory record". The record is somewhere else and stimulation of the temporal lobe somehow arranges for the record to be brought to consciousness. As with the primary areas, vertical cuts around the temporal regions in no way affect the results, so once again the phenomenon is not due to transcortical pathways but to some subcortical structure—the centrencephalic system.

I

Note that temporal lobe hallucinations are not properly described as the elicitation of *memories*. The patient does not merely remember a song being sung; he *hears* the song. One of Penfield's patients refused to believe that there was not a record player in the theatre. What happens when the appropriate part of the temporal lobe is stimulated is that the patient has an instant of *consciousness* that he had once before. From these findings Penfield put forward an explanation of consciousness. Afferent sensory impulses are received by the primary sensory areas of the cortex. These project information down to a subcortical structure that is functionally common to both hemispheres. In some way the centrencephalic system records the informational pattern received from the cortex and in the process of doing so projects the pattern onto the temporal cortex. Consciousness, in this view, consists in the making of a sensory record. What the subject is conscious of at any instant is what is being recorded at that instant, and if the pattern of neuronal activity that corresponds to that instant of consciousness is reactivated, then the subject has an identical instant of consciousness.

General Mechanism

As far as the matter of remaining conscious is concerned, we have evidence and interpretations from three independent lines of approach which we can conceive in one general mechanism of consciousness. From the Magoun system we have the constant bombardment of the cerebral cortex by sensory information that has been amplified and spread out by the RAS. At the same time, on the Bremer system, the cerebral cortex is examining its data and sending fresh information to the RAS. This structure could be said to represent Penfield's centrencephalic system, which is recording all this information including that from purely cortical activity so that we record what we feel about what we sense, and the RAS–centrencephalic system projects to the temporal lobe cortex. It is this process of recording and projecting that *is* consciousness.

If all this be true, then it is easy to see how natural sleep occurs. Part of the mechanism is the reduction of sensory input, removing the Magoun system. Another part is the reduction of cortical activity—thinking—removing the Bremer system. With these systems inactive there can be none of Penfield's recording and projecting, and when there is no recording and projecting there is no consciousness. Naturally, this is by no means an all-or-none mechanism. Common sense observations show degrees of unconsciousness or levels of drowsiness. Evidently the various subdepartments of the consciousness mechanism vary in extent of excitation both conjointly and separately. It is again a matter of familiar experience that consciousness or attention can mainly involve thinking processes to the relative exclusion of external stimuli, or, conversely, may be so dominantly involved with environmental changes that thinking is reduced to a minimum. Only when both kinds of attention are simultaneously reduced does sleep come.

THE TROPHOTROPIC CENTRE

On the above general view of consciousness, sleep is associated with decreasing neuronal activity. Accordingly to Hess, sleep can be induced by an *increase* of neuronal activity. No great problem is involved in postulating that activation of the trophotropic region causes inhibition of other structures, such as RAS and cerebral cortex. But what, under physiological conditions, would be likely to excite the hypnogenic centre? It is a matter of common observation that even if the sensory input is artificially maintained at a high level by continued external stimulation, the organism eventually becomes unconscious, with or without an intervening period of insanity. Such familiar occurrences as people going to sleep on noisy trains or when marching, suggest that the mechanism outlined in earlier paragraphs does not always apply. Perhaps it is under these extreme conditions that Hess's region becomes involved. It is possible that the sensory input all the time produces increasing facilitation of Hess's region. If the sensory input is not reduced or cannot be voluntarily reduced, then this facilitation may reach threshold level and the trophotropic region fires off inhibitory impulses which command unconsciousness. According to this view, Hess's region may play little or no part in normal sleep but may exert an important role as a safety device under extreme conditions. The matter is open to cogitation.

The preceding account is a simplified and incomplete survey of the experimental data available in the field of consciousness. Several facets have been ignored altogether. Some of these are dealt with in Chapter 16, pp. 267–290. At this point it is enough if this section has demonstrated that an apparently subjective phenomenon is capable of objective study.

CHAPTER 15

MEMORY

As mentioned in the preceding section, it is not easy to draw a warrantable distinction between memory and learning. Quite clearly, memory is an essential feature of any learning process, and yet there seems to be more to memory than just this. From our own experience we know that we can recall past experiences for a sort of internal inspection rather than for the performance of any learned act. This section is concerned with examining the available knowledge about the characteristics of memory, the places in the CNS where it might occur and the mechanism by which engrams are stored.

Characteristics of Memory

MEANINGFUL STIMULI

For memory to occur there must be something to be memorized. That is, there must be some external stimulus or set of stimuli that are dealt with by memory mechanisms. The astonishing amount of recall that can be induced under hypnosis led some workers to conclude that the whole of the sensory input is recorded. An excellent example is the elderly retired bricklayer who was able, under hypnosis, to describe features of some bricks he had laid when a young man. Subsequent checks on the actual building showed his descriptions to be accurate. Even more remarkable, perhaps, are the individuals who reveal under hypnosis memories of conversation among the surgical team when the patient was under general anaesthesia. Nevertheless, when even the most remarkable recollections are considered impartially, it is evident that still only a part of the total input has gone into memory storage. This is not really surprising, for at any waking instant the amount of sensory information entering the nervous system is enormous. What seems to happen is that parts of the sensory input that have some significance, i.e. to which attention is being directed, are the ones that are recorded. The organism is not *conscious* of a good deal of the sensory input that is occurring so continually. It has been mentioned in the section on Sensation (p. 62) that there are several mechanisms by which the CNS is able to reduce the amount of information coming to it in any particular mode. It is this economy of attention that seems to be at the source of what is memorized and what is not. Naturally it is not possible to make out a list of which stimuli are memorized. This will change from time to time according to the organism's shifting estimates of significance. During the exploratory activity of an animal a whole mass of stimuli must be experienced that have no meaning for the creature. It is not unreasonable to assume that the animal promptly forgets them. If, suddenly, a particular stimulus—say an illuminated circle—is found to coincide with food, then by its mere juxtaposition in space and time this stimulus will take on a special meaning and will be recorded.

REPETITION

Only when a stimulus (a) is highly charged with meaning, and (b) falls into a category similar to what has previously been memorized, is it recorded at one presentation. Far more common is the necessity for considerable repetition before a stimulus is safely tucked into the memory store. This is familiar in the number of trials required when teaching animals and is distressingly apparent to those preparing for examinations. Sometimes, as in the latter case, there is a conscious determination to memorize something which in itself carries very little interest to the student. We are all familiar with the extra difficulty, i.e. larger number of repetitions, associated with these attempts to memorize rather insignificant things. It seems as though whatever constitutes the basic mechanism of engram storage needs to be activated a number of times to make it endurable.

TIME REQUIRED

Quite apart from the need for repetition of stimuli, there is no doubt that a certain amount of time is necessary after each presentation for storage to occur. In many, if not all, cases of severe head injury with loss of memory, there is a period of permanent retrograde amnesia that covers the few minutes or seconds immediately prior to the trauma. It seems as though the accident brought to an end the memory mechanisms, which included the laying down of records of what had been recently experienced. Similarly, it has been shown several times that if an animal is subjected to convulsant electroshock some hours after it has been put through a training schedule, this procedure does not affect its retention of the response. However, if the convulsions are produced within a few minutes of training then no such recall occurs. Evidently, as will be shown later, the basic

physico-chemical mechanisms of memory storage are of such a kind
that they do not occur rapidly but require a definite time for completion.

TYPES OF RECALL

Given that a series of engrams have been stored, there are differences in the degree to which they can be brought to consciousness.
By and large the degrees seem to fall into short-term, medium-term
and long-term categories. Short-term ones are those that have a little
but not much significance; for example, the name of someone rather
unimportant to us introduced for the first time, or a telephone number
taken without much intention of ever using it. Most of us would be
able to reproduce these stimuli if called upon to do so within a few
minutes (or sometimes only seconds), but would fail dismally if
required to do the recalling hours or days later. When, however, the
stimulus has rather more meaning, such as the name of someone being
introduced to us, whom we shall *have* to communicate with in the near
future, then this stimulus seems to go into the medium-term storage
and we are able to recall it over a period of days or weeks. Every now
and then, representing only a tiny fraction of the total input, stimuli
occur that have some very extra-special significance to us. These go
into the long-term memory and are retained for immediate recall
over very many years. The contents of an examination syllabus
usually contains examples of all three of these types, differing to a
fair degree with individual student make-up.

CONSOLIDATION OF ENGRAMS

There seems to be a mechanism whereby once a memory is stored
it acquires greater tenacity with the passage of time. In other words,
at any given instant the engrams that are most intact are the ones that
were memorized long ago; those that were most recently memorized
are the most insecure. Again, human post-traumatic amnesia provides
many examples. As temporary retrograde amnesia wears off so, in
every case, the first memories to return are those that were acquired
in the distant past. Shrinkage of the amnesic period regularly occurs
from the past up to the time of trauma, never the other way round.
Similarly, in the aged when powers of memory are fading, the ones that
are clearest and most easily recallable are frequently those from the
individual's early years; it is the happenings of yesterday that are
not retained. Of course, one must also bear in mind that to the elderly
the things that are happening *now* are not nearly as interesting, valuable or important as the things that happened *then*!

Brain Regions Involved in Memory

A good deal of what has been said about the brain regions involved in learning is applicable also to memory. But there are some rather more specific data available for memory, although still not enough to give anything like a clear picture of what is happening. Both subcortical and cortical regions are involved, with many people placing considerable emphasis upon the cerebral cortex. As with learning, so with memory, this latter attitude does not seem to be entirely justified for there is clear evidence that memories are (a) formed with the essential help of subcortical structures and (b) formed in the total absence of cerebral cortex. These points will be examined below. At the moment we are concerned only with those regions that can be shown to play a part in memory to the extent of degree of record and recall. The matter of where engrams are stored will come later.

SUBCORTICAL STRUCTURES

One of the earliest pieces of evidence relating a part of the brain to memory loss was when Korsakow described the pathology of the psychosis that now bears his name. In this condition there is selective damage to the mammillary bodies, with no detectable damage elsewhere, probably due to avitaminosis consequent upon the anorexia of alcoholism. One of the constant and dominant features of the disease is a loss of the ability to memorize. Stored engrams are more or less readily recalled, but the happenings of the last few minutes or hours are either not stored or are stored in a manner that prevents recall. In animals, lesions of the mamillary bodies have produced an apparently similar effect, viz. the inability to remember new training situations.

On the basis of further lesions in regions known to be anatomically related to the mammillary body, some workers have proposed a subcortical circuit scheme. This runs from hippocampus to mammillary body to anterior thalamic nuclei to the cingulate gyrus. Lesions at any point on this circuit—which is highly reminiscent of the Papez scheme for emotional behaviour (see Behaviour, pp. 267–290)—have profoundly deleterious effects upon the ability to memorize. Clearly, the limbic system is again involved, especially when taking account of the fact that electrical stimulation of the amygdala in man causes a similar loss of recent memory.

CEREBRAL CORTEX

In both animals and man there is clear implication of the frontal lobes in the memory mechanism. Frontal lobotomy in the human is routinely followed by impairment of the power to memorize, though this may not be too apparent in daily life. Such patients exhibit very clearly, however, their inability to benefit from practice runs in psychometric testing. Similar conditions are found in the rare cases of bilateral frontal pathology in man and after ablation of the frontal lobes in cat and monkey. In view of the connexions between the hypothalamus and the frontal lobes, some workers consider that the limbic circuit described above works in conjunction with the frontal lobes in a *diencephalo-frontal* mechanism for at least some types of memorizing.

It may also be necessary to include parts of the temporal lobe in the scheme, for several saddening pieces of information are available that implicate the uncal region of the temporal pole in memory in man. Epileptic patients whose EEGs revealed foci in the temporal poles were operated upon for removal of the focus. With unilateral removal of the uncal region only rare cases showed an immediate and permanent loss of the ability to memorize. In each of these rare cases it was later found that a spontaneous lesion of the temporal pole was present on the unoperated side. With bilateral removal of the uncal regions loss of recent memory was the rule. These patients retained all engrams that had been stored prior to the operation but on emergence from the anaesthetic they could remember nothing new for more than a few minutes or in some cases seconds. It needs no emphasis that these results, which leave the patient almost completely incapacitated, were a great shock to the surgeons, who lost no time in issuing a warning to their neurosurgical colleagues. Careful preoperative EEG studies rule out the possibility of such disasters recurring.

Damage to the posterior parietal regions has also been found to be accompanied by impairment of memorizing power coupled with a more or less gradual loss of memories already stored. These areas and the occipital lobe are, of course, intimately involved with vision. With regard to loss of visual memory, Nielson (1958) studied many cases of brain damage and came to some conclusions that include the following. In some people memory patterns for animate objects are located in one occipital lobe and those for inanimate objects are located in the opposite side. Other people have both types of object located in just one hemisphere. The rest of the population has both types of object located in both hemispheres. Incidentally, it is rather interesting that when brain damage results in loss of the power to revisualize, there is also a loss of dreaming capacity (Nielson, 1958).

Site of Storage

Until fairly recently only inspired guesses could be made about the possible sites of storage of engrams, some workers favouring various limbic and subcortical structures and some preferring parts of the cerebral cortex, especially the temporal pole. Even now it is not possible to state precisely where memories are lodged, but at least some good experimental data are available and it seems that more will come very soon. It began with the split-brain preparation. Myers (1955 *et seq.*) found that if a cat was prepared by sectioning the optic chiasma and corpus callosum (so that visual input from each eye was restricted to the ipsilateral hemisphere) it could learn a task through one eye, the other eye being blinkered, but could not carry out that task if the blinker was put over the eye through which the task was learned. This indicated clearly that the stimuli entering one eye under these conditions was "remembered" in one hemisphere. Since the integrity of only a small amount of corpus callosum was sufficient for the task to be performed with both eyes, it seems safe to assume that in the normal animal memory traces are passed between the hemispheres by this route. Indeed, there now seems to be no cause to doubt this, for transfer of memory occurs quite normally if the corpus callosum is sectioned some time after the training period; evidently the transfer occurs during or shortly after the learning process. The work has since been extended to monkeys and to other sense modalities, including tactile, with essentially similar results.

Moreover, another route to much the same conclusions but without the necessity for surgical intervention became available when Bures (1959) utilized the property of spreading inhibition. It was found that if dilute potassium chloride (KCl) was applied to the cerebral cortex, its spontaneous activity and its power to be excited were both depressed. Thus, when KCl was applied to one hemisphere, that half of the cortex was reversibly inactivated and was no longer able to take part in neurological events. Bures found that a tactile task, learned through one paw while one hemisphere was inactivated, was remembered only in the untreated hemisphere. Even though the corpus callosum was intact, the messages that were presumably being sent across it from the untreated hemisphere (contralateral, of course, to the paw being used) were not able to exert their normal effects upon the depressed hemisphere. So far, this work parallels the findings in the surgically prepared monkey.

These two groups of workers then addressed themselves to the problem of the exact site of memory storage in the cortex. One group used surgical ablation to eliminate all but small islands in various parts of the trained hemisphere. The other group took advantage of the power of magnesium chloride ($MgCl_2$) to protect cortical tissue from the effects of KCl; small islands of cortex were treated with $MgCl_2$ prior to treatment of the whole hemisphere with KCl so that the small island retained its activity. Both groups found that a tactile task was remembered if only the paw region of the sensorimotor area was (a) left unablated or (b) left uninactivated. This work seemed to lead to two conclusions. First, that at least with a fairly simple tactile task, vast regions of the cortex are inessential to both the remembrance and the performance of the task. Second, that at least for tactile tasks, the engram was lodged in the sensorimotor cortex corresponding to the part of the body used in the task. These results were duplicated when a visual task was given, only here (in the chiasma-sectioned animal) it was the ipsilateral visual areas that had to be intact.

Unfortunately, the concept that memories are stored in the corresponding part of the cortex suffered a serious blow when tasks involving synthesis of multimodal stimuli were studied. Using both of the above techniques, monkeys were trained to discriminate between paired visual (e.g. circle, cross) and tactile (e.g. rough and smooth) stimuli presented in such a way that only a particular combination of stimuli produced the reward. Under the preparative conditions described above, the visual stimulus would go into the ipsilateral hemisphere and the tactile stimulus into the contralateral hemisphere with no connexion between them. Nevertheless, the monkeys showed no difficulty in relating the stimuli to each other or in remembering how to perform the task. As intimated earlier, these findings raise serious doubts about the justification for assigning an essential or even dominant role in memory to the cerebral cortex. It seems highly likely that subcortical structures mediate the comparison of tactile and visual information under these experimental conditions, and there is no reason to assume that this is not the case in the untreated animal. Indeed, Bures et al. (1964), using passive avoidance tests, have reached the conclusion that memories are stored in the tectal region and in the reticular formation. They also feel that the exact site of storage and the precise mechanism of recall depends to a very large extent upon the detailed character of the engram to be memorized. Bures cites the fact that whereas active avoidance responses can be transferred during unilateral spreading depression, passive avoidance responses are not transferred under identical conditions. Evidently a good deal more work with more careful analysis of the external situation and more attention to subcortical structures is required before these anomalies are resolved.

Mechanisms of Storage

Through the years ideas on mechanisms of memory storage have come and gone, but one has remained all through. This is the belief that there has to be some permanent or at least nearly permanent *change* in the CNS for engrams to be stored. No one has yet elaborated a theory based upon a mechanism whereby memories are evoked by the mere activation of certain preferred circuits. Offhand it would seem that if the passage of an impulse or set of impulses over a particular network of neurones give rise to a particular instant of consciousness, there is no reason to suppose that re-excitation of that network would not evoke a memory of the past instant of consciousness, in much the same way as stimulation of the temporal lobe may induce organized hallucinations (see Consciousness, p. 253). However, the experts in the field do not seem to favour such a simple account, and it does seem as though the available evidence supports the concept of actual enduring change. Agreement has by no means been reached as to the character, let alone the precise form of such changes. Broadly, there are those who support morphological mechanisms and there are those who prefer biochemical reactions.

MORPHOLOGICAL MECHANISMS

In almost every respect the matters dealt with in the section on Learning (see p. 243) apply equally to memory. Increase in number of dendrites, increase in size of synaptic junctions, increase in axon diameter, increase in area of perikaryon and so on have all been cited as being part of the enduring neuronal change that goes with deposition of an engram. Although it has been easy to demonstrate the occurrence of such phenomena with repetitive stimulation of a given region, it has not so far been possible unequivocally to relate them to memory, especially loss of memory. Given that these morphological changes represent the actual form in which memories are stored, it is difficult to see how so many of them would (a) suddenly disappear and (b) gradually return without retraining, after a mere blow upon the head. More specifically, it does not seem easy to explain post-traumatic retrograde amnesia if the lost engrams were represented by increased size of neuronal elements. There just does not seem to be enough time available for this increased size to be lost or atrophied. Nevertheless, hypertrophy with great use and atrophy with great disuse are unassailable facts of observation. The interpretation of these facts is still rudimentary.

BIOCHEMICAL REACTIONS

One of the most fertile and intriguing of recent developments in this field is the application of biochemical methods to the study of memory and learning. A good deal of it centres around the molecule of ribonucleic acid (RNA). This has been shown, in other fields, to be intimately concerned not so much with protein synthesis as such, but with controlling the specific amino acids or nucleotides that are used in the synthesis of any particular protein. Nerve cells contain RNA and it is believed that the function of it is to control the protein synthesis of the perikaryon. Hence, considerable interest was attached to the demonstration that when neurones are activated in a learning process, i.e. repetitively and over longish periods, their RNA content increases. Again, the experimental formation of an epileptogenic mirror focus parallels an increase in the RNA content of the neurones in the focus. Further, animals treated with a compound (8-azaguanine) that causes the formation of defective RNA, are not able to memorize new tasks but are able to recall engrams already laid down. In humans with brain disease accompanied by impairment of memory, it is rather remarkable that administration of RNA (in the form of yeast) has been claimed to effect considerable improvement of the memory (Cameron and Solyom, 1961). How far experiments on invertebrates can be extrapolated to mammals is highly debatable, but it is nevertheless interesting in this context that an untreated planarian tail retains conditioned reflexes established in the un-damaged organism unless treated with ribonuclease—an enzyme that breaks down RNA. Even more astonishing is the claim (McConnell, 1962) that one planarian can acquire the learning of another one by eating it!

So far we have considered RNA and the neurone, but the picture is complicated by concurrent studies of the neuroglia. These cells have long been looked upon as mere supportive elements in the nervous system, with a possible nutritional biochemical role. Ideas along these lines are having to be changed. Quite likely, the neuroglia that are in close association with brain blood vessels—the capillary glia—may have limited functions of this kind. But the glia that are far removed from blood vessels and whose processes are closely applied to nerve cells—the neuronal glia—cannot now be looked upon in this light. When animals were trained in a balancing task, it was found that as the RNA content of the neurones in Deiter's nucleus increased, so the RNA of associated glial cells decreased. The proportions of nucleotides (adenine to uracil) was changed in a manner that was reciprocal among these elements of the region. No such changes were found in adjoining capillary glia. From these and other data, many workers now believe that memory engrams are represented by specific protein molecules, the formation of which is determined by the activities of the neuroglia. A note of caution has been introduced by Dingman and Sporn (1964) who raise some objections to this theory and ask for attention to be paid to other chemical aspects of memory, for example, lipids. They set out three criteria that must be satisfied before we can accept anything as the basis of a memory engram: (1) the molecule must undergo a change in state in response to experience; (2) this altered state must persist as long as the memory can be demonstrated; (3) specific destruction of the altered state must result in permanent loss of the memory. It is unfortunately evident that none of these criteria is as yet adequately satisfied by any theory.

UNRECALLABLE ENGRAMS

It seems to have been quite definitely established that each individual possesses a set of engrams that are not available to voluntary recall. This memory store is usually called the subconscious mind. Special techniques such as hypnosis, narcosis or psychoanalysis are necessary to bring these memories to consciousness. Under these conditions the subconscious mind is found to contain anti-social, anti-religious and traumatic memories. But all psychoanalysts would agree that the subconscious mind contains a great deal that is simply trivial or quite nice. In fact, one would be hard put to draw any clearly demonstrable distinction between the kind of memories in the subconscious mind and those in the conscious mind, because the conscious mind also contains anti-social, anti-religious and traumatic memories. There is no evidence whatever for the claim that the engrams in the subconscious mind have been repressed. The only evidence available is that they have been forgotten, in the perfectly ordinary and understandable sense of the word.

Since both the conscious and the unconscious minds contain material that is too anti-social to spill over into behaviour, and since both types of mind are possessed by the normal and the abnormal, there is no basis for drawing a distinction between the mentally abnormal and the mentally normal on the basis of the *content* of the subconscious mind. On the other hand, it may well be that some people have a (poorly detectable) fault of memory and are not able to deposit memories in such an easily recallable way as other people. These might well be the group that benefit from a special technique that resurrects such memories. In the normal individual, experiences occur in succession and are memorized. These memories are recallable and are compared with each other and with new experiences, this whole process leading to the integration of the personality. The person who is unable properly to recall past experiences is in a poor condition for incorporating new ones into a generalized, acceptable pool. Such a person's behaviour will reflect the "missing pieces" in his experiential inventory and such behaviour will be improved by bringing the missing pieces into availability by some such technique as psychoanalysis.

The above paragraphs are inserted for the cogitation of psychiatrically minded readers, in the hope that this approach might remove some of the mystique from psychoanalysis and similar processes, and show that there is a straightforward neurophysiological basis for all of them.

CHAPTER 16

BEHAVIOUR

Behaviour is one of those vague terms that cannot have a precise meaning given to it, but yet we all know more or less what it means. In this section it will be taken in its widest possible sense. Anything that an organism *does* in terms of movement will be included. Initially the treatment will be of experimental work showing which parts of the CNS must remain intact or which parts can be stimulated in order to have "normal" behaviour. By normal we shall mean the kind of behaviour that is not unexpected by the experienced observer.

Chronic Decerebration

Much of the fundamental work in this field stems from the studies of Bard and his associates (see Bard, 1956) who made a systematic approach to the problem. At the lowest level of decerebration, in the *pontile* preparation, there was removal of the interpeduncular and red nuclei, rostral quarter of the pons, tegmentum, the whole of the mesencephalon, the rostral third of the tectum and the caudal part of the hypothalamus. Cats prepared in this way were examined by faradization of the tail. They exhibited only the rudiments of a fear or rage reaction, with no biting, hissing or ear retraction. There was some degree of vocalization, protrusion of the claws and piloerection. Head-righting was possible, but not of the body. At a more anterior level, in the *low mesencephalic* preparation, a section was made through the rostral part of the superior colliculus to the exit of the oculomotor nerve. These animals responded to stimulation of the tail with a much more complete fear/rage reaction, with hissing and lashing of the tail in addition to the features seen in the pontile preparation, but no biting. In the *high mesencephalic* preparation a section was made through the rostral midbrain, but sparing the red nucleus and the oculomotor nucleus. Stimulation of the tail in these animals produced all of the reactions seen in the other preparations with the addition of clawing and biting. All of these preparations could be conditioned but the response disappeared the same day, even with constant reinforcement. The investigators point out that even in the high mesencephalic preparation several normal components of the fear/rage reaction are missing, e.g. arching of the back and, most important, the *integrated* attack with teeth and claws in a directed fashion. It is clear, however, that some of the brain stem regions are sufficient for the rudiments of protective behaviour. In more recent work on the mesencephalic preparation (Woods, 1964) the whole forebrain was removed from rats with the exception of the hypothalamus. Connexions between the hypothalamus and the mesencephalon were also severed. These animals suffered permanent loss of tactile placing reactions, temporary loss of righting and loco-motory reflexes and no loss of hopping reactions. Unlike carnivores subjected to this operation, the rats nibbled at objects held near to them (edible or inedible), grasped and drank from proferred pipettes and groomed themselves well. Painful stimuli evoked highly accurate and complete rage/fear responses in sharp distinction to the reactions of the similarly operated cat. Whether these distinctions are based upon essential differences between carnivores and herbivores, or upon differences in level of phylogenetic advance, remains for further research to clarify.

Hypothalamus

When cats are decerebrated below the mammillary bodies, they do not show *sham rage*. Cuts made above the tuberal region of the hypothalamus do produce this condition, which can be defined as an intense attack response to stimuli that would not normally be expected to have such an effect, e.g. merely touching the animal or even talking to it. It was later shown that electrical stimulation of the lateral hypothalamus (but not of nearby regions) in the intact animal routinely evoked a rage response. Then it was found that specific destruction of the ventromedial nuclei of the hypothalamus had the same effect, which was of course permanent. Hence, it may be concluded that the hypothalamic control of rage reactions is mediated by an excitatory lateral area and an inhibitory effect from the ventromedial nucleus. The reverse effect of *placidity*, with an almost complete absence of emotional responsivity has been reported by several workers to follow lesions in the posterior part of the hypothalamus, dorsal to the mammillary bodies. Destruction of the ventromedial nucleus in rats, cats and dogs has also been found to produce the behaviour of *hyperphagia*. In this condition the animals eat almost continually and become remarkably obese. Destruction of the lateral hypothalamic area is followed by the reverse effect of hypophagia, in which the animals cannot be induced to eat and suffer a tremendous weight loss. This evidence suggests again that with regard to eating behaviour the hypothalamus contains a lateral excitatory control and an inhibitory mechanism in the ventromedial nucleus. However, the phenomenon of eating does not seem to be entirely under neurological control, as might be expected in something with so many metabolic implications. First, it has been shown that if two rats are given the same amount of food (i.e. not *ad lib.* but restricted) and one of them has a lesion in the ventromedial nucleus, then the lesioned rat becomes larger than the intact animal, indicating, perhaps, a difference in intermediary metabolism. Second, if a pair of rats are parabiosed and one of the pair given a lesion in the ventromedial nucleus, the unlesioned animal loses a good deal of weight while the other grows fat. If the intact partner is now given a lesion, then it, too, increases in weight. Evidently, then, the hypothalamic mechanisms are reinforced or modulated by some kind of metabolic component that probably feeds back upon the hypothalamus. These findings bring to mind some of the features of Frohlich's syndrome in man. Destruction of parts of the hypothalamus has given rise to *hypodipsia*, a disinclination to drink. On the other hand, electrical stimulation of the lateral hypothalamic area evokes polydipsia. In this situation animals (goats) that have normally satiated themselves with water will drink voluminously and compulsively when the current is switched on. So also with regard to drinking behaviour the hypothalamus exerts both excitatory and inhibitory effects. If the hypothalamus is sectioned immediately posterior to the mammillary bodies, *sexual behaviour* (as seen in oestrous responses in guinea-pigs) is virtually abolished. This effect is not obtained if the cut is made anterior to the mammillary bodies. Lesions made in the ventral (but not dorsal) regions of the hypothalamus as well as lesions in the posterior region also abolish oestrous responses. Thus there appears to be an area in the postero-ventral region of the hypothalamus that activates or maintains the mechanisms of sexual behaviour. The role of hormones in these mechanisms is discussed in the section on neuroendocrinology (p. 173). An inhibitory effect upon sexual behaviour seems to be located in the anteroventral part of the hypothalamus, for lesions in this region in rats are frequently followed by continuous oestral responses. In man there are several records where damage of various sorts to this area is accompanied by sexual precocity. Lesions in this region have induced precocious endocrinological puberty in rats and ferrets (see p. 163).

In a rather different category of behaviour, and one that is difficult to label, come the results of Olds (1962) on self-stimulation. Rats are provided with electrodes in various parts of the brain which deliver a small shock when the rat presses a lever. Under these conditions the animal is able to decide for itself how much shocking it will get. The presumption is that the rat will press the lever if the shock pleases it—gives a *reward*—and will keep away from the lever if the shock is unpleasant. It was found that about 60% of the brain is neutral in this respect; with the electrode in such sites, the rat presses the bar only as many times as if no current were flowing. Five per cent. of the brain showed negative characters inasmuch as the animals actively avoided pressing the lever. Positive responses were obtained in about 35% of the brain. The most rewarding site found was in the ventral hypothalamus (dorsal and lateral regions were negative). With the electrodes in the anterior part of the hypothalamus, the rats pressed the bar about 400 times per hour. When the electrodes were in the postero-ventral region, the pressing rose to 5 000 times per hour. Indeed, under these conditions the rats continued pressing the lever until they collapsed from fatigue. On recovery they immediately began pressing the lever again. This behaviour occurred also in rats that were deprived of food and sexual satisfaction inasmuch as they preferred pressing the lever to eating or mating when given the choice of all three. One may cogitate cautiously that when various types of rewarding stimuli are encountered, their common feature is that they evoke excitation of this hypothalamic region.

Not exactly in the field of behaviour, but impinging upon it, is the loss of recent memory that follows damage to the mammillary bodies (see p. 259). This and the other features of hypothalamic involvement in behaviour described above have been reported to occur in much the same form in humans with trauma, vascular accidents, tumours and other damage to the hypothalamus. From all these data it is quite clear that the hypothalamus has a considerable part to play in the control of several types of behaviour. One should not, however, assume that under normal circumstances the hypothalamus actually initiates behaviour. It is apparent that although the hypothalamus may exert a strong control of autonomic function, it is very much under the influence of higher structures where behaviour is concerned.

Thalamus

This region is, of course, the main relay and integration centre for sensory information on its way to the cortex. Therefore the thalamus must contribute to all forms of behaviour that have a sensory antecedent. But whether it has any special role in behaviour above and beyond this is a moot point. It has been claimed that lesions of the dorsomedial nucleus in the monkey result in outbursts of motor activity and distractibility; in cats it was reported that similar lesions cause hostility and something rather like sham rage. However, on repetition by other workers this was not confirmed, dorsomedial lesions in monkeys resulting, if anything, in rather more placid and aimless behaviour. The generally agreed view seems to be that the thalamus has no specific role to play in behaviour. Even the finding that lesions of the posteromedial nucleus result in hypodipsia and apparent loss of taste may be explained simply by the interruption of sensory pathways. Some of the other reported effects of thalamic stimulation upon behaviour can be presumed to be due to excitation of pathways from the dorsomedial thalamus and the frontal cortex and from the anterior thalamus to the cingulate gyrus.

Reticular Formation

As time goes by it seems that the reticular formation is involved in just about everything that goes on in the CNS, and behaviour is no exception. Consciousness and memory are essential ancillaries of behaviour and the role of the reticular formation in these phenomena is discussed in the appropriate sections (see pp. 248–259). A good deal of behaviour is conditioned and the reticular formation is involved in this, too (see p. 221). With regard to *sexual* behaviour there seems to be a clear relationship between strength of libido and threshold of the reticular formation. When the latter is measured throughout the oestrous cycle, it is found to fall precipitately at full oestrus and becomes 200–300% higher during the dioestrous phase. On the basis of this and other evidence, it has been proposed that the hormones and the sensory input both act upon the reticular formation to maintain an unconscious "vigilance" that leads to the initiation of instinctual behaviour. It is also worth noting that most of the tranquillizers that reduce the general level of behaviour also have a depressant effect upon the reticular formation.

Amygdaloid Nucleus

We shall come across this component of the limbic system again when dealing with the role of the cerebral cortex in behaviour, but it deserves a few words at this point. A great deal of work has been done on this structure (for review, see Gloor, 1960), yet its place in the general scheme of neurophysiology is by no means clear. Bard and Mountcastle (1947) found that bilateral ablation of the amygdala in cats and dogs evoked a *rage* response of considerable ferocity to the point of savageness. Yet in monkeys similar treatment results in removal of the signs of fear and anger (Kluver and Bucy, 1939) and wild rats became as docile as tame animals after this operation (Woods, 1956). This species difference is highly puzzling, but quite incontrovertible and may be related either to the carnivorous as against the herbivorous habit or to the degree to which the species can be domesticated. It should be borne in mind that there is a definite anatomical pathway from the ventromedial nucleus of the hypothalamus (p. 236) and it is likely that the amygdala is not so much a centre as a way station in the diencephalo-limbic system that is concerned with the cruder forms of behaviour. Hence, it is not surprising that amygdaloid lesions give rise to enhanced *sexual behaviour* and *hyperphagia* in cats. Again there is a species difference, for in the laboratory rat lesions of the amygdala lead to aphagia and adipsia. It appears that the amygdaloid complex does not, by its own excitation, occasion pleasure, for in self-stimulation experiments (see p. 269) the rats press the lever about 600 times per hour, putting this region into the neutral category as far as *reward* is concerned. It is important to note that the hypersexuality induced by amygdalectomy in cats is abolished by castration and returns when sex hormones are administered. Hence, the blood level of endocrine secretions plays a part in the mediation of behavioural responses (see p. 172).

Cerebral Cortex

Whereas the various subcortical structures seem to have close structural and functional similarity in the lower animals and man, this is by no means true of the cerebral cortex. Hence, we must all beware of extrapolating to man in our minds the results obtained on the role of the cerebral cortex in behaviour in lower animals.

The effect upon *maze-learning* behaviour of removal of various amounts of cortex has already been mentioned (see p. 196) where it was shown that, at least in the rat, some degree of mass action seems to be present. That is, in some behavioural respects each part of the cortex has some influence above and beyond any specific role it may have by virtue of sensorimotor functions. Other studies that involved large scale cortical ablations have been concerned with *sexual behaviour*. The female of many species—rabbits, rats, guinea-pigs, cats—can suffer removal of the whole neocortex and parts of the rhinencephalon (olfactory bulbs) and yet still exhibit normal mating behaviour during spontaneous or induced oestrus. Males are rather more susceptible, as are female mice. In these forms removal of the olfactory bulbs alone (mouse) or together with neocortex (rabbit) abolishes mating behaviour. The male cat and rat show a loss of mating behaviour that is proportional to the amount of neocortex ablated, total abolition occurring when 60% is removed, irrespective of site of ablation, so that here again is evidence of mass action. Once more it is most important to bear in mind the small proportion of "association" cortex in these species compared with higher forms (Fig. 57). Sixty per cent. loss of cortex in a rat or cat means that a good deal of the motor area is removed. Since sexual behaviour in the male is rather more active than in the female, this reduction in motor power may at least partly explain the male's enhanced sensitivity to cortical ablations.

With respect to *rage* reactions, a series of studies by Bard and Mountcastle (1947) has established the situation fairly clearly. Removal of various fairly small parts of the neocortex did not result in sham rage, whereas total corticectomy did produce this condition. When the whole neocortex was ablated, leaving intact the limbic system and amygdaloid nuclei, the cats became more docile than normal, requiring much stronger stimuli to evoke hostility. Such placid animals were transformed into the full sham-rage condition either by removal of the amygdaloid nuclei or by ablation of the limbic system. It should be recollected that removal of the amygdala from intact cats evokes sham rage; ablation of the limbic system in normal cats does not have this effect. Hence, from all these data one may conclude (where cats are concerned) that (a) the amygdala exerts a strong inhibitory influence upon rage responses, and (b) the limbic cortex has a weak inhibitory effect upon them. One might also be led to conclude that the neocortex is not involved in rage responses. This would, perhaps, be true if only the rather artificial condition of sham rage is considered. Under natural conditions the neocortex is essential for rage reactions in response to auditory or visual stimuli and it is essential for the integration, timing and direction of the components of the normal rage response. Thus, when the amygdala is lesioned the sham rage produced closely approaches normal rage, but if the neocortex is now ablated the hostility responses lose direction, accuracy and timing.

LIMBIC SYSTEM

In view of the above results it would not be out of place to consider the limbic system a little more closely. In the present context the limbic system is taken to comprise the gyrus cinguli, the isthmus of the gyrus fornicatus, the hippocampal gyrus and the uncus. This is what is frequently called the "smell-brain", a misnomer because of its considerable size in animals with a poor (microsmatic, man) or absent (anosmatic, porpoise) sense of smell. However, it seems to be essential for the establishment of olfactory *conditioned reflexes*, and, strangely enough, stimulation of the hippocampus or fornix stops the performance of conditioned responses even when they are of the avoidance kind. In the field of *sexual* behaviour Green (1958) has shown that lesions in the pyriform cortex—where olfactory gyrus and hippocampal gyrus meet—induce a marked hypersexuality. Such lesions result in a much slower loss of sexual drive after castration and the overall effects are of a chronic nature. It is Green's belief, shared by many, that the pyriform cortex exerts a tonic restraining effect upon the brain stem mechanisms that mediate sexual behaviour.

One of the largest components of the limbic system is the cingulate gyrus, very old and with many connexions with both neocortex and subcortical structures, including the thalamus, hypothalamus, basal ganglia and reticular formation. It has already been pointed out that the cingulate gyrus has motor functions (see p. 117) and it has been known for some twenty years that it is involved in autonomic mechanisms. Stimulation of the anterior part of the cingulate gyrus in animals and man has given cardiovascular changes, piloerection, shivering and alterations in respiration rate. By and large the more posterior regions are inhibitory while the rostral parts are excitatory. Extensive lesions of the cingulate gyrus in monkeys cause them to become extremely placid and to show little signs of fear. Conversely, electrical stimulation of this gyrus induces hostility that is by no means savage, yet is unmistakeably a sort of rage. Bilateral destruction of the cingulate gyrus in man (mainly the anterior part) has resulted in a kind of placidity, represented in extreme form by catatonic stupor and akinetic mutism. Epileptic seizures have been induced in man and monkey by electrical stimulation of the cingulate gyrus, but this may, of course, be due to transfer of excitation to other regions. Data of this kind led Papez (1937) to put forward a theory of control of emotional behaviour that dropped out of favour but is returning with the new information that is accumulating. According to this theory, "emotion" is accumulated in the hippocampus, and is transferred via the fornix to the mammillary bodies, from which it is passed along the mammillo-thalamic tract to reach the dorsal group of thalamic nuclei. The final stage in the proposition is the transfer of emotion from the thalamus to the cingulate gyrus. Thus, the cingulate gyrus is looked upon as integrating the emotional content of experience into appropriate action, both somatic and visceral. We have already seen that the neocortex plays a guiding role in effective action and one can apply Hughlings Jackson's idea of levels to this whole system. At the brain stem level there is apparatus for crude responses of a purely emotional character. These are dominated by diencephalic-limbic mechanisms that give more complete and more effective responses. Above these, the cingulate gyrus brings the integrative powers of cortical organization to bear upon the hypothalamic-amygdaloid mechanisms. Finally, the neocortex with its greater complexity of organization and its associative powers, is able to consider past experience and modify the purely emotional and instinctive behaviour into action that is effective on a more long-term basis.

TEMPORAL LOBE

After this rather long digression into the limbic system, we now return to the neocortex and consider the temporal lobes, although it will be seen that limbic structures are still involved. Functional knowledge of this lobe really began with the description of the "temporal lobe syndrome" by Kluver and Bucy (1939). This syndrome was produced when sexually mature monkeys had their temporal lobes ablated (including the amygdala, hippocampus and uncus), so that the syndrome may not be entirely due to removal of neocortex. The animals exhibited the following characteristics. (a) Visual agnosia: their ability to discriminate visually was lost, even to the point of being unable to detect the difference between animate and inanimate objects. (b) Orality: a strong inclination repetitively to place objects in the mouth and manipulate them with the lips and teeth. (c) Hypermetamorphosis: preoccupation with visual and tactile stimuli, repeatedly looking at and touching every object in sight. (d) Placidity: marked emotional indifference to stimuli that would normally produce rage or fear, such as a snake, which the lobectomized monkey picks up and examines with no sign of affect but curiosity. (e) Hypersexuality: a strong sexual drive that is directed indiscriminately at inanimate objects, males, females and the animal itself. These are undoubtedly very severe defects of behaviour and they have been paralleled in some degree in the human (Falconer *et al.*, 1955) after a similar operation. The problem has been to explain this syndrome, to discover why all of these varied disturbances of behaviour should follow removal of such a small part of the brain. The following scheme is put to the reader for his own consideration.

We have already seen (p. 260) the disastrous effect upon recent memory in the human when the hippocampal-uncal regions are removed bilaterally. It seems possible that the Kluver-Bucy syndrome could be explained by invoking this finding. Let us suppose that the lobectomized monkeys have a defect of recent memory, and are unable to memorize anything. They will not be able to remember what they have looked at lately; will not remember that some particular objects are animate and others inanimate; they will have visual agnosia. They will remember for only a few seconds what things taste like and feel like when touched by the lips and tongue; they will be constantly putting things in their mouths (orality). Everything around such monkeys is new from minute to minute; their instinctive exploratory drive will make them pick things up and look at surrounding objects; they will exhibit hypermetamorphosis. Rage and fear are evoked by things that are known to be harmful; these monkeys cannot remember whether any particular stimulus is harmful, so they demonstrate placidity. The basic sexual drive is still operative in these monkeys, but because they cannot remember under what conditions they obtain satisfaction, they keep trying to get it from anything that is in the offing, including themselves; they show hypersexuality. Thus the major symptoms of the temporal lobe syndrome can be explained on the basis of loss of the power to memorize. If this be true, then the syndrome is not really part of the field of behaviour, except in so far as it is a reflection of loss of memory. Nor is the temporal lobe neocortex to be necessarily involved in these behaviour changes. Support for the latter statement comes from the studies of Blum *et al.* (1950) who removed the lateral surfaces of the temporal and preoccipital cortex and found practically no effects on emotional behaviour. Nevertheless, as mentioned above, it is dangerous to extrapolate from species to species. Emotional changes that occur during flicker stimulation (see p. 208) produce fairly specific changes in the EEG records from the temporal lobes in man. As with so much of cortical function, the role of the temporal neocortex in behaviour has yet to be defined.

PARIETAL LOBES

Obviously the parietal lobes play a considerable part in the mediation of all behaviour, inasmuch as they contain primary areas for somatic sensation and for much motor co-ordination. But several association areas (see p. 202) are also present in this lobe and these have a rather more special part to play. Lesions of the primary areas lead to behavioural changes that are merely reflections of sensorimotor losses—various types of paralyses, aphasias and faults of stereognosis. Damage to the association areas is accompanied by much more serious behavioural deficits involving speech and body image. Most important seems to be the region where parietal, temporal and occipital lobes meet. With large lesions in this region, even unilaterally if in the dominant hemisphere, the patient is frequently unable to comprehend words in any form, written or spoken and is unable to write sensibly himself. Such an inability leads to the appearance of demented behaviour. With regard to the spoken word, an elaborate cortical mechanism is involved that is by no means properly understood yet.

No harm will come from a digression into this subject, though it involves more than the parietal lobes. At least six cortical areas are implicated. (1) The posterior end of the third frontal convolution. (2) The posterior part of the temporal lobe. (3) The inferior parietal lobule. (4) The superior frontal convolution. (5) The inferior part of the precentral gyrus. (6) The inferior end of the postcentral gyrus. Electrical stimulation of 1, 2 and 3 inhibits the mental formation of words and also prevents their utterance. Stimulation of 4, 5 and 6 only prevents their utterance. It is easy to presume that stimulation of these latter areas causes interference with the direct motor mechanisms of speech, since these are the regions that control the appropriate muscles. Evidently the areas designated by 1, 2 and 3 above have a dual function. They connect with the areas designated by 4, 5 and 6 thus influencing the muscles of articulation. Their second function is to aid in the mental formulation of the words that are going to be spoken by those muscles. Hence, they are concerned both with verbal apraxia and with language aphasia. The picture is a little more complicated, however, by the fact that stimulation over various parts of the inferior regions of the pre- and postcentral gyri elicits vocalization. The patient emits some sort of vowel sound and cannot voluntarily stop while the stimulus is on. It is possible that these different effects of activating the same region are due to different frequencies of stimuli, a point that does not seem to have been examined. There is also some evidence that the temporo-parietal region is involved in the understanding of the spoken word. One can see the importance of this association area (lying about midway between primary auditory and primary visual areas) for the comprehension of things seen and heard. It is obvious that various subcortical regions are also involved in speech, because they are way-stations for the sensory (proprioceptive) or motor components of this function. Medullary lesions affecting portions of the nucleus of the vagus, for example, will cause slight difficulties in speech if unilateral and serious difficulties of speech if bilateral, due to paralysis of the laryngeal muscles. Damage in midbrain regions has led to initial absence of voice followed by speech of a highly disorganized kind. Explosive, syllabic speech frequently follows lesions to the vermis of the cerebellum, presumably the laryngeal counterpart of the general asynergy of the musculature under these conditions. More detailed treatment, with extensive bibliography has been presented by Zangwill (1960).

Returning now to our consideration of the parietal lobe, one of its most remarkable features should, perhaps, be included in the field of behaviour. This is its role in the concept of body image. MacDonald Critchley (1953) has given a careful analysis of the earlier observations on this aspect of the somato-psyche and is careful to point out that our awareness of the body scheme is probably a function of the brain as a whole. Nevertheless, there is strong evidence that the posterior part of the parietal lobe in the non-dominant hemisphere has a specially marked importance in this respect. Small lesions in this region do not seem to have much effect, but larger lesions lead to the strange and distressing condition in which the patient believes that some part or even one side of his body is missing (hemidepersonalization). Klein and Ingram (1958) describe a case of tumour in the right parietal lobe accompanied by loss of awareness of the left-hand side of the body, with no motor or sensory loss. Rare cases have occurred in which the patient is convinced that he has no body at all (total depersonalization). It is Critchley's view (1953) that damage to the dominant hemisphere produces an effect on body image that is obscured by concomitant apraxias, both motor and vocal. According to Schilder (1935) the body image is built from sensory units in the tactile, visual, labyrinthine and kinaesthetic modalities. If this be true, and there is no reason to think it is not, then we may look upon the posterior parietal lobe as having wide associative powers leading to the synthesis of a variety of stimuli. Schilder also considered that some degree of depersonalization occurs in the development of all neuroses. Certainly it is reported to be a frequent, or at least not uncommon, accompaniment to anxiety states, hysterias, obsessions, schizophrenia and endogenous depression.

FRONTAL LOBES

It is extremely difficult to pin down any precise function for the frontal lobes. Recourse has to be made to such vague terms as biological intelligence, moral values, ethical sense and so on. Certainly, complete removal of this part of the forebrain seems to have little effect. Even in man, where many suppose it has reached its (so far) highest development, bilateral loss of the frontal lobes has no detectable effect upon the activity of vision, visual discrimination, perception time, response time or discrimination of weight. Many reports, however, describe changes in personality after frontal leucotomy or lobotomy. Clinical textbooks should form the source of such information and here we may simply note that, by and large, loss of frontal mechanisms seems to make many people treat all others as if they were well known to the patient. Strangers are told, for example, quite directly that they have a dirty face. Such an accusation may be true, but most intact individuals would approach the matter more obliquely where total strangers are concerned. In general terms it seems more or less agreed that the frontal lobes exert some kind of tonic inhibition on the less socially acceptable tendencies of the effect. The cynic might well, with some justification, consider the frontal lobes as the seat of hypocrisy. Even with some visceral functions there appears to be an inhibitory action, for in both monkeys and man frontal lobe damage has been associated with hyperphagia, mild but definite. In conditioning studies the evidence is clear that lesions of the frontal lobes reduce an animal's ability to learn delayed responses, irrespective of the modality of the stimulus. Another interesting aspect of frontal lobe function comes from experiments on the split-brain preparation (see p. 194). If the frontal lobe is removed on one side in a monkey treated in this way, then a snake viewed through the contralateral eye induces the usual marked fear reaction, whereas the same reptile seen through the ipsilateral eye produces no effect at all. Apart from the intriguing psychometric possibilities of such "schizophrenic" animals, they clearly show that the frontal lobes play a role that is not purely inhibition. More truly, they mediate a "caring" attitude. In their absence there is a tendency not to care about the consequences of either internal or external events.

SUMMARY

Generalizations are just as dangerous in the field of behaviour as elsewhere, but bearing this in mind it might still be useful to have a tentative overall view of behaviour. Such a view will need many modifications as new research gradually clarifies the situation. At the moment it seems that (a) the basic equipment of behaviour is lodged in the spinal effector mechanisms (and their bulbar equivalents involving the cranial nerves); (b) lower brain stem regions can manipulate this basic system to evoke the cruder, more emotional, more non-specific components of behaviour; (c) upper subcortical structures such as the hypothalamus and parts of the limbic system integrate more sources of information and more parts of the effector mechanisms, to produce a more co-ordinated but incomplete response which is still predominantly of a rather primitive kind; (d) limbic structures are functionally linked to old cortical regions, such as cingulate gyrus, to bring a higher level of association to bear upon the workings of the lower structures; (e) with special respect to the higher animals including man, the neocortex is concerned with the highest level of integration of new and old sensory data in such a way that highly complex, multiple stimuli are transformed into highly complex, multiple responses. Less emotion, more reason is brought into behaviour at this final level.

Supplement on Higher Functions

CORTICAL ORGANIZATION

The impression may have been given in earlier sections that sensory information is projected from the thalamus to the primary sensory areas of cortex and from these to the association areas. This is true, but is not the whole truth. There is evidence that sensory information can reach association areas without relay from the primary areas. In the cat four main cortical association fields have been mapped (Fig. 61) and it has been found that activation of any sense modality evokes electrical activity in all four association areas. Stimulation of the eye by a flash of light, the ear by a click, or a peripheral cutaneous nerve by an electric shock produces not merely evoked responses in the four association areas but also the same topographical distribution of amplitude variations (Thompson et al., 1963). This indicates that there is some common central mechanism for the transmission of sensory information. Moreover, when stimuli in two modalities are given in succession the second evoked response in the association regions is attenuated, pointing to occlusion and a common neuronal

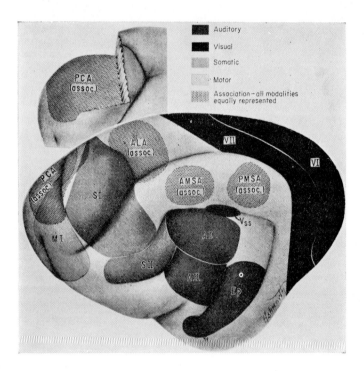

FIG. 61. Lateral view of cat's brain showing distribution of cortical functional regions. Roman numerals indicate first and second sensory areas. Stippled regions are the four association areas. These have the same distribution of responses to all modalities of stimulation. (From Thompson *et al.*, 1963.)

network for all modalities. These results are still obtained when all the cortex except the association regions is removed, so that they are evidently not due to relays from the primary sensory area. Additional evidence of this is that in the association areas the recovery cycle (roughly, the refractory period) is much longer than in the primary cortex. It has been repeatedly pointed out here and elsewhere that it is dangerous to extrapolate the results obtained in a lower species to man. Hence it must be emphasized that none of the above results have been found or, it seems, looked for in the human. In the absence of such data, however, there is no reason to believe that the human brain is organized differently and one may in the meantime reflect upon the significance of such an arrangement.

To begin with one may speculate as to the anatomical pathways involved in these phenomena. Since the sensory input to the four association areas was diffuse and non-specific, it would seem likely that it passed through either the reticular nucleus of the ventral thalamus (see p. 60) or via the midbrain reticular formation (see p. 66). Of the two the latter is more probable because, unlike the reticular nucleus of the thalamus, its output is usually *excitatory* and widespread. It becomes a reasonable hypothesis, then, to believe that the non-specific excitation of association areas described above forms the neurological basis of the alerting reaction. In this way the whole association cortex is prepared by any sensory input to receive and interpret the specific sensory information that will be sent to it by the primary area that corresponds to the modality of the stimulus. Further research will be necessary before this concept can be accepted.

Throughout this book references have been made to active inhibition of neurones without any details being given as to its mechanism. Although speculation about the mechanism has been rife in the past, only recently has any experimental evidence been adduced to support conjecture. When a cortical neurone is stimulated electrically at suprathreshold strength, it can be shown that many or all of the neurones within about 1 cm radius are inhibited inasmuch as they are less easily (or not at all) excited by the local application of glutamate (Krnjevic *et al.*, 1964). Undercutting of the cortex does not abolish the effect so it is unlikely that the inhibition is caused by a reflexive chain involving a subcortical structure. The possibility that the excited cortical neurone inhibits adjacent neurones by recurrent collaterals seems unlikely because antidromic impulses produced by stimulation of the pyramidal tract are known to have only a weak inhibitory effect upon the cortex. A much more likely mechanism is based upon the assumption that the cortex contain neurones whose processes lie entirely within the cortex and whose function is to produce inhibition of the cortical cells with which their axons connect. The Golgi Type II or "short axon" cells of the cerebral cortex (see p. 189) would seem to be likely candidates for this role. That a neuronal component is involved is shown by the fact that close circumsection of an excited cell reduces the area of inhibition. Cortical inhibition produced in this way lasts for periods in the region of 200 msec and therefore probably includes a chemical component in addition to the neuronal one. Many anti-inhibitory compounds have been found to be without effect upon this form of inhibition. Investigators in this field hold the opinion that γ-aminobutyric acid may be the compound involved since it is known to depress the activity of cortical cells and has been found to occur in the brain in fair quantity. However, in view of the fact that this type of cortical inhibition shows temporal radiation to regions more remote from the stimulated cell, the possibility should be borne in mind that it may be due to some form of ionic transport and may indeed represent the fundamental mechanism of the spreading depression produced in the cortex by application of potassium chloride solution (see p. 261). In trying to imagine what role is played in the functioning brain by this mechanism, one could suppose that, once having taken a decision for action, the cortex arranges for the production of an inhibitory zone around the effector pyramidal cells so that for a short time there will be no possibility of a second action interfering with the first, unless the stimulus for such a second action is so urgent and strong as to overcome the increased threshold of the inhibited cells. In other words, cortical spreading depression "clears the lines" and keeps them clear so that a definitive action is given priority and proceeds unhindered.

There seems to have been some misunderstanding in the past about the time of appearance of electrical activity of the cerebral cortex. It was a widespread belief that the EEG records of newborn humans reveal only a minimum of electrical activity. This is effectively disproved by the findings of Liberson and Frazier (1962), who examined 196 babies during the first few hours after birth. It was found that the α-rhythm was present in a large number of cases, especially among those delivered by caesarean section. If long anaesthesia was used on the mother during birth the percentage incidence of α-rhythm fell from 91 to 71, whereas the percentage incidence of δ-silence rose from 0 to 57. It rather looks as though the anaesthetic reached the mother's brain in doses high enough to cause neuronal depression, but reached the foetal brain in a low enough concentration to exert a stimulatory effect. In the adult, the effect of hypnotic anaesthesia has been studied. Recordings were taken from the cortex before, during and after subjects were hypnotized and given suggestions of sensory loss (Fig. 62). Electroshock to the hand, mechanical taps to the finger and click stimuli were reported by the subjects to be non-existent even though the specific (somatic) and non-specific (auditory) cortical responses to the stimuli were normal. Hence, as with many another higher function, the activity of the cerebral cortex does not seem to be of paramount importance in the phenomenon of hypnotic anaesthesia any more than with regard to chemical anaesthesia (see p. 251). Once again, it seems likely that subcortical structures play a larger part in higher functions than is

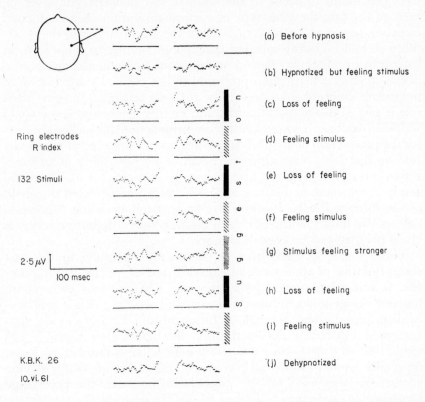

FIG. 62. Averaged cerebral evoked responses in a subject (KBK) to 132 electrical stimuli to the right index finger, given once per sec. Responses were recorded (a) before hypnosis and (b) after hypnosis. Thereafter the subject could be made to feel or not to feel the stimulus at will, by direct suggestion under hypnosis. The nature of the suggestion given before each record is indicated on the right and its success was in each case confirmed by the subject's reports. Before record (g) it was suggested that the stimulus would feel much stronger than before, though its objective strength was in fact unaltered. The final record (j) is a control taken after hypnosis had been abolished when the subject was reporting as feeling the stimuli normally. (From Halliday and Mason, 1964.)

frequently believed to be the case. The importance of subcortical structures in the maintenance of sleep is also seen when records are taken from dreaming subjects. Under these conditions, even though the subject is not easily aroused, the EEG traces show a low voltage rapid activity in the cortex "which is indistinguishable from periods of intense alertness" (Goldensohn, 1963).

CONDITIONING

Psychiatrists who prefer neurophysiological rather than psychological explanations of at least some mental disorders may care to ponder on the theory of neuroses put forward by Mackay (1962). He divides all neuroses into two classes: (a) conditioned or character neuroses, and (b) conflict neuroses. The first type is considered to result from (known or unknown) conditioning procedures that have acted upon the unconditioned immature individual's genetic affective bias to produce a character that makes responses which are unacceptable in the given social milieu. Such "conditioned misbehaviour" disorders include the compulsions, the hysterias and the anxieties. Theoretically, relief should be obtained by reconditioning, deconditioning or negative conditioning, using classical Pavlovian methods. In the second type of neurosis it is proposed that an individual with a conditional history that has produced acceptable responses, undergoes additional conditioning that demands impossible discriminations or evokes responses that conflict with the already established responses. Again, a more "localized" type of conditioning should improve the malady. Such therapeutic use of conditioning procedures recalls the modern technique of behaviour therapy. A good example is seen in the case of transvestism treated (and cured) by administration of emetics concurrently with projection of transparencies of the patient in various forms of female attire (Lavin et al., 1961).

At this point the reader's attention might be directed to page 282 where a mechanism of cortical inhibition is discussed. Consideration of this mechanism should be coupled with a re-reading of the account of irradiation of inhibition as a feature of conditioning phenomena (p. 217). It seems quite likely that when a conditioned stimulus is made inhibitory by extinction, the transcortical spread of defacilitation described above forms an essential feature of the process. Certainly, its proposed anatomical basis and its temporal characteristics make it a suitable candidate for this role.

LEARNING

It may perhaps be thought that in the earlier section under this heading too much emphasis was given to the concept that the cerebral cortex should not be looked upon as the most important structure concerned in learning. Evidence for the involvement of subcortical structures was only lightly touched upon, but we may now look more closely at this matter, when we shall see the great need for a precise and workable classification of the different types of learning. Rats in which the posterior cerebral cortex was bilaterally removed showed a deficiency in performance in the Hebb–Williams maze, whereas rats with bilateral lesions of the caudate nucleus were not different from normal animals in this situation. It would be easy to conclude from such an experiment that the caudate nucleus is not involved in learning. However, when the investigators (Chorover and Gross, 1963) tested rats with lesions in the caudate nucleus by exposing them to spatial alternation tasks, it was found that they had a marked impairment for the acquisition and retention of such habits. The importance of the caudate nucleus for this type of learning is not restricted to the lower forms in which the cerebral cortex is more rudimentary. It has been shown to be just as essential for the proper performance of alternation tasks in the monkey (Dean and Davis, 1959). A similar need for careful observation in learning experiments is highlighted in investigations where an absence of a particular form of learning is apparently due to the presence of a new form of behaviour. Cats in which the mammillo-thalamic tract has been severed do not carry out conditioned avoidance responses which they learned pre-operatively. It would have been tempting to infer that the mammillo-thalamic tract plays an essential role in this type of learning, but the investigators noticed that the operated cats were not quite unresponsive to the conditioned stimulus but exhibited a different and unfortunately ineffective defensive reaction. When the conditioning stimulus was given the animals "froze"—tense, crouched and immobile (Thomas et al., 1963). Presumably, in the intact cat the mammillo-thalamic tract plays a part in learning to the extent that it mediates inhibition of the "freezing" reaction in order to allow a more active defensive response to develop. It is to be hoped that these indications of the importance of subcortical structures will not go unheeded by future investigators in the field of learning.

CONSCIOUSNESS

In the earlier section under this heading considerable attention was paid to the midbrain portion of the reticular formation which was referred to as the reticular activating system (RAS, see p. 248ff.). It is now necessary to look rather more analytically at reticular mechanisms. Until recently it was considered that the reticular formation was essentially composed of (a) an ascending activating division, and (b) a descending inhibitory division, the latter being of great importance in the extrapyramidal control of postural reactions (see p. 138). Deactivation of the higher regions, in drowsiness or sleep was considered to result from diminution of ascending impulses, coupled under some conditions with widespread inhibitory influences from some diencephalic region. It has recently become apparent that this is not the full story. To the above mechanisms must be added an *ascending* defacilitating division of the reticular formation. Morphologically this division is ill-defined. It has elements at least as low as the obex region of the medulla and appears to run forward coextensively with the RAS and has been traced as high as the rostral parts of the midbrain. Excellent reviews of the earlier work on the ascending deactivating system (ADS) have been prepared by Cordeau (1962) and Moruzzi (1963). Some of this experimental evidence will now be dealt with briefly. When, as mentioned in the earlier section (p. 248), a lesion is made in the midbrain region of the reticular formation, a state of sleep appears both behaviourally and in terms of the EEG anterior to the lesion. Such lesions destroy the influence of the RAS. However, when the reticular region is destroyed at the pontine level, the reverse effect of continued alertness occurred during which any quite slight peripheral stimulus would produce a state of frenzied activity. These results suggest that at the pontine level or below there are elements of the ADS which in the intact animal exert a tonic inhibitory action upon the higher alertness equipment. Again, injection of adrenaline into the RAS has for quite a time been known to induce a long-lasting state of alertness. It is now known that injections of acetylcholine into the reticular formation are followed by behavioural and EEG manifestations of sleep. While the regions responding in these ways to the injected materials were of considerable and overlapping extent, adrenaline was most effective in the rostral midbrain area whereas acetylcholine gave its maximal effect when injected into the caudal pontine or bulbar regions of the reticular formation. Evidence along other lines was obtained by a study of cortical evoked potentials. Compounds known to inhibit neuronal activity, such as pontocaine, produced the expected observation of reduced evoked potentials when injected into midbrain regions of the reticular formation. The existence of an inhibitory system was indicated by increased amplitude of cortical evoked potentials when pontocaine was injected into the pontine or bulbar regions of the reticular formation. More recently it has been shown (Berlucchi *et al.*,

K

1964) that localized cooling as far down as the medullary floor of the
fourth ventricle evokes an EEG and behavioural arousal response.

Thus, there can be no doubt that there is a concentration in the more
caudal parts of the reticular formation of reticular elements which
exert tonic and phasic inhibitory influences upon the electrical activity
of the cerebral cortex. The anatomical disposition of this inhibitory
system is not yet clear nor are its afferent and efferent connexions
established. Physiologically there appears to be a clear difference
between the two ascending systems inasmuch as low-frequency
electrical stimulation of the reticular formation results in synchroniza-
tion of the EEG and behavioural signs of sleep, whereas faster frequencies cause desynchronization of the EEG and behavioural
alertness.

Important as the ADS may be, it is not the only neural mechanism
that has an inhibitory effect on cortical activity. Injections of acetylcholine into the preoptic region elicit a sleeping state, provided that
the medial forebrain bundle is intact (Hernandez-Peon et al., 1963).
Thus it should be borne in mind that the mechanisms of consciousness include a limbic component.

Stimulus parameters are seen to be of importance in connexion
with studies of the role of other brain regions in consciousness.
Stimuli composed of 30 c/s square wave pulses of subliminal
intensity, given repetitively, produce EEG and behavioural signs of
sleep when applied to regions of the brain that would not be expected
to be closely related to this state. Structures that have been shown to
respond in this way to subliminal stimulation include the cerebellum,
hippocampus, amygdaloid nuclei, visual and motor cortices (Roelofs
et al., 1963).

As with so many of the higher functions, it seems that there is a
dominant hemisphere with regard to consciousness, which is the
same hemisphere that is dominant for speech and handedness.
Injection of barbiturate (via the internal carotid artery) into the
dominant hemisphere resulted in loss of consciousness more often
and more rapidly than when injected into the non-dominant hemisphere (Serafetinides et al., 1964). This is not to be interpreted as
meaning that consciousness is *located* in the dominant hemisphere,
but simply that the latter, perhaps by virtue of its importance in
symbolic processes, plays the major cortical role in consciousness.
This finding recalls the postulation by Efron (1963) of a possible
mechanism underlying the subjective phenomenon of *déjà vu*. It is
suggested that the vague feeling of having had an experience before

without a clear memory of it, may be due to a temporary defect in interhemispheric transfer of experience. In the absence of such a defect it may be assumed that quanta of sensations reach the non-dominant hemisphere both directly and also indirectly via the dominant hemisphere at such an interval of time that the quanta are recorded as one experience. If, however, the temporal gap is widened a little the direct input will be partially recorded before the indirect input arrives. The recording of the indirect input will be automatically compared with the ill-defined recording of the direct input, generating the impression that the same sensory quanta have been experienced twice.

Before leaving the subject of consciousness, it may be useful at this point to refer the reader to the beginning of this Supplement where a possible neurological basis for the alerting reaction is given. There it will be seen that some evidence is now available which indicates the role of association areas in this response.

Behaviour

Although the topic overlaps into neuroendocrinology, it is convenient at this point to deal with behavioural responses elicited by the application of chemicals to various parts of the brain. Minute injections of testosterone into hypothalamic areas in the male rat causes the animal to carry out a pattern of behaviour that is characteristic of the post-parturient female. This maternal behaviour ceased after about half an hour, but recurred with a subsequent injection of testosterone. These were injections in the midline, but when testosterone was injected more laterally in the hypothalamus, vigorous male behaviour was evoked in both male and female rats (Fisher, 1964). It should be noted for later reference that these patterns of behaviour were not elicited by electrical stimulation of the same sites. In much the same way, eating and drinking behaviour has been evoked by chemical stimulation of various brain regions. Well-fed rats begin to eat ravenously when noradrenaline is injected just above the hypothalamus. Acetylcholine caused rats to drink excessively when injected into the same region. Many parts of the brain have been shown to respond in a similar way to acetylcholine, some of them being associated with a water intake of forty-to-fifty times normal. A consideration of all these regions leads to the view that several circuits in the limbic system mediate drinking responses. The complexity of this mechanism is believed to reflect the vital nature of the water intake; several parts of it could be damaged without the animal's drive to drink being abolished.

Some regions of the brain seem to be specifically involved in a particular function, inasmuch as only one kind of behaviour can be elicited by stimulation of them. Such regions also respond only to a particular compound, so that the particular chemical is also specific for a given form of behaviour. Other parts of the brain do not have behavioural specificity but do exhibit chemical specificity. It is possible, for example, by careful choice of injection site, to find a region that will evoke maternal behaviour with testosterone, eating with noradrenaline and drinking with acetylcholine. This type of non-specificity suggests that in some areas of the brain there are heterogeneous pools of neurones concerned with behaviour. A high level of a particular compound in the blood reaching that area will activate only a portion of the cells in the pool, while high blood levels of some other compound will activate a different set of neurones in the same pool. It seems to be more than a coincidence that many of the regions that give behavioural responses upon chemical stimulation are the same as those which have been shown to be concerned both in consciousness and in the Papez circuit for emotionally-based behaviour. There can be little doubt that in more primitive forms of behaviour the limbic system plays a fundamental co-ordinating role.

REFERENCES

Adrian, E. D. (1937). Synchronized reactions in the optic ganglion of *Dytiscus*. *J. Physiol.* **91**, 66–89.

Adrian, E. D. (1943). Afferent areas in the cerebellum connected with the limbs. *Brain* **66**, 289–315.

Albe-Fessard, D. and Kruger, L. (1962). Duality of unit discharges from cat centrum medianum in response to natural and electrical stimulation. *J. Neurophysiol.* **25**, 1–20.

Andy, O. J. and McChinn, R. (1957). Cingulate gyrus seizures. Correlations of electroencephalographic and behavioural activity in cat. *Neurology* **7**, 56–68.

Angel, A. (1963). Evidence for cortical inhibition of transmission at the thalamic sensory relay nucleus in the rat. *J. Physiol.* **169**, 108–109P.

Arduini, A. and Arduini, M. G. (1954). Effect of drugs and metabolic alterations on brain stem arousal mechanism. *J. Pharmac. exp. Ther.* **110**, 76–85.

Bard, P. (1956). *In* "Medical Physiology", chap 71, p. 1056. Kimpton, London.

Bard, P. and Mountcastle, V. B. (1947). Some forebrain mechanisms involved in expression of rage with special reference to suppression of angry behaviour. *Proc. Ass. res. nerv. ment. Dis.* **27**, 362–404.

Barraclough, C. A. (1961). Production of anovulatory, sterile rats by single injections of testosterone propionate *Endocrinology* **68**, 62–67.

Becht, F. C. (1920). Studies of the cerebrospinal fluid. *Am. J. Physiol.* **51**, 1–125.

Berger, H. (1929). Uber das Elektrenkephalogramm des Menschen. *Arch. Psychiat.* **87**, 527–570.

Bergstrom, R. M. (1962). Prenatal development of motor functions. *Annls Chir. Gynaec. Fenn.* **51**, Suppl. 112, 1–48.

Bergstrom, R. M. and Bergstrom, L. (1963). Prenatal development of stretch reflex functions and brain stem activity in the human. *Annls Chir. Gynaec. Fenn.* **52**, Suppl. 117, 1–21.

Berlucchi, G., Maffei, L., Moruzzi, G. and Strata, P. (1964). EEG and behavioural effects elicited by cooling of medulla and pons. *Archs ital. Biol.* **102**, 372–392.

Berman, A. L. (1961). Interaction of cortical responses to somatic and auditory stimuli in anterior ectosylvian gyrus of cat. *J. Neurophysiol.* **24**, 608–620.

Bishop, G. H. (1961). The organization of cortex with respect to its afferent supply. *Ann. N. Y. Acad. Sci.* **94**, 559–569.

Blum, J. S., Chow, K. L. and Pribram, K. H. (1950). A behavioural analysis of the organization of the parieto-temporo-preoccipital cortex. *J. comp. Neurol.* **93**, 53–100.

Boyd, I. A. (1962). The structure and innervation of the nuclear bag muscle fibre system and the nuclear chain muscle fibre system in mammalian muscle spindles. *Phil. Trans. R. Soc.* B, **245**, 81–136.

Boyd, J. D. (1957). Intermediate sympathetic ganglia. *Br. med. Bull.* **13**, 207–212.

Bremer, F. (1935). Cerveau "isolé" et physiologie du sommeil. *C. r. Séanc. Soc. Biol.* **118**, 1235–1241.

Bremer, F. (1953). "Some problems in Neurophysiology." University of London Press.

Brodal, A. (1963). Some data and perspectives on the anatomy of the so-called "extrapyramidal system". *Acta neurol. scand.* **39**, Suppl. 4, 17–38.

Brookhart, J. M., Moruzzi, G. and Snider, R. S. (1951). Origin of cerebellar waves. *J. Neurophysiol.* **14**, 181–190.

Brooks, V. B., Rudomin, P. and Slayman, C. L. (1961). Peripheral receptive fields of neurons in the cat's cerebral cortex. *J. Neurophysiol.* **24**, 302–325.

Bucy, P. C. and Keplinger, J. E. (1961). Section of the cerebral peduncles. *Archs Neurol.* **5**, 132–139.

Buller, A. J., Eccles J. C. and Eccles, R. M. (1958). Controlled differentiation of muscle. *J. Physiol.* **143**, 23–24P.

Bures, J. (1959). Reversible decortication and behaviour. *In* "The Central Nervous System" (M. A. B. Brazier, ed.). Josiah Macy Jr. Foundation, New York.

Bures, J., Buresova, O. and Fifkova, E. (1964). Interhemispheric transfer of a passive avoidance reaction. *J. comp. physiol. Psychol.* **57**, 326–330.

Burnstock, G. and Holman, M. E. (1963). Smooth muscle: Autonomic nerve transmission. *A. Rev. Physiol.* **25**, 61–90.

Buser, P., Bruner, J. and Sindberg, R. (1963). Influences of the visual cortex upon posteromedial thalamus in the cat. *J. Neurophysiol.* **26**, 677–691.

Cajal, Ramon y (1909). "Histologie du systeme Nerveux." Maloine, Paris.

Cajal, Ramon y (1955). "Studies on the Cerebral Cortex (Limbic Structures)" (L. M. Kraft, trans.). Year Book Publishers, Chicago.

Cameron, D. E. and Solyom, L. (1961). Effects of ribonucleic acid on memory. *Geriatrics* **16**, 74–81.

Campbell, H. J. (1959). The effect of partial hypophysectomy in the rabbit. *J. Physiol.* **149**, 394–409.

Campbell, H. J. (1963). Endocrine secretion and the central nervous system. *In* "Recent Advances in Physiology" (R. Creese, ed.). Churchill, London.

Campbell, H. J. (1964a). Androgen-induced reversal of parental behaviour in the female rabbit. *Nature, Lond.* **204**, 809–810.

Campbell, H. J. (1964b). The effects of neonatal hormone treatment on reproduction in the rabbit. *J. Physiol.* **176**, 29–30P.

Campbell, H. J. and Eayrs, J. T. (1965). Influence of hormones on the central nervous system. *Br. med. Bull.* **21**, 81–86.

Campbell, H. J. and Harris, G. W. (1957). The volume of the pituitary and median eminence in stalk-sectioned rabbits. *J. Physiol.* **136**, 333–343.

Campbell, H. J., George, R. and Harris, G. W. (1960). The acute effects of injection of thyrotrophic hormone or of electrical stimulation of the hypothalamus on thyroid activity. *J. Physiol.* **152**, 527–554.

Campbell, H. J., Feuer, G. and Harris, G. W. (1964). The effect of intrapituitary infusion of median eminence and other brain extracts on anterior pituitary gonadotrophic secretion. *J. Physiol.* **170**, 474–486.

Cannon, W. B. (1939). "The Wisdom of the Body", 2nd ed. W. W. Norton, New York.

Celesia, G. G. (1963). Segmental organization of cortical afferent areas in the cat. *J. Neurophysiol.* **26**, 193–206.

Chambers, W. W. and Sprague, J. M. (1955). Functional localization in the cerebellum. *Archs Neurol. Psychiat.* **74**, 653–680.

Christ, J. (1962). The early changes in the hypophysial neurosecretory fibres after coagulation. *Mem. Soc. Endocr.* No. 12, 125–147.

Chorover, S. L. and Gross, C. G. (1963). Caudate nucleus lesions: behavioural effects in the rat. *Science* **141**, 826–827.

Clare, M. H. and Bishop, G. H. (1955). Dendritic circuits: the properties of cortical paths involving dendrites. *Am. J. Psychiat.* **111**, 818–825.

Clarke, F. J. J. and Belcher, S. J. (1962). On the localization of Troxler's effect in the visual pathway. *Vision Res.* **2**, 53–68.

Cordeau, J. P. (1962). Functional organization of the brain stem reticular formation in relation to sleep and wakefulness. *Rev. canad. Biol.* **21**, 113–125.

Crevel, H. van and Verhaart, W. J. C. (1963). The exact origin of the pyramidal tract. *J. Anat.* **97**, 495–515.

Critchley, M. (1953). "The Parietal Lobes." Edward Arnold, London.

Critchley, M. (1956). Congenital indifference to pain. *Ann. intern. Med.* **45**, 737–747.

Critchlow. V. (1958). Blockade of ovulation in the rat by mesencephalic lesions. *Endocrinology* **63**, 596–610.

Cushing, H. (1914). Studies on the cerebrospinal fluid. *J. med. Res.* **31**, 1–19.

Dandy, W. E. (1919). Experimental hydrocephalus. *Ann. Surg.* **70**, 129–142.

Dartnall, H. J. A. and Tansley, K. (1963). Physiology of vision: retinal structure and visual pigments. *A. Rev. Physiol.* **25**, 433–458.

Dean, W. H. and Davis, G. D. (1959). Behaviour changes following caudate lesions in Rhesus Monkey. *J. Neurophysiol.* **22**, 524–537.

Dempsey, E. W. and Morison, R. S. (1943). The electrical activity of a thalamo-cortical relay system. *Am. J. Physiol.* **138**, 283–296.

Dingman, W. and Sporn, M. B. (1964). Molecular theories of memory. *Science* **144**, 26–29.

Ditchburn, R. W. and Ginsborg, B. L. (1953). Involuntary eye movements during fixation. *J. Physiol.* **119**, 1–17.

Dow, R. S. (1939). Cerebellar action potentials in response to stimulation of various afferent connections. *J. Neurophysiol.* **2**, 543–555.

Dow, R. S (1961). Some aspects of cerebellar physiology. *J. Neurosurg.* **18**, 512–530.

Downman, C. B. B. (1955). Skeletal muscle reflexes of splanchnic and intercostal nerve origin in acute spinal and decerebrate cats. *J. Neurophysiol.* **18**, 217–235.

Eayrs, J. T. (1960). The influence of the thyroid on the central nervous system. *Br. med. Bull.* **16**, 122–127.

Eayrs, J. T. (1965). *In* "Proceedings of the Second International Congress of Endocrinology" (S. Taylor, ed.), pp. 779–784. Excerpta Medica, Amsterdam.

Eayrs, J. T. and Lishman, W. A. (1955). The maturation of behaviour in hypo-thyroidism and starvation. *Br. J. Anim. Behav.* **3**, 17–24.

Eccles, J. C., Eccles, R. M. and Lundberg, A. (1957). The convergence of mono-synaptic excitatory afferents on to many different species of alpha motoneurones. *J. Physiol.* **137**, 22–50.

Efron, R. (1963). Temporal perception, aphasia and déjà vu. *Brain* **86**, 403–424.

Endroczi, E., Lissak, K., Bohus, B. and Kovacs, S. (1959). The inhibitory in-fluence of archicortical structures on pituitary adrenal function. *Acta physiol. hung.* **16**, 17–22.

Engstrom, H., Ades, H. W. and Hawkins, J. E. Jr. (1962). Structure and functions of the sensory hairs of the inner ear. *J. acoust. Soc. Am.* **34**, 1356–1363.

Enroth-Cugell, C. and Jones, R. W. (1963). Responses of cat retinal ganglion cells to exponentially changing light intensities. *J. Neurophysiol.* **26**, 894–907.

Euler, U. S. von (1959). Autonomic neuroeffector transmission. *In* "Handbook of Physiology. Section 1. Neurophysiology", Vol. 1, pp. 215–237. American Physiological Society, Washington.

Evans, D. H. L. and Schild, H. O. (1953). Reaction of nerve-free chronically denervated plain muscle to drugs. *J. Physiol.* **122**, 63P.

Faivre, E. (1854). Structure du conarium et des plexus choroides chez l'homme et les animaux. *Gaz. Méd.* **9**, 555–556.

Falconer, M. A., Hill, D., Meyer, A., Mitchell, W. and Pond, D. A. (1955). Treatment of temporal-lobe epilepsy by temporal lobectomy. *Lancet* **1**, 827–835.

Fex, J. (1959). Augmentation of cochlear microphonic by stimulation of efferent fibres to the cochlea. *Acta oto-lar.* **50**, 540–541.

Fisher, A. E. (1964). Chemical stimulation of the brain. *Sci. Am.* **210**, 60–68.

Fritsch, G. and Hitzig, E. (1870). Uber die elektrische errogbarkeit des grosshirns. *Arch. Anat. Physiol. wiss. Med.* **37**, 300–332.

Galambos, R. (1960). *In* "Neural Mechanisms of the Auditory and Vestibular Systems" (G. L. Rasmussen and W. F. Windle, eds.). Thomas, Springfield.

Ghent, L., Weinstein, S., Semmes, J. and Teuber, H.-L. (1955). Effect of unilateral brain injury in man on learning of a tactile discrimination. *J. comp. physiol. Psychol.* **48**, 478–481.

Gillespie, J. S. (1961). The membrane potential and mechanical response o smooth muscle cells of the rabbit colon to stimulation of the extrinsic sympathetic nerves. *J. Physiol.* **156**, 32–33P.

Giuliani, G., Martini, L. and Pecile, A. (1961). Midbrain section and release o ACTH following stress. *Acta neuroveg.* **23**, 21–34.

Gloor, P. (1960). Amygdala. *In* "Handbook of Physiology. Section 1. Neurophysiology", Vol. 2, pp. 1395–1420. American Physiological Society, Washington.

Goldensohn, E. S. (1963). *In* "EEG and Behaviour" (G. H. Glaser, ed.), pp. 293–314. Basic Books, New York and London.

Gordan, G. S. (1956). Influence of steroids on cerebral metabolism in man. *Recent Progr. Hormone Res.* **12**, 153–170.

Granit, R. (1955). "Receptors and Sensory Perception." Yale University Press.

Granit, R., Henatsch, H. D. and Steg, G. (1956). Tonic and phasic ventral horn cells differentiated by post-tetanic potentiation in cat extensors. *Acta physiol. scand.* **37**, 114–126.

Green, J. D. (1951). The comparative anatomy of the hypophysis, with special reference to its blood supply and innervation. *Am. J. Anat.* **88**, 225–312.

Green, J. D. (1958). The rhinencephalon and behaviour. *In* "Ciba Foundation Symposium on the Neurological Basis of Behaviour" (G. E. W. Wolstenholme and C. M. O'Connor, eds.). Churchill, London.

Green, J. D. (1960). *In* "Handbook of Physiology. Section 1. Neurophysiology", Vol. 2, pp. 1373–1389. American Physiological Society, Washington.

Halliday, A. M. and Mason, A. A. (1964). The effect of hypnotic anaesthesia on cortical responses. *J. Neurol. Neurosurg. Psychiat.* **27**, 300–312.

Harn, G. L. van (1963). Responses of muscles of cat small intestine to autonomic nerve stimulation. *Am. J. Physiol.* **204**, 352–358.

Harris, G. W. (1948). Neural control of the pituitary gland. *Physiol. Rev.* **28**, 139–179.

Harris, G. W. (1955). "Neural Control of the Pituitary Gland." Edward Arnold, London.

Harris, G. W. (1960). Central control of pituitary secretion. *In* "Handbook of Physiology. Section 1. Neurophysiology", Vol. 2, pp. 1007–1038. American Physiological Society, Washington.

Harris, G. W. (1964). Female cycles of gonadotrophic secretion and female sexual behaviour in adult male rats castrated at birth. *J. Physiol.* **175**, 75–76P.

Hassler, R. (1961). Motorische und sensible Effekte umschreibener Reizungen und Ausschaltungen im menshlichen Zwischenhirn. *Dt. Z. NervHeilk.* **183**, 148–171.

Hassler, R. (1962). New aspects of brain functions revealed by brain diseases. *In* "Frontiers in Brain Research" (J. D. French, ed.). Columbia University Press.

Hawkins, J. E. Jr. (1964). Hearing. *A. Rev. Physiol.* **26**, 453–480.

Hensel, H. (1953). *Acta physiol. scand.* **29**, 109.

Hernandez-Peon, R., Chavez-Ibarra, G., Morgane, P. J. and Timo-Iaria, C. (1963). Limbic cholinergic pathways involved in sleep and emotional behaviour. *Expl. Neurol.* **8**, 93–111.

Hess, W. R. (1929). Hirnreizversuche uber den Mechanismus des Schlafes. *Arch. Psychiat. NervKrankh.* **86**, 287–292.

Hines, M. (1936). The anterior border of the monkey's (*Macaca mulatta*) motor cortex and the production of spasticity. *Am. J. Physiol.* **116**, 76.

Hodgkin, A. L. (1957). Ionic movements and electrical activity in giant nerve fibres. *Proc. R. Soc.* B **148**, 1–37.

Hoff, E. C. and Hoff, H. E. (1934). Spiral terminations of the projection fibres from the motor cortex of primates. *Brain* **57**, 454–474.

Holmes, G. (1939). The cerebellum of man. *Brain* **62**, 1–30.

Hubel, D. H. (1963). Integrative pathways in central visual pathways of the cat. *J. opt. Soc. Am.* **53**, 58–66.

Hubel, D. H. and Wiesel, T. N. (1963). Receptive fields of cells in striate cortex of very young, visually inexperienced kittens. *J. Neurophysiol.* **26**, 994–1002.

Humphrey, T. (1964). *In* "Growth and Maturation of the Brain" (P. M. Dominick and J. P. Schade, eds.). Elsevier, London.

Hunt, C. C. (1955). Monosynaptic reflex response of spinal motorneurones to graded afferent stimulation. *J. gen. Physiol.* **38**, 813–852.

Hunt, C. C. (1961). On the nature of vibration receptors in the hind limb of the cat. *J. Physiol.* **155**, 175–186.

Hunt, C. C. and Perl, E. R. (1960). Spinal reflex mechanisms concerned with skeletal muscle. *Physiol. Rev.* **40**, 538–579.

Hunt, C. C. and Takeuchi, A. (1962). Responses of the nerve terminal of the pacinian corpuscle. *J. Physiol.* **160**, 1–21.

Hyden, H. and Egyhazi, E. (1962). Nuclear RNA changes of nerve cells during a learning experiment in rats. *Proc. natn. Acad. Sci. U.S.A.* **48**, 1366–1373.

Iggo, A. (1955). Tension receptors in the stomach and the urinary bladder. *J. Physiol.* **128**, 593–607.

Iggo, A. (1962). New specific sensory structures in hairy skin. *Acta neuroveg.* **24**, 173–180.

Jasper, M. M. (Ed.) (1958). "Reticular Formation of the Brain." Churchill, London.

Job, C. and Lundberg, A. (1952). Reflex excitation of cells in the inferior mesenteric ganglion on stimulation of the hypogastric nerve. *Acta physiol. scand.* **26**, 366–382.

John, E. R. (1961). Higher nervous functions. Brain functions and learning. *A. Rev. Physiol.* **23**, 451–484.

Jung, R. and Hassler, R. (1960). *In* "Handbook of Physiology. Section 1. Neurophysiology", Vol. 2, pp. 863–927. American Physiological Society, Washington.

Kennard, M. (1949). Autonomic function. *In* "The Pre-central Motor Cortex", 2nd ed. (P. C. Bucy, ed.), pp. 293–306. University of Illinois Press, Urbana.

Kety, S. S. (1948). "Methods in Medical Research" Vol. 1, pp. 204–217. Year Book Publishers, Chicago.

Klein, R. and Ingram, I. M. (1958). Functional disorganisation of the left limbs in a tumour of the corpus callosum infiltrating the hemispheres. *J. ment. Sci.* **104**, 732–742.

Kluver, H. and Bucy, P. C. (1939). Preliminary analysis of functions of the temporal lobes in monkeys. *Archs Neurol. Psychiat.* **42**, 979–1000.

Krnjevic, K., Randic, M. and Straughan, D. W. (1964). Cortical inhibition. *Nature, Lond.* **201**, 1294–1296.

Kuntz, A. (1953). "The Autonomic Nervous System", 4th ed. Lea, Philadelphia.

Landau, W. M. (1953). Autonomic responses mediated via the corticospinal tract. *J. Neurophysiol.* **16**, 299–311.

Larrabee, M. G. and Bronk, D. W. (1952). Metabolic requirements of sympathetic neurons. *Cold Spring Harb. Symp. quant. Biol.* **17**, 245.

Lashley, K. S. (1929). *In* "Brain and Behaviour" (M. Brazier, ed.), Vol. 1. American Institute of Biological Sciences, Washington.

Lassek, A. M. and Evans, J. P. (1945). The effect of hemispherectomies on the fiber components of the pyramids. *J. comp. Neurol.* **83**, 113–119.

Lavin, N. I., Thorpe, J. G., Barker, J. C., Blakemore, C. B. and Conway, C. G. (1961). Behaviour therapy in a case of transvestism. *J. nerv. ment. Dis.* **133**, 346–353.

Lende, R. A. (1963). Cerebral cortex. A sensorimotor amalgam in the Marsupialia. *Science* **141**, 730.

Liberson, W. T. and Frazier, W. H. (1962). Evaluation of EEG patterns of newborn babies. *Am. J. Psychiat.* **118**, 1125–1131.

Loewenstein, W. R. (1961). Excitation and inactivation in a receptor membrane. *Ann. N. Y. Acad. Sci.* **94**, 510–534.

Lorenz, K. (1954). "Man meets Dog" (M. K. Wilson, trans.). Methuen, London.

Lundberg, A., Norrsell, V. and Voorhoeve, P. (1963). Effects from the sensorimotor cortex on ascending spinal pathways. *Acta physiol. scand.* **59**, 462–473.

McConnell, J. V. (1962). Memory transfer through cannibalism in planarians. *J. Neuropsychiat.* **3**, Suppl. 1, S.42–S.48.

McCullogh, W. S. (1947). Some connections of the frontal lobe established by physiological neuronography. *Proc. Ass. Res. nerv. ment. Dis.* **27**, 95–105.

McIlwain, H. (1959). "Biochemistry and the Central Nervous System," 2nd ed. Churchill, London.

Mackay, R. P. (1962). Neurologic theory of neuroses. *Neurology* **12**, 657–664.

McLennan, H. (1963). "Synaptic Transmission." Saunders, Philadelphia.

Magee, K. (1963). Congenital indifference to pain. *Archs Neurol.* **9**, 635–640.

Magoun, H. W. (1950). The ascending reticular activating system. *Ass. Res. nerv. ment. Dis.* **30**, 480–492.

Matthews, B. M. (1931). The response of a single end organ. *J. Physiol.* **71**, 64.

Mehler, W. R. (1957). The mammalian 'pain tract' in phylogeny. *Anat. Rec.* **127**, 332.

Meyers, R. (1953). The extrapyramidal system. An inquiry into the validity of the concept. *Neurology* **3**, 627–655.

Moll, J. (1959). Localization of brain-stem lesions inhibiting compensatory adrenal hypertrophy following unilateral adrenalectomy. *Z. Zellforsch.* **49**, 515–524.

Morison, R. S. and Dempsey, E. W. (1943). Mechanism of thalamo-cortical augmentation and repetition. *Am. J. Physiol.* **138**, 297–308.

Moruzzi, G. (1963). Active processes in the brain stem during sleep. *Harvey Lect.* **58**, 233–297.

Mountcastle, V. B. (1961). "Brain and Behaviour" (M. Brazier, ed.), Vol. 1. American Institute of Biological Sciences, Washington.

Myers, R. E. (1955). Interocular transfer of pattern discrimination in cats following section of crossed optic fibres. *J. comp. physiol. Psychol.* **48**, 470–473.

Myers, R. E. (1962). Commissural connections between occipital lobes of the monkey. *J. comp. Neurol.* **118**, 1–10.

Myers, R. E. and Henson, C. O. (1960). Role of corpus callosum in transfer of tactuokinesthetic learning in chimpanzee. *Archs Neurol.* **3**, 404–409.

Nachmansohn, D. (1959). "Chemical and Molecular Basis of Nerve Activity." Academic Press, New York.

Neff, W. D. (1961). *In* "Sensory Communication" (W. A. Rosenblith, ed.). Massachusetts Institute of Technology Press, Cambridge, Mass.

Neilson, J. M. (1958). "Memory and Amnesia." San Lucas Press, Los Angeles.

Nieman, E. A. (1961). The electroencephalogram in congenital hypothyroidism. A study of ten cases. *J. Neurol. Neurosurg. Psychiat.* **24**, 50–57.

Nelson, P. G. and Erulkar, S. D. (1963). Synaptic mechanisms of excitation and inhibition in the central auditory pathway. *J. Neurophysiol.* **26**, 908–923.

Olds, J. (1962). Hypothalamic substrates of reward. *Physiol. Rev.* **42**, 554–604.

Ortman, R. (1960). Neurosecretion. *In* "Handbook of Physiology. Section 1. Neurophysiology", Vol. 2, pp. 1039–1065. American Physiological Society, Washington.

Papez, J. W. (1937). A proposed theory of emotion. *Archs Neurol. Psychiat.* **38**, 725–743.

Penfield, W. (1951). Mechanism of memory. *Trans. Am. clin. climat. Ass.* **62**, 165–169.

Penfield, W. and Rasmussen, T. (1950). "The Cerebral Cortex of Man." Macmillan, New York.

Perl, E. R. (1963). Somatosensory mechanisms. *A. Rev. Physiol.* **25**, 459–492.

Petrie, A., Holland, T. and Walk, J. (1963). Sensory stimulation causing subdued experience: audio-analgesia and perceptual augmentation and reduction. *J. nerv. ment. Dis.* **137**, 312–321.

Pfalz, R. K. J. (1962). Centrifugal inhibition of afferent secondary neurons in the cochlear nucleus by sound. *J. acoust. Soc. Am.* **34**, 1472–1477.

Polyak, S. (1941). *In* "The Retina", p. 270. University of Chicago Press.

Pribram, K. H. (1955). Lesions of "Frontal Eye Fields" and delayed responses of baboons. *J. Neurophysiol.* **18**, 105–112.

Pribram, K. H. (1963). The new neurology: memory, novelty thought and choice. *In* "EEG and Behaviour" (G. H. Glaser, ed.). Basic Books, New York and London.

Roelofs, G. A., van den Hoofdakker, R. H. and Prechtl, H. F. R. (1963). Sleep effects of subliminal brain stimulation in cats. *Expl. Neurol.* **8**, 84–92.

Rose, J. and Mountcastle, Y. B. (1959). Touch and kinaesthesis. *In* "Handbook of Physiology. Section 1. Neurophysiology", Vol. 1, pp. 387–429. American Physiological Society, Washington.

Sawyer, C. H. (1960). Effect of brain lesions on estrual behaviour and reflexogenic ovulation in the rabbit. *J. exp. Zool.* **142**, 227–246.

Sawyer, C. H. and Kawakami, M. (1961). Interactions between the central nervous system and hormones influencing ovulation. *In* "Control of Ovulation" (C. A. Villee, ed.), pp. 79–97. Pergamon Press, Oxford.

Schally, A. V., Andersen, R. N., Lipscomb, H. S., Long, J. M. and Guillemin, R. (1960). Evidence for the existence of two corticotrophin-releasing factors, α and β. *Nature, Lond.* **188**, 1192–1193.

Scharlock, D. P., Tucker, T. J. and Strominger, N. L. (1963). Auditory discrimination by the cat after neonatal ablation of temporal cortex. *Science* **141**, 1197–1198.

Schilder, P. (1935). "The Image and Appearance of the Human Body." Keegan, Trench, Trubner, London.

Schreiber, V. (1961). A hypothalamic factor activating pituitary acid phosphatases and the secretion of TSH. *Acta Univ. Carol. Med.* **7**, 33–87.

Schreiber, V. (1963). "The Hypothalamo-hypophysial System." Czechoslovak Academy of Sciences, Prague.

Serafetinides, E. A., Hoare, R. D. and Driver, M. V. (1964). A modification of the intracarotid amylobarbitone test: findings about speech and consciousness. *Lancet* **1**, 249–250.

Sherrington, Sir Charles (1906). "The Integrative Action of the Nervous System." Yale University Press.

Showers, M. J. (1959). The cingulate gyrus. *J. comp. Neurol.* **112**, 231–287.

Slusher, M. A. and Hyde, J. E. (1961). Inhibition of adrenal corticosteroid release by brain-stem stimulation in cats. *Endocrinology* **68**, 773–782.

Smelser, G. K. (Ed.) (1961). "The Structure of the Eye." Academic Press, New York.

Smith, C. E. (1962). Is memory a matter of enzyme induction? *Science* **138**, 889–890.

Smith, C. A. and Rasmussen, G. L. (1963). Recent observations on the olivo-cochlear bundle. *Ann. Otol. Rhinol. Lar.* **72**, 489–506.

Snider, R. S. and Eldred, E. (1949). Maintenance of spontaneous activity within the cerebellum. *Proc. Soc. exp. Biol. Med.* **72**, 124–127.

Snider, R. S. and Stowell, A. (1942). Evidence of a projection of the optic system to the cerebellum. *Anat. Rec.* **82**, 448–449.

Snider, R. S. and Stowell, A. (1944). Receiving areas of the tactile, auditory and visual systems in the cerebellum. *J. Neurophysiol.* **7**, 331–357.

Sokoloff, L. (1960). Metabolism of the central nervous system *in vivo*. *In* "Handbook of Physiology. Section 1. Neurophysiology", Vol. 3, pp. 1843–1864. American Physiological Society, Washington.

Sperry, R. W. (1945). The problem of central nervous reorganization after nerve regeneration and muscle transplantation. *Q. Rev. Biol.* **20**, 311–369.

Sperry, R. W., Stamm, J. S. and Minter, N. (1956). Relearning tests for inter-ocular transfer following division of optic chiasma and corpus callosum in cats. *J. comp. physiol. Psychol.* **49**, 529–533.

Swank, R. L. and Brendler, S. J. (1951). The cerebellar electrogram: effects of anaesthesia, analeptics and local novocaine. *Electroenceph. clin. Neurophysiol.* **3**, 207–212.

Szentagothai, J. and Mess, B. (1958). Zur zentralen steuerung der thyreotropen Activitat des Hypophysenvorderlappens. (Die funktionelle Bedeutung des Nucleus medialis Habenulae.) *Wien. klin. Wsch.* **70**, 258–261.

Tasaki, I. (1959). Conduction of the nerve impulse. *In* "Handbook of Physiology. Section 1. Neurophysiology", Vol. 1, pp. 75–121. American Physiological Society, Washington.

Teuber, H. L. (1960). Perception. *In* "Handbook of Physiology. Section 1. Neurophysiology", Vol. 3, pp. 1595–1668. American Physiological Society, Washington.

Thomas, G. J., Fry, W. J., Fry, F. J., Slotnick, B. M. and Krieckhaus, E. E. (1963). Behavioural effects of mammillothalamic tractotomy in cats. *J. Neurophysiol.* **26**, 857–876.

Thompson, R. F., Smith, E. H. and Bliss, D. (1963). Auditory, somatic sensory and visual response interactions and interrelations in association and primary cortical fields of the cat. *J. Neurophysiol.* **26**, 365–378.

Tower, D. B. (1960). Chemical architecture of the central nervous system. *In* "Handbook of Physiology. Section 1. Neurophysiology", Vol. 3, pp. 1793–1813. American Physiological Society, Washington.

Tower, S. S. (1935). The dissociation of cortical excitation from cortical inhibition by pyramid section and the syndrome of that lesion in the cat. *Brain* **58**, 238–255.

Verjaal, A. (1947). Physiologie en pathologie van de liquordruk. (Physiology and pathology of the fluid pressure.) *Geneesk. Bl. Klin. Lab. Prakt.* **41**, reeks XI.

Walter, W. Grey (1953). "The Living Brain." Duckworth, London.

Walter, W. Grey (1959). Intrinsic rhythms of the brain. *In* "Handbook of Physiology. Section 1. Neurophysiology", Vol. 1, pp. 279–298. American Physiological Society, Washington.

Weddell, G. (1945). The anatomy of cutaneous sensibility. *Br. med. Bull.* **3**, 167–172.

Weddell, G. (1961). "Brain and Behaviour" (M. Brazier, ed.), Vol. 1. American Institute for Biological Sciences, Washington.

Wells, C. E. (1963). Electroencephalographic correlates of conditioned responses. *In* "EEG and Behaviour" (G. H. Glaser, ed.). Basic Books, London.

Wiener, N. and Schade, J. P. (Eds.) (1963). "Nerve, Brain and Memory Models." Elsevier, London.

Woods, J. W. (1956). International Physiological Congress, Abstracts of Communications, p. 978.

Woods, J. W. (1964). Behaviour of chronic decerebrate rats. *J. Neurophysiol.* **27**, 635–644.

Woolsey, C. N. (1961). *In* "Sensory Communication" (W. A. Rosenblith, ed.). Massachusetts Institute of Technology Press, Cambridge, Mass.

Woolsey, C. N., Settlage, P. H., Meyer, D. R., Spencer, W., Hamuy, T. and
Travis, A. M. (1950). Patterns of localization in precentral and "supplementary"
motor areas and their relation to the concept of a premotor area. *Proc. Ass. Res.
nerv. ment. Dis.* **30**, 238–264.

Young, W. C. (1961). The hormones and mating behaviour. *In* "Sex and Internal
Secretions" (W. C. Young, ed.), Vol. 2, pp. 1173–1239. Williams and Wilkins,
Baltimore.

Zangwill, O. L. (1960). Speech. *In* "Handbook of Physiology. Section 1. Neurophysiology", Vol. 3, pp. 1709–1722. American Physiological Society, Washington.

BIBLIOGRAPHY

THE ANATOMY OF THE CEREBROSPINAL FLUID
  J. W. Miller and D. H. M. Woollam (1962). Oxford University Press, London.
THE BASAL GANGLIA
  D. Denny-Brown (1962). Oxford University Press, New York.
BRAIN MECHANISMS AND INTELLIGENCE
  K. S. Lashley (1963). Dover Publications, New York.
CONDITIONED REFLEXES
  I. P. Pavlov (1960). Dover Publications, New York.
THE ELECTRICAL ACTIVITY OF THE NERVOUS SYSTEM
  2nd ed., M. A. B. Brazier (1960). Macmillan, London.
ELECTROENCEPHALOGRAPHY
  D. Hill and G. Parr, eds. (1963). Macdonald, London.
EVOLUTION OF NERVOUS CONTROL FROM PRIMITIVE ORGANISMS TO MAN
  A. D. Bass, ed. (1959). American Association for the Advancement of Science,
  Washington.
THE EYE
  H. Davson, ed. (1962). Academic Press, New York.
HIGHER CEREBRAL FUNCTIONS AND THEIR CLINICAL DISORDERS
  B. Schlesinger (1962). Grune and Stratton, New York and London.
THE HYPOTHALAMO-HYPOPHYSIAL SYSTEM
  V. Schreiber (1963). Czechoslovak Academy of Sciences, Prague.
INFORMATION STORAGE AND NEURAL CONTROL
  W. S. Fields and W. Abbott, eds. (1963). Thomas, Springfield.
THE INTEGRATIVE ACTION OF THE NERVOUS SYSTEM
  Sir Charles Sherrington (1961). Yale University Press.
THE LIVING BRAIN
  W. Grey Walter (1961). Penguin Books, London.
MEMORY AND AMNESIA
  J. M. Nielsen (1958). San Lucas Press, Los Angeles.
NEURAL CONTROL OF THE PITUITARY GLAND
  G. W. Harris (1955). Edward Arnold, London.
PERCEPTION
  R. R. Blake and G. V. Ramsey, eds. (1951). Ronald Press, New York.
THE PHYSIOLOGICAL BASIS OF MENTAL ACTIVITY
  R. Hernandez-Peon, ed. (1963). Elsevier, Amsterdam.
RECEPTORS AND SENSORY PERCEPTION
  R. Granit (1962). Yale University Press.
STUDIES IN TOPECTOMY
  N. D. C. Lewis, ed. (1956). Grune and Stratton, New York.
THE SUBMICROSCOPIC ORGANISATION AND FUNCTION OF NERVE CELLS
  H. Hernandez-Moran and R. Brown, eds. (1958). Academic Press, New York.

INDEX

Audition *contd.*
  reticular formation and, 249
  spiral ganglion, 53, 79
  superior colliculus, 92
  superior olivary nuclei, 80
  thalamus and, 58, 63
  visual pathway, connexions, 62
Auditory nerve, 51, 53, 79, 93, 124, 135,
    136
Autonomic mechanisms
  antagonistic actions, 155
  central control of, 117
  cerebellum and, 146
  cerebral cortex and, 156, 201
  conditioning and, 223
  general features, 149
  joint actions, 154
  sensory nerves and, 177
  special features, 175
  spinal cord and, 179
  thalamus and, 156
Avoidance responses, 212, 223, 231,
    238

B

β-rhythm, 209
Balance, 127
Basal ganglia, 120, 143
Basilar membrane, 51
Behaviour, 267
  cerebellum and, 180
  decerebration and, 267
  emotional, 201, 205, 228, 259
  endocrines and, 172
  fear, 267
  general mechanism, 280
  hyperphagia, 268, 272
  hypodipsia, 269
  hypothalamus and, 268
  Kluver–Bucy syndrome, 275
  learning and, 228
  misbehaviour, 285
  placidity, 268, 272
  rage, 267, 272
  reticular formation and, 271
  self-stimulation and, 269
  sequential, 233
  sexual, 173, 269
  special features, 289

Behaviour *contd.*
  thalamus and, 270
  unusual, 205, 275
Blind spot, 48
Blocking reaction, 207, 241, 249
Blood vessels, 17
Blushing, 157
Body scheme, 202
Brachium conjunctivum, 59, 124
Brachium pontis, 124
Brain
  activity, 23
  blood flow, 20
  blood supply, 17
  composition, 15
  learning, regions involved, 234
  metabolism, 16, 170, 172
    blood flow and, 22
    electrical activity and, 17
    thyroid gland and, 170
  method of study, 19
  rhythms, 205

C

Carbohydrates, 14
Carbon dioxide
  brain blood flow and, 22
  in brain, 16
  sleep and, 246
Caudate nucleus
  athetosis and, 120
  effector receptors, 69
  extrapyramidal system and, 143
  motor phenomena and, 118
  posture and, 137
Central excitatory state, 38
Centrencephalic system, 252
Cerebellum
  anatomy, 122
  archicerebellum, 123, 124, 127
  audition and, 84
  autonomic mechanisms and, 146
  behaviour and, 180
  connexions with cerebral cortex, 66,
      124
  connexions with spinal cord, 55, 124
  dentate nucleus, 59
  effect on receptors of, 69
  electrical activity, 132